Pharmacy Practice for Technicians

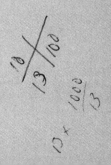

Pharmacy Practice for Technicians

Second Edition

SR. JANE M. DURGIN
ZACHARY I. HANAN
JANET MASTANDUONO

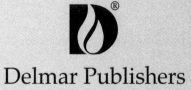

Delmar Publishers

I(T)P® International Thomson Publishing

Albany • Bonn • Boston • Cincinnati • Detroit • London • Madrid
Melbourne • Mexico City • New York • Pacific Grove • Paris • San Francisco
Singapore • Tokyo • Toronto • Washington

Notice to the Reader

Publisher does not warrant or guarantee any of the products described herein or perform any independent analysis in connection with any of the product information contained herein. Publisher does not assume, and expressly disclaims, any obligation to obtain and include information other than that provided by the manufacturer.

The reader is expressly warned to consider and adopt all safety precautions that might be indicated by the activities herein and to avoid all potential hazards. By following the instructions contained herein, the reader willingly assumes all risks in connection with such instructions.

The publisher makes no representation or warranties of any kind, including but not limited to, the warranties of fitness for particular purpose or merchantability, nor are any such representations implied with respect to the material set forth herein, and the publisher takes no responsibility with respect to such material. The publisher shall not be liable for any special, consequential, or exemplary damages resulting, in whole or part, from the readers' use of, or reliance upon, this material.

Cover Design: Charles Cummings Advertising/Art Inc.

Delmar Staff:
Publisher: Susan Simpfenderfer
Acquisitions Editor: Marlene McHugh Pratt
Production Manager: Linda Helfrich
Project Editor: Stacey Prus
Developmental Editor: Marge Bruce
Art & Design Coordinator: Rich Killar
Editorial Assistant: Maria Perretta
Marketing Manager: Darryl L. Caron

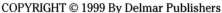

COPYRIGHT © 1999 By Delmar Publishers

an International Thomson Publishing company I(T)P®

The ITP logo is a trademark under license
Printed in Canada
For more information contact:

Delmar Publishers
3 Columbia Circle, Box 15015
Albany, New York 12212-5015

International Thomson Publishing Europe
Berkshire House
168-173 High Holborn
London, WC1V7AA
United Kingdom

Nelson ITP, Australia
102 Dodds Street
South Melbourne,
Victoria, 3205 Australia

Nelson Canada
1120 Birchmont Road
Scarborough, Ontario
M1K 5G4, Canada

International Thomson Publishing France
Tour Maine-Montparnassc
33 Avenue du Maine
75755 Paris Cedex 15, France

International Thomson Editores
Seneca 53
Colonia Polanco
11560 Mexico D.R. Mexico

International Thomson Publishing GmbH
Königswinterer Strasβe 418
53227 Bonn
Germany

International Thomson Publishing Asia
60 Albert Street
#15-01 Albert Complex
Singapore 189969

International Thomson Publishing Japan
Hirakawa-cho Kyowa Building, 3F
2-2-1 Hirakawa-cho, Chiyoda-ku,
Tokyo 102, Japan

ITE Spain/Paraninfo
Calle Magallanes, 25
28015-Madrid, Espana

2 3 4 5 6 7 8 9 10 XXX 03 02 01 00 99

Library of Congress Cataloging-in-Publication Data
Pharmacy practice for technicians / [edited] by Jane M. Durgin, Zachary Hanan,
    and Janet Mastanduono. – 2nd ed.
        p.   cm.
    Includes bibliographical references and index.
    ISBN 0-7668-0458-5
    1.   Pharmacy technicians –Handbooks, manuals, etc. 2. Pharmacy-Handbooks,
    Manuals, etc. I. Durgin, Jane M. II. Hanan, Zachary III. Mastanduono, Janet
    [DNLM: 1. Pharmacy handbooks. 2. Pharmacists' Aides handbooks.
    2.   Pharmaceutical Preparations handbooks. QV 735 P536 1999]
    RS 122.95.P43   1998
    615'.1—dc21
DNLM/DLC
for Library of Congress   98-54627
                                                                    CIP

Contents

Chapter 4   Long-Term Care   53

Janet M. Unger

Chapter 5   Regulatory Standards in Pharmacy Practice   59

Zachary I. Hanan

PART II　THE PROFESSION OF PHARMACY

APPENDICES

Preface

Introduction

The practice of pharmacology has evolved into a knowledge profession in which the need for knowledgeable, technically skilled, and competent supportive personnel is paramount. This need is significantly illustrated by today's increased demand for trained, supportive personnel in institutional and community practice, the accreditation of a training program for supportive personnel by the American Society of Health System Pharmacists, the establishment of the American Association of Pharmacy Technicians, and the recognition of technicians by many state boards of pharmacy and state pharmaceutical organizations.

It is our objective that this book will be a useful reference and practical guide for pharmacy practitioners, practicing pharmacy technicians, and pharmacy technician students and their instructors in the formal teaching environment, as well as for self-instruction. The framework provides a stepwise approach for learning and understanding the various components of the profession of pharmacy and the meaningful role of supportive personnel in the practice of contemporary pharmacy. Job opportunities abound in institutional and community pharmacy practice and will continue to offer challenging career options for pharmacy technicians in the future.

Organization of the Text

This textbook is divided into the following major sections: Overview of Health Care, The Profession of Pharmacy, Administrative Aspects of Pharmacy Technology, and Professional Aspects of Pharmacy Technology. Several of the chapters in this text deal with contemporary pharmacy activities that are acknowledged to be beyond the scope of the technician's responsibilities and function. Chapters such as "Basic Biopharmaceutics" and "Administration of Medications" are essential for an overview and appreciation of the practice of contemporary pharmacy. Other chapters give the technician an understanding of the health care system and the use of drugs.

The Author Team

The editors wish to note the professional and clinical expertise of an outstanding cadre of authors. Included are presidents and deans of colleges of pharmacy, directors of institutional pharmacy practice, pharmacy leaders in institutional and community practice, executives in health care organizations, scientific researchers and teachers in colleges of pharmacy, hospital administrators, a physician expert in medical ethics, and clinical and administrative nurse practitioners. Each author has enhanced this text with his or her knowledge, experience, and dedication in support of the education and training of pharmacy technicians.

New to This Edition

The second edition reflects the expanding influence of pharmacy practice and the many roles of the pharmacy technician within this practice. Following is a summary of the major changes and additions to this edition.

- **Chapter 1 Historical Developments in Pharmacy and Health Care**
  This chapter was expanded to provide more comprehensive coverage of the development of pharmacy from ancient times to the present. Content from Chapters 1 and 8 of the previous edition was combined in this new chapter. Major contributions by individuals and cultures are briefly described.

- **Chapter 3 Home Health Care**
  Major revisions in this chapter describe the evolution and future of pharmacy's role in the home health care industry, particularly in home infusion therapy and home care pharmacy practice. The chapter includes a detailed discussion of drugs most commonly used in home infusion therapy and the infusion control devices used. The roles of the pharmacy technician in the home infusion industry are discussed.

- **Chapter 4 Long-Term Care**
  This chapter includes new content on types of long-term care facilities, regulation of facilities, sources of funding for services provided by the facilities, pharmaceutical services required by facility residents, and pharmaceutical personnel providing services.

- **Chapter 5 Regulatory Standards in Pharmacy Practice**
  Revisions include the addition of the MedWatch Reporting Program form (for reporting adverse effects and product problems by health professionals), a new section on the Omnibus Budget Reconciliation Act (OBRA) with particular attention to three main provisions that affect the pharmacy profession, and new content on the JCAHO survey process.

- **Chapter 6 An Ethical Pharmacy Concern: The Informed Drug Consent**
  This new chapter deals with an important aspect of pharmacotherapy—the patient's right to know the benefits and risks involved in the prescribed drug therapy, whether for healing, alleviating symptoms, or long-term replacement therapy.

- **Chapter 7 Drug-Use Control: The Foundation of Pharmaceutical Care**
  This revision includes information on pharmaceutical care plans and an updated code of ethics.

- **Chapter 8 Information and Resources: Drug Information and Clinical Services**
  Extensive revisions in this chapter update content to reflect the continuing development of drug information services. The purpose of these services is to collect, evaluate, and disseminate drug information with the goal of improved patient care through rational drug therapy. The chapter discusses the expanded role of the pharmacy technician in drug information services.

- **Chapter 9 Organizations in Pharmacy**
  Updated content includes information on the Pharmacy Technician Certification Board (PTCB).

■ **Chapter 10   Pharmacy Practice in the Third Millennium**

This completely rewritten chapter describes the major influences that resulted in the most significant changes in pharmacy practice and health care to date, explores the current forces that will shape future changes and opportunities in pharmacy practice, identifies career path options that will be available to pharmacists and pharmacy technicians, and describes the educational and training requirements to meet professional needs in the third millenium.

■ **Chapter 11   The Policy and Procedure Manual**

Revisions include the addition of a sample technician evaluation form (evaluation of job performance), a sample job description for a pharmacy technician, content on multidisciplinary policies and procedures with a sample of the sign-off process for a multidisciplinary policy or procedure, brief discussion of computerization of policies and procedures to improve availability to personnel, and use of institution-wide computer networks.

■ **Chapter 12   Materials Management of Pharmaceuticals**

This chapter includes added discussion of cost-benefit analysis in reaching a decision on the addition of a drug to institutional formulary, new content on the safe handling and storage of oncology drugs, and expanded content on drug repackaging and labeling considerations.

■ **Chapter 13   The Pharmacy Formulary System**

This chapter includes added content on the impact of new drug therapy as part of the decision-making process in revising the institution's formulary, with a flowchart and sample cases illustrating possible decision alternatives. This chapter also has new content on the ability to track adverse drug reactions.

■ **Chapter 14   Computer Applications in Drug-Use Control**

This completely rewritten chapter covers the following topics: applications facilitated by computer automation, how computer systems interact within the pharmacy and with other systems in the health care delivery process, project management relating to the implementation of a computer system, and the roles of the pharmacist and pharmacy technician in the management of a pharmacy information system.

■ **Chapter 15   Medication Errors**

This new chapter covers the role of the pharmacy technician in preventing medication errors, causes of medication errors, types of medication errors that may occur during the ordering and dispensing process, guidelines for the proper dispensing of medications, commonly used drugs that may result in medication error deaths, and guidelines for minimizing errors when taking verbal orders.

■ **Chapter 16   Pharmaceutical Terminology and Medical Abbreviations**

Updated sections of this chapter include common medical pharmacy abbreviations and brand/trade names of drugs and generic names.

■ **Chapter 20   Parenteral Admixture Services**

Revisions include addition of information on the effect desired for the routes of administration for injectable drugs, addition of the intracardiac route of administration, new content on the types of class II vertical laminar airflow hoods used in the pharmacy, added needle gauge ranges for subcutaneous, intradermal, and intramuscular injections, new content on the safe handling of cancer chemotherapy agents (cytotoxic drugs), and an updated list of pharmacy technician roles.

■ **Chapter 21   Basic Biopharmaceutics**

This completely rewritten chapter includes a definition of bioavailability of drugs (rate and extent of absorption following administration), factors affecting drug bioavailability (pharmaceutical factors, route of administration, and anatomic and physiologic considerations), and methods of measuring bioavailability. The chapter also discusses gene therapy.

■ **Chapter 22 The Actions and Uses of Drugs**

This completely rewritten chapter covers the factors that modify drug action, including routes of administration, food-drug and drug-drug interactions and their effects, and patient-associated factors. The chapter also thoroughly describes the major classifications of drugs and presents primary drugs (generic and trade names) for each classification.

■ **Chapter 23 Administration of Medications**

This chapter includes added content on patient teaching relating to drug therapy and the factors that affect patient compliance with drug therapy.

■ **Chapter 24 Drug Distribution Systems**

Expanded discussion of systems, including an individual prescription system, combined floor stock and patient prescription system, unit-dose distribution system, centralized dispensing, and decentralized dispensing; expanded information under physician's original order to include basic requirements of a complete medication order and methods of transmitting orders to pharmacy; updated section on computerization of medication orders and record keeping; updated and expanded discussion of the roles of the pharmacist and pharmacy technician in the order process; updated guidelines for labeling and dispensing medications; expanded content on medication delivery systems, including unit-dose system and robotics.

■ **Chapter 25 The Pharmacy and Infection Control**

This completely rewritten chapter covers work practice controls for the prevention of infection and of sterile products prepared in the pharmacy, responsibilities of the pharmacy in infection control, quality control, modes of transmission of pathogens, universal and standard precautions, and transmission-based precautions.

Supplements

An Instructor's Manual (IML) accompanies the text. Answers to chapter assessments are provided. In addition to the answers, each chapter of the IML includes learning activities, evaluation methods, and additional learning references.

Acknowledgments

Sincere thanks to our professional colleagues, personal friends, peers, and associates whose time, effort, and contributions to the textbook made this publication possible.

We thank the administrative staff and department of pharmacy of Mercy Medical Center. Our thanks also to the administrative and teaching faculty of St. John's University, College of Pharmacy and Allied Health Professions. Together they provided their approval and support for this professional endeavor.

We thank our developmental editor, Marjorie Bruce, for her enthusiasm and encouragement and Larry Goldberg of Carlisle Publishers Services for his invaluable assistance during the production of this textbook. Special thanks to Annette Danaher of Danaher Editorial Services for managing the contributors during the final draft revision stage.

Last, we thank Cleo Tamis, our secretarial assistant, for her diligence and gracious assistance in the coordination of the numerous details of this comprehensive project.

Reviewers

We wish to thank the following individuals for providing valuable assistance in the development of this second edition.

Patricia K. Anthony, BSPhS, BS Biology, MS, PhD
Pima Medical Institute
Tucson, AZ

Carolyn Bunker, RPh
Salt Lake Community College
Salt Lake City, UT

Jane Doucette, RPh
Salt Lake Community College
Salt Lake City, UT

Emery C. Fellows, Jr., CPhT
Pima Medical Institute
Denver, CO

Tova R. Wiegand-Green
Ivy Tech State College
Fort Wayne, IN

Percy M. Johnson
Bidwell Training
Pittsburgh, PA

Elizabeth Johnson
Houston Community College System
Southeast College
Houston, TX

Kathy Moscou, BS Pharmacy
North Seattle Community College
Seattle, WA

Larry Nesmith, BS Ed
Academy of Health Sciences, AMEDD Center & School
Pharmacy Branch, Fort Sam Houston, U.S. Army
San Antonio, TX

Glen E. Rolfson, RPh
Salt Lake Community College
Salt Lake City, UT

Peter E. Vonderau, RPh
Cuyahoga Community College
Highland Falls Village, OH

Sharon Burton-Young, RN
POLYtech Adult Education
Woodside, DE

Jane M. Durgin
Zachary I. Hanan
Janet Mastanduono

Introduction

As we approach the upcoming millennium, all of us who are currently associated with health care or who aspire to be a part of the health care sector must acknowledge one unassailable truth—that the health care industry within the last decade has undergone unprecedented changes which have redefined the roles and expectations of those who provide, pay for, and receive health care services. In large part, these changes are due to continuous and dramatic advances in the science and technology of our understanding of disease and its treatment, a more demanding and expectant patient population, rising costs of health care services, and limits on the extent and willingness of public and private sectors to pay the true economic costs of health care.

At the same time, drug therapy has become a mainstream modality in the treatment and prevention of diseases. Moreover, drug therapy is acknowledged as a major determinant of outcome in the treatment and/or management of many diseases. In fact, in some instances, advances in drug therapy have virtually eliminated or greatly reduced morbidity and mortality for millions of Americans.

The growing centrality and importance of drug therapy in health care, in turn, has had a major impact on pharmacy. It has redefined the roles of pharmacist and pharmacy, the purpose of pharmacy as a profession, and the education and training of all those engaged in the practice of pharmacy. For today and tomorrow, pharmacy's mission as a profession is helping people make the best use of medications, focusing on the *consequences* of drug therapy and providing drug products. This change in purpose has evolved over the last three decades. What began as "clinical pharmacy" in the mid-1960s (a new function for pharmacy), has gradually evolved into a mandate for pharmaceutical care. Pharmacy's focus is now on patients and the improvement of their health care status through proactive pharmacist involvement and assumption of responsibility for identifying, resolving, and preventing drug-related problems that improve the quality of patients' lives.

Unfortunately, pharmaceutical care is still a concept in formation, since much of current-day pharmacy practice is still consumed by the traditional dispensing role of the pharmacist. Pharmacy's new purpose of pharmaceutical care can only be realized through reengineering practice to enable pharmacists to assume their new roles as patient advocates in drug therapy. The role of pharmacy technicians has now become pivotal in achieving pharmacy's destiny of pharmaceutical care, especially in light of the enormous changes in the health care sector. Without a cadre of well-qualified and trained pharmacy technicians, the future of pharmacy as a valued health profession will be mired in uncertainty at best and perhaps even hopelessness. From the mid-1940s through the early 1980s, the role of pharmacy technicians in pharmacy practice evolved at a glacial pace. Many forces both within and outside of pharmacy have, since the 1980s, converged to shed new light on and a heightened sense of urgency in the recognition and development of well-qualified, trained technicians. In fact, a historical watershed was reached during the late 1980s and the 1990s with virtually all sectors of the profession (through their respective organizations) separately acknowledging and endorsing the role, legitimacy, and strategic importance of technicians in pharmacy's current and future mission.

More recently, both the American Society of Health System Pharmacists and the American Pharmaceutical Association have officially endorsed recommendations on the functions, training, and regulation of technicians.[1] The recent establishment and success of the Pharmacy Technician Certification Board (PTCB) as a consolidated voluntary national certification body for technicians is further evidence of a concept reaching maturity and broad professional endorsement. Currently, there are well over 18,000 PTCB-certified pharmacy technicians in the United States.

The critical role of the pharmacy technician has now come to pass. It is axiomatic that the profession of pharmacy's future in a newly landscaped health care scenario is, in large measure, highly dependent on the roles and functions of well-educated and trained pharmacy technicians.

In short, the major thrust of any discourse on pharmacy technicians today and in the future will be not on role definition and/or legitimacy, but on competency and the means of achieving the same.

This second edition of *Pharmacy Practice for Technicians* represents a major contribution to the educational and training matrix for contemporary pharmacy technicians. The authors trust that readers and students will find the text both relevant and useful in preparation for their key roles in pharmacy practice.

Paul G. Pierpaoli

---

[1](1996). White paper on pharmacy technicians: Recommendation of pharmacy practitioner organizations on the functions, training and regulation of technicians. *Am J Health-System Pharm, 53,* 1793–1796.

Contributors

Chapter 1

Jane M. Durgin, CIJ, RN, RPh, EdD
Former Professor, Pharmacy and
    Administrative Sciences
St. John's University
College of Pharmacy and Allied Health
    Professions
Jamaica, NY

Chapter 2

Kevin M. Spiegel, MS, MBA, CHE
Deputy Commissioner
Westchester Medical Center
Valhalla, NY

Chapter 3

Darryl S. Rich, Pharm D, MBA
Associate Director
Home Care and Long Term Care Pharmacy
    Accreditation Services
Joint Commission on Accreditation of
    Healthcare Organizations
Oakbrook Terrace, IL

Barbara Limburg-Mancini, Pharm D, BCNSP
President
Infusion Solutions, Inc.
Indian Head Park, IL
and
Pharmacist Surveyor
Joint Commission on Accreditation of
    Healthcare Organizations
Oakbrook Terrace, IL

Chapter 4

Janet M. Unger, MPA, LNHA
Administrator
Chapin Home for the Aging
Jamaica, NY

Chapter 5

Zachary I. Hanan, MS
Director, Pharmaceutical Services
Mercy Medical Center
Rockville Centre, NY

Chapter 6

Edmund D. Pellegrino, MD
Professor of Medicine and Medical Ethics
School of Medicine
Georgetown University
Washington, DC

Chapter 7

William N. Kelly, Pharm D
Professor and Chairman
Department of Pharmacy Practice
School of Pharmacy
Mercer University
Atlanta, GA

Chapter 8

William J. Tomasulo, RPh, MS
Former Assistant Director of Pharmaceutical
    Services
Mercy Medical Center
Rockville Centre, NY

Chapter 9

Kenneth W. Miller, PhD
Vice President for Graduate Education, Research
    and Scholarship
American Association of Colleges of Pharmacy
Alexandria, VA

Herman L. Lazarus, MS
Regional Vice President
Pharmacy Practice
Cardinal Health Inc.
Syracuse, NY

Chapter 10

Paul G. Pierpaoli, MS
Vice President, Pharmacy Practice
McKesson MedManagement
Minneapolis, MN

Gary W. Schwartz, RPh, MBA
Assistant Director of Pharmacy
Production Support Services
Rush–Presbyterian–St. Luke's Medical Center
Chicago, IL

Chapter 11

Seymour Katz, MS, RPh, FASHP
Director, Pharmacy Services
Brookdale University Hospital and
    Medical Center
Brooklyn, NY
and
Clinical Associate Professor
Arnold & Marie Schwartz College of Pharmacy &
    Health Sciences of Long Island University
Brooklyn, NY

Chapter 12

Steven J. Ciullo, RPh, MS, MPS
Regional Director, New York Metropolitan Area
Owen Healthcare, Inc.
Morris Plains, NJ

Chapter 13

Joseph N. Gallina, Pharm D
Director of Pharmacy
University of Maryland Medical System
Department of Pharmacy Services
Baltimore, MD

Chapter 14

Martin A. Bieber
Senior Vice President
Chief Operating Officer
St. Francis Hospital
Roslyn, NY

Chapter 15

Susan M. Proulx, Pharm D
Vice President, Operations
Institute for Safe Medication Practices
Warminster, PA

Michael R. Cohen, MS, FASHP
President
Institute for Safe Medication Practices
Warminster, PA

Chapter 16

Christine Martin, MS, RPh
Pharmacy Department
Good Samaritan Hospital Medical Center
West Islip, NY

Chapter 17

P. L. Madan, PhD
Professor of Pharmacy and Administrative
    Sciences
St. John's University
College of Pharmacy and Allied Health
    Professions
Jamaica, NY

Chapter 18

Barry S. Reiss, BS, MS, PhD, RPh
Professor, Department of Pharmacy Practice
Albany College of Pharmacy
Albany, NY

Ronald L. McLean, RPh, MS
Interim Director of Office of Postgraduate
    Professional Education
Albany College of Pharmacy
Albany, NY

Chapter 19

Joseph A. DuPrey, RPh, MS
Inpatient Supervisor
Lancaster General Hospital
Lancaster, PA

Chapter 20

Michael J. Ficurilli, RPh, MS
Assistant Director
Department of Pharmaceutical Services
Mercy Medical Center
Rockville Centre, NY

Chapter 21

Andrew B. C. Yu, PhD, RPh
John S. Lee, BS Pharm

Chapter 22
Janet J. Mastanduono, PhD, RPh
Director of Drug Information, Clinical and
    Education Services
Mercy Medical Center
Rockville Centre, NY

Chapter 23
Jean H. Rogers, RN, MSN
Vice President, Patient Care Services
Mercy Medical Center
Rockville Centre, NY

Chapter 24
Fred S. Gordon, RPh, MS
Director of Purchasing
St. Francis Hospital/Mercy Medical Center
Brookville, NY

R. David Anderson, BS
Director of Pharmacy (Retired)
Waynesboro Community Hospital
Waynesboro, VA

Chapter 25
Joanne Selva, RN, BS, CIC
Director, Infection Control
Nassau County Medical Center
East Meadow, NY
and
Co-President
Infection Control Consultants, Inc.
Islip, NY

Maria Ninivaggi, RN, MSN, CIC
Assistant Director, Infection Control
Nassau County Medical Center
East Meadow, NY
and
Co-President
Infection Control Consultants, Inc.
Islip, NY

Chapter 26
Donald E. Letendre, Pharm D
Director of Accreditation Services
American Society of Health-System Pharmacists
Bethesda, MD

Lisa S. Lifshin, RPh, BCNSP
Senior Accreditation Services Associate
American Society of Health-System Pharmacists
Bethesda, MD

Pharmacy Practice for Technicians

PART

I

Overview of Health Care

Historical Developments in Pharmacy and Health Care

COMPETENCIES

After completion and review of this chapter, the student should be able to

1. Explain his or her understanding of this statement: Hospitality and care of the sick have been and continue to be cultural concerns wherever communities of persons gather.

2. Describe the foundation of health care institutions as found in Greece and Rome.

3. Explain the evolution of health care from a religious perspective as demonstrated by Hippocrates, Maimonides, Basil, Camillus, and the Crusaders.

4. Name the father of medicine, father of botany, father of toxicology, and father of pharmacology.

5. List six dosage forms described in the Hippocratic Corpus.

6. Explain why Gheel in Belgium is considered remarkable in the care and treatment of the mentally ill.

7. List a contribution to pharmacy or health care by the following: Dioscorides, Galen, Shen-Nung, Sirach, Theophrastus, Benjamin Franklin, Abraham Lincoln, King George III, Louisa May Alcott, Crawford Long, and Benjamin Rush.

8. Distinguish between the treatment of persons with tuberculosis at the beginning of the twentieth century and today.

9. Describe the cause and effects of the deinstitutionalization of persons with emotional and behavioral problems.

10. State the person who discovered, isolated, or synthesized each of the following drugs: codeine, smallpox vaccine, arsphenamine, digitalis, quinine, insulin, penicillin, streptomycin, prontosil, and diphtheria antitoxin.

Introduction

The objective of this chapter is to provide the student with knowledge and an appreciation of the values, the evolution, and the development of the healing arts and health care.

Literature records remarkable developments in the evolution of health care facilities and methods of treatment over many centuries. Hospitality and care for the sick have been and continue to be cultural concerns wherever communities of persons gather. The facilities designed to carry out these functions have gone through architectural, administrative, and clinical changes. They have been modified by environmental factors and diagnostic treatment needs brought about by wars, **epidemics,** and scientific discoveries.

From the beginning of time, individuals have searched for remedies to heal the various maladies that affect the mind and the body. The history of the search is fascinating. Healing often requires the help and intervention of others. Originally provided almost exclusively in the family or within the clan or tribe, eventually places were established dedicated to the care of the sick (e.g., monastic infirmaries, almshouses, and later, hospitals). Remedies for nearly 2000 years were found in plants and minerals. The last part of this century has achieved healing remedies so remarkable that they are called "miracle drugs."

This chapter briefly describes the evolution of health care facilities at home and abroad. The historical development and present-day trends in drug therapy are also highlighted to give a mosaic of health care from a historical perspective.

The approach is based on the contribution of the various cultures from early Greece through modern-day America.

Greek Influence

The Greek temple dedicated to Aesculapius, the mythical god of medicine, and the temple on the Greek Island of Cos where **Hippocrates,** the renowned father of medicine, practiced medicine and pharmacy (400–300 B.C.) are early examples of healing centers where gods were implored, physicians practiced medicine, and apprentices learned the art of healing. Patients who came to these temples were diagnosed, treated, and cared for until they were able to return home. Treatments included herbal remedies, mineral baths, exercise, fresh sea air, and sunshine. Archaeologists have found admission records and other medical records inscribed in the columns of these temples.

Hippocrates, circa 400 B.C.

For thousands of years the writings of Hippocrates, the famous philosopher, physician, and pharmacist, occupied a place in medicine corresponding to that of the Bible in the literature and ethics of Western people. Through the use of rational concepts based on objective knowledge he liberated medicine from the mystic and the demonic. The concept of **homeostatis**—the attainment and retainment of equilibrium in the body through appropriate drugs and diet—was the traditional benchmark of his numerous practices and writings. Hippocrates is considered to be the "father of medicine."

Hippocratic Corpus

Through the writings and practice of Hippocrates and his colleagues, medicine moved from the magical to the rational. The theory of humoral **pathology** considers disease as a disturbance of a body fluid (e.g., blood, **phlegm,** and yellow and black **bile**). Disease is treated by restoring equilibrium. Health is preserved by care for the internal environment (e.g., diet, sleep, exercise) and the external environment (e.g., rain, excess sun, climate changes) to enhance the physical harmony of the body. Over 200 herbal remedies and a dozen minerals are recommended. These drugs were available as **pills, troches, gargles,** eye washes, **ointments,** and inhalants. In the Corpus, the word for *drug*—pharmakon—was defined as a purifying remedy; later it was described as a healing remedy.

To purify the body of excess fluids, drugs were frequently used as **expectorants, emetics, cathartics, diuretics,** and **sudorifics.** The common cold, seen as cold and damp, was treated with mustard, which is hot and dry. This example conveys the concept of allopathy employed by the Greeks. The juice of the poppy, which today we recognize as opium, was among the 200 drugs mentioned in the Hippocratean Corpus.

Theophrastus

Theophrastus was a Greek philosopher botanist who lived circa 300 B.C. Botany, the study of plants, is closely related to **pharmacognosy,** the science that deals with the medicinal ingredients in living plants. Theophrastus classified plants by their leaves, roots, seeds, and stems. His accurate pharmaceutical and pharmacologic observations related to the classification and action of medicinal plants won for him the title of "father of botany."

Pedanios Dioscorides (A.D. 100)

The noted botanist and pharmacologist Dioscorides was the major authority on drugs for sixteen centuries. He added to the work of Hippocrates the knowledge he gained while accompanying the Roman armies on their conquests. A major focus of his studies and writings was the use and biological effects of these early remedies. For this reason, perhaps he should be called the "father of pharmacology."

Dioscorides's herbal

The information in Dioscorides's herbal, known in Latin as *De Materia Medica,* was the major authority on drugs for sixteen centuries. More than 600 plants and ninety minerals were included. Knowledge was collected by Dioscorides from his extensive travels in Africa, Gaul, Persia, Armenia, and Egypt. The remedies of these countries were incorporated into the herbal, which gave plant/mineral descriptions, instructions for growing and preservation, dosage, medicinal uses, and side effects. Considered the most important pharmaceutical guide of antiquity, thirty-five translations and commentaries had been issued by 1540.

Roman Influence

In early Rome (A.D. 200–500), hospitals were often endowed by wealthy citizens who frequently cared for the sick as volunteers. Fabiola, a wealthy Roman woman, donated her palace for the care of the sick and injured and personally cared for their needs. With the fall of the Roman Empire, major changes occurred. The care of the sick became a civil responsibility and prostitutes and prisoners were assigned health care tasks.

Claudius Galen (A.D. 130–200)

Until 1950, pharmacy students took a course entitled "Galenical Pharmacy." Galen practiced and taught both pharmacy and medicine in Rome. His principles, derived from Hippocratean theory for the preparation and compounding of medicines, were followed in the Western world for 1500 years. This Greek-born physician who practiced in Rome organized the **pharmacotherapy** of humoral pathology into a scientific system.

On the Art of Healing (A.D. 1500)

Galen compiled and added to drug information available in Rome in the most famous of his writings, *On the Art of Healing.* The properties and mixtures of simple remedies and compounded drugs are described. Pharmacotherapy of humoral pathology was systemically classified according to the theories of Hippocrates. The treatments described such **galenicals** as **tinctures, fluidextracts, syrups,** and ointments. This class of drugs has only recently lost popularity due to the present use of synthetic chemicals, antibiotics, and **biologicals.**

Jewish Influence

Biblical Records (1200 B.C.)

The Old Testament book of Sirach (38:4–8) states, "The Lord created medicines from the earth and a sensible man will not despise them. Was not water made sweet with a tree in order that His power might be known? And he gave skill to men that He might be glorified in His marvelous works. By them He heals and takes away pain; the pharmacist makes of them a compound. His works will never be finished; and from Him health is upon the face of the earth." Genesis, the first book of the Bible, mentions myrrh, a remedy used throughout history as an appetite stimulant, **carminative,** and a skin protective with healing properties. Olibanum (frankincense) is gum-resin mentioned in the books of Exodus, Ezra, Jeremiah, Ezekiel, and the Song of Solomon. The pharmacist's role, professional norms, and many drug examples are included in the Old Testament of the Bible.

Ancient Hebrews (1200 B.C.)

"God hath created medicines out of the earth and let not a discerning man reject them" (Sirach 38:4). Several drugs mentioned in the Old Testament are still in use today. Garlic (Numbers 11:5), with a history of thousands of years, is currently being investigated as a means to reduce blood pressure, lower cholesterol, and possibly inhibit growth of cancer cells. Aloe, mentioned in the New Testament (John 19:39) but available much earlier, is an official ingredient in compound benzoin tincture. Acacia (Exodus 26:15), used earlier for building purposes, is now commonly used as an emulsifying agent. Other items still in use include coriander, myrrh, almond, and anise. Presently they are mainly used as foods or flavors.

The Jewish influence on health care is demonstrated by the teachings and works of the famous rabbi and physician, **Moses Maimonides.** The Prayer of Maimonides for many years continued the pledge of service made by pharmacists as they completed school and began professional practice.

Moses ben Maimon (Maimonides) (1135–1204)

For many decades pharmacy students were presented with a scroll at graduation containing the Prayer of Maimonides, a Spanish rabbi and scientist. Included are the phrases, "May I be filled with love for my art. Preserve my strength that I may be able to preserve the strength of (others) may there never rise in me the notion that I know enough." Although Maimonides is best known for this document, he also published a glossary of drug terms and a manual of poisons.

Christian Influence

The spread of Christianity brought the teachings of Jesus to the care of the sick and infirm. At the Council of Nicaea in the fourth century A.D., bishops were required to provide a shelter for the care of the sick in each diocese. The Basilius, built by St. Basil the Great in the fourth century, has influenced hospital design to this day. Bishop Landry founded the Hotel Dieu in Paris in A.D. 660. This hospital still cares for the sick from its location on the Seine River in Paris.

Cosmas and Damian (d. A.D. 303)

While the early Greeks had their mythical gods and goddesses of healing (e.g., Aesculapius, Hygeia, and Panacea), the early Christians venerated those saints who significantly contributed to healings. Cosmas was a physician; Damian, his twin brother, practiced pharmacy. They were among many who were martyred for their Christian beliefs during Diocletian's persecutions (303–313). Over the years they have been honored as the patron saints of medicine and pharmacy.

The early Christian **monasteries** included an infirmary in their structural design. These infirmaries served the sick monks and persons in the neighborhood who required special care. During periodic plagues, the monks cared for persons with deadly and frightening diseases. Monasteries also contributed to health service by growing, preserving, and preparing herbal medicines and retaining and printing drug information available at the time. These early manuscripts were the medical textbooks of the day.

Monastic Manuscripts (A.D. 500–1200)

The impact of political, intellectual, religious, social, and cultural upheavals of the Middle Ages gave rise to medieval monasteries as centers of learning and science, including medical/pharmacy knowledge. Manuscripts from throughout the world were translated or copied in the famous monastic scriptoria (libraries). Among the most famous treaties are *De Viribus Herbarum* ("herbs used by people") composed in a French abbey by Abbott Odo; and *Causae et Curae* written by the Abbess Hildegard in a monastery in Bingen, Germany. Both manuscripts were completed during the eleventh to twelfth centuries. In addition to compiling existing knowledge, the monks added to the knowledge through studying the effects of the numerous plants grown in the monastery gardens.

Christian Renaissance Period

At the beginning of the Renaissance, several encouraging events occurred. In 1586 St. Camillus de Lellis founded a religious order, Clerics Regular Servants of the Sick, at the Hospital of St. James in Rome. Through his efforts the deplorable, filthy conditions in hospitals and miserable treatment by civil servants were scrutinized. St. Camillus took his new community of men and centered their activities in the Hospital of the Holy Spirit, which had been founded in 717 and was one of the largest hospitals in Europe. The brothers provided personal care for the patients, with special attention to diet. Holy Spirit Hospital soon became a major site for the education of lay physicians, with nearly 100 physicians in attendance. The hospital still contains an impressive library of medical literature. Thus, hospitals were beginning to emerge from the Dark Ages.

After St. Camillus founded his religious order, Pope Sixtus V authorized the red cross as a special insignia designating the special service provided by the order in the care of patients, many with diseases. To this day, a fourth vow of service at the time of pestilence is made by members of this order who wear the red cross on the breast of their habit. The red cross was soon seen on battlefields and ultimately became the insignia of the famous relief organization, the International Red Cross (recently renamed the International Movement of the Red Cross and Red Crescent).

Eastern Influence

Clay Tablets of Mesopotamia (3000–2500 B.C.)

Among thousands of clay tablets unearthed in the present Persian Gulf region, over 800 tablets contained materia medica information. These first pharmaceutical texts contained over 500 remedies from plant, mineral, and other sources. The Code of Hammurabi was also discovered containing a section on ethical standards for health practitioners.

Pen T'sao (3000 B.C.)

The Chinese document *Pen T'sao,* freely translated as "the botanical basis of pharmacy," describes over 1000 plants and 11,000 prescriptions handed down by oral tradition from Shen-Nung, considered the father of Chinese pharmaceutics. The early Chinese texts were inscribed on bamboo slats. They indicated the name of the drug, the **dosage,** and the symptoms it was used to treat.

About 500 B.C., Lao-tsu, a Taoist philosopher, composed a herbal compendium called "Tao te Ching" (The Way).

China (500 B.C.)

Drugs used in early China include ephedra, cassia, rhubarb, camphor, and ginseng. Yin drugs were cold and wet, and yang drugs were warm and dry. Red drugs treated heart conditions and yellow drugs were used to treat liver problems.

Mithradates VI (d. 63 B.C.)

Early in history the adverse or poisonous effects of drugs were a matter of concern. Mithradates might be called the "father of toxicology" for his investigation and writings related to the prevention and counteraction of the poisonous effects of drugs through the use of appropriate **antidotes.**

Arabia and Persia (A.D. 700–800)

In Arab countries, attitudes were humane and compassionate. Asylums for **psychiatric** patients were built that provided gardens, fountains, pleasant music, and a healthy setting where drugs, baths, and good nutrition were given to the patients.

New **dosage forms** were introduced as syrups and jams that contained active ingredients such as aloes, senna, nutmeg, clover, camphor, and musk. The *Minhaj (Handbook for the Apothecary Shop)* stated that a pharmacist "ought to have deep religious convictions, consideration for others, especially the poor and needy, a sense of responsibility and be careful and God-fearing."

Avicenna (Ibn Sina) (A.D. 980–1037)

Avicenna, also known as Ibn Sina, is called the "Persian Galen." His Arabic writings unified pharmaceutical and medical knowledge known at the time. His teachings were accepted in the West until the seventeenth century and to this day remain influential in the East.

India (1000 B.C.)

More than 2000 drugs are mentioned in Charaka's writings, including cinnamon, cardamom, ginger, pepper, aconite, and licorice. These condiments and spices are in use today. Mercury was used in numerous preparations and is used today as Mercurochrome and Merthiolate as an external antiseptic.

Egyptian Influence

The great Al-Mansur Hospital in Cairo, Egypt, is an example of the Arabs' interest and dedication to health care. The hospital had special wards for particular diseases, outpatient clinics, convalescent areas, diet kitchens, and a large medical library. Both men and women were trained to provide care for the sick.

Ebers papyrus (1500 B.C.)

The parchment (papyrus) scroll, found in Egypt by George Ebers (1837–1898), is one of eleven medical scrolls that preserve the knowledge of early Egyptian medicine. Over 700 drugs are mentioned, with formulas for more than 800 remedies. According to these scrolls, the pharmacist selected the drugs, prepared them in a magically correct way, and then said prescribed benediction over them. The use of mortars and pestles, hand mills, sieves, and weighing scales is mentioned in the papyrus.

Military Influence

Wars accelerate the need for health care. Military medicine throughout history has provided the stimulus for improvement in infection control, surgical interventions, and trauma management. The Crusaders brought personal and financial support to the hospitals in the areas of conquest between A.D. 1096 and 1291. The Crusaders built hospitals in the Holy Lands. During this period the Hospitalers of the Order of St. John of God were established to staff the hospitals and care for the wounded on the battlefield. This order continues to maintain health facilities throughout the world.

Hospitals began to take shape in what is now the United States in approximately the same way. It is known that military hospitals functioned during the Revolutionary War in New York (Manhattan), Pennsylvania (Lititz), Massachusetts, and other areas of battle. For the most part these were temporary field hospitals.

A historic example of a hospital formulary was compiled in Pennsylvania during the Revolutionary War. Known as the "Lititz Pharmacopoeia," it was used in preparing medications for the military hospital located in that town.

During the Civil War in the United States, Louisa May Alcott served as a volunteer and observed the wanton conditions of poor sanitation, depressing environment, and patient and staff misery at the Union Hospital in Georgetown, Virginia. She describes these conditions in detail in her published book, *Hospital Sketches.* This book influenced President Abraham Lincoln to establish the U.S. Sanitary Commission, which has as its goal "a single desire and resolute determination to secure for the men who have enlisted in this war and that care which it is the duty of the nation to give them."[1] Lincoln also requested the Sisters of Charity to care for the wounded on the battlefields in the Civil War.

During the ensuing decades rapid changes took place. The wars of the twentieth century have seen significant changes in hospitals and health care delivery systems. World War I brought about the need to care for patients suffering from major trauma, burns, poison gas, and infections of all kinds. Hospital design reflected these needs in dealing with the masses of the injured, maimed, and sick. Ships designed as floating hospitals (begun during the Civil War) were in great demand to handle large numbers of casualties away from the immediate battlefield. They were also used to transport the sick under treatment to land-based institutions. World War II saw major advances in trauma surgery, the introduction of systemic sulfonamides, penicillin, and the wide use of blood and plasma for transfusion. The volume of injured increased and very large hospitals were built to provide the services needed. The Cadet Nurse Corps was developed in the early 1940s to answer the need for large numbers of professionally trained people to nurse the sick. Because of the kinds of injuries, new forms of treatment of war injuries were developed. The professions of occupational therapist and physical therapist came into being. Emotional problems resulting from the war gave new impetus for hospital facilities to deal with war-related psychiatric problems. One vivid reminder of the Korean conflict was the television series *M.A.S.H.* The weekly series brought us the experience of war through the eyes and emotions of a mobile army surgical hospital staff. It was the close proximity of these mobile operating rooms and support resources that resulted in saving the lives of hundreds if not thousands of victims.

European Influences

Western Europe (A.D. 500–1200)

Medieval physicians prescribed approximately 1000 natural substances, most of plant origin. **Herbs** were the main source of medication. Materia medica was derived from the Greeks, Romans, and Arabs. The monasteries in England, Germany, and France preserved this information and added to it the medicinal herbs grown in the monastery gardens.

During the Middle Ages, medical advancement came close to a standstill. A church edict in 1163 forbade clerics from performing any surgery that caused a loss of blood. At this time, monks were the primary health care practitioners, so surgical procedures were eliminated. Between 1347 and 1350, the **Black Plague** killed almost one-third of the inhabitants of Europe. Although most people were cared for and/or died in their own homes, many either died on the street or were brought to overcrowded hospitals. Hotel Dieu, one of the finest hospitals in Europe at the time, was reported to dismiss up to 500 bodies a day to be buried during the height of the plague.

Throughout the centuries, persons afflicted with mental health problems were often secluded from society in confined custodial care. The poor conditions of care are reflected in the story of Bethlehem Hospital in London, called Bedlam. (The word continues in the English language to convey the idea of confusion and disorder.) Modern health care requires concern for those afflicted with mental disorders.

In Italy, mental hospitals were built in Metz, Uppsala, Bergamo, and Florence in which patients were treated in a humanistic way. Outstanding in the care of psychiatric patients was the town of Gheel in Belgium, where the focus of town employment and activities was on the care of psychiatric patients who were given residence in the homes of the townspeople. It was in this town that St. Dymphna, the patron saint for mental disorders, was murdered by her deranged father who was king of Ireland and who pursued his daughter in rage after she had fled his abuse.

To this very day, the town of Gheel is given over to the care of the mentally ill, with support from the Belgian government.

Swiss influence

Paracelsus (1493–1541). Born Philippus Aureolus Theophrastus Bombast von Hohenheim, this Swiss alchemist changed his name to indicate the superiority over the great herbalist, Celsus. A product of Renaissance, Paracelsus revolutionized pharmacy from a botanical science to the beginnings of a chemical orientation in the profession. He replaced the four body fluids identified by Hippocrates (blood, phlegm, yellow bile, and black bile) with three chemical constituents of the body. Paracelsus was the prime mover in bringing pharmacy from a botanical to a chemical science. Sulfur, mercury, and salt were the materials of the body, and drugs were used to overcome excess acid or alkalinity in the body. Alcohols, spirits, acids, and oils were used, and mercurials and other minerals.

German influence

The Magna Carta of pharmacy. For the first time in the history of Western Europe, pharmacy was declared an independent profession separate from medicine through the official Edict of 1231. Emperor Frederick II of Germany was the author of this edict, known as the Magna Carta of pharmacy. By it, pharmacies were subject to government inspections; the pharmacist was obliged, under oath, to prepare drugs as prescribed in a reliable and uniform method. This edict influenced the practice of pharmacy across all of Western Europe.

Pharmacopoeias. Books that contain official drug standards have been known through the ages as recipe books, formularies, **dispensatories,** and pharmacopoeias. The distinction of having the first legal pharmacopoeia goes to the city of Nuremberg, Germany, where the municipal authorities in 1546 made it the official book of drug standards for that city. This book, known as *Dispensatorium Pharmacopolarum,* also became official in Augsburg, Cologne, Florence, and Rome.

Frederick Serturner (1783–1841), a pharmacist, won international recognition when he prepared salts of morphine (1804), a drug of universal acclaim in the control of intractable pain.

Johannes Buchner (1783–1852), a pharmacist and professor of pharmacy in Munich, discovered salicin in the willow bark and nicotine in tobacco. These discoveries paved the groundwork for aspirin (acetylsalicylic acid) and nicotinic acid. The latter was synthesized from nicotine in 1867 and is used today as niacin, a member of vitamin B complex.

Rudolph Brandes isolated hyoscyamine (1819) and, with fellow pharmacist Philipp Geiger (1785–1836), collaborated in research to discover atropine (1835). Atropine, used to this day, is a prototype for antispasmodic drugs.

Although Emil von Behring (1854–1917) was a physician and not a pharmacist, his contribution to pharmacy was a landmark. His work with antitoxin to combat the effects of diphtheria, and later tetanus, initiated serum therapy. Diphtheria antitoxin (1892) created a whole new category of pharmaceuticals.

The concept of chemotherapy was introduced by Paul Ehrlich (1854–1915), who researched 606 chemical combinations until he found an arsenical that would be effective in combating the contemporary **pandemic,** syphilis. Arsphenamine was patented in 1907 and achieved fame as the "magic bullet" against syphilis. Ehrlich was a German physician and a pioneer in cellular pathology. Specific remedies, many of a chemical nature, were targeted at specific microbial and specific human cells. An intensive warfare against infection had begun.

Gerhard Domagk (1895–1964), a German scientist, discovered a sulfa drug, Prontosil, to be effective against hemolytic streptococci. The use of this drug became widespread as its effectiveness against a wide range of microorganisms became evident.

Swedish influence

Karl Scheele (1742–1786) was a Swedish pharmacist who made numerous chemical discoveries in the laboratory of his pharmacy shop. Among his discoveries were arsenic (1771), chlorine (1774), glycerin (1783), and numerous organic acids.

English influence

During the eighteenth century, many hospitals were built in England to provide diagnosis and treatment of the poor. The Bristol Royal Hospital claims to be the first voluntary hospital in the provinces. One of the most famous hospitals, Guy's Hospital in London, was built in 1740 and provided free care through a ticket admission system.

William Withering (1741–1799), a clinician and a botanist in England, investigated the active ingredient in a folk remedy used to cure dropsy (an accumulation of fluids due to heart impairment). He called attention to digitalis (1741) as the active **alkaloid** in the foxglove plant. Digoxin, a form of digitalis, is widely used today as a cardiotonic drug.

Edward Jenner (1749–1823), an English physician, vaccinated against smallpox with the cowpox vaccine (1789). This discovery in turn led to the eradication of smallpox in the twentieth century.

Ten years later a new class of anti-infective drugs became available in limited quantities. Penicillin (1942), the first antibiotic to be used in therapy, was available to treat 100 patients. It was first observed as an inhibitor of microbial growth by Alexander Fleming at St. Mary's Hospital in London in 1928. Later Howard Florey (1898–1968) and his coworkers succeeded in first isolating and then making available this lifesaving antibiotic to treat gram-positive infections.

French influence

Bernard Courtois (1777–1838) discovered iodine (1811) in marine algae. In 1826, the year he graduated from pharmacy school in Montpellier, Antoine Balard discovered bromine in sea water. He later became a faculty member of the same school.

Joseph Caventou (1795–1877), a pharmacist, collaborated with Pierre Pelletier (1788–1842) in the discovery of quinine (1820) which has become a worldwide treatment for **malaria.** He made other discoveries as well, including the identification of caffeine (1821).

Pierre Robiquet (1788–1840), a pharmacist who was also a phytochemist, made a number of significant discoveries, including codeine (1832). Codeine, an analgesic weaker than but similar to morphine, is a drug widely used to control pain.

Henri Moissan (1852–1907) obtained free fluorine (1886) by electrolytic methods, thus completing the elements in the halogen family of drugs.

International Influence

Canadian Contribution

Another dramatic and lifesaving discovery was made by Frederick Banting (1891–1941) and Charles Best (1899–1978) when they collaborated to discover insulin (1922). The lives of millions of diabetic patients have been saved and enhanced by this major therapeutic breakthrough.

World Health Organization

The World Health Organization (WHO) published the first *International Pharmacopoeia* in Geneva, Switzerland, in 1951. This book was published in English, French, and Spanish and later in German and Japanese. Although not a legal document, it assists in setting internationally acceptable drug standards. Drugs that are included in any pharmacopoeia are those of proven pharmaceutic and therapeutic value.

Developments in the United States Related to Health Care and Drug Therapy

Hospitals have emerged over the years from **almshouses** for the sick poor, **asylums** for the care and confinement of orphans and the mentally ill, **sanatoriums** for long-term care of tuberculosis patients and the victims of other chronic diseases, **hospices** for the terminally ill, and infirmaries for short-term acute care.

Nonmilitary Hospitals

Nonmilitary hospitals came into existence in New Amsterdam, New York; Salem, Massachusetts; and Philadelphia, Pennsylvania. Philadelphia General Hospital was started in 1713 by the Quakers as an almshouse to give relief to the sick, the incurables, the poor, orphans, and abandoned infants.

Benjamin Franklin obtained a grant in 1751 to found the first American hospital, known as the Pennsylvania Hospital. Jonathan Roberts was recruited as the pharmacist and enjoys the reputation of being the first American hospital pharmacist. This institution has had a reputation for excellence from its earliest beginnings. The New York Cornell Medical Center was initially supported by King George III in a charter granted in 1771. The apothecary-in-chief was one of the four administrative officers named in the original charter.

Psychiatric Care

In the United States, Benjamin Rush, who is a physician, introduced new methods of treatment for psychiatric patients based on moral principles. His concerns and methods were outlined in a treatise on the topic that he published in 1812. Dr. Rush was a friend of Benjamin Franklin and cared for the mentally ill at Pennsylvania Hospital. The hospital was a forerunner in the care of the mentally disturbed in a general hospital, although at that time psychiatric patients were housed in the lower level of the hospital and separated from the medical treatment areas.

Custodial care

The nineteenth century continued the manner of dealing with mental patients by separating them from family and society. At the same time, the term *asylum* was substituted for the term *hospital*. The growth in the number and size of mental hospitals after the turn of the century was tremendous. Custodial care in gigantic facilities became the norm, with half the hospital beds in the United States occupied by mental patients. During the middle of the twentieth century, the trend reversed.

Deinstitutionalization

Appropriate use of psychiatric drugs and various psychiatric treatment methods allowed many patients to leave custodial care and assume the activities of daily living in society. Under this concept of **deinstitutionalization,** large numbers of persons were discharged to communities and in some cases to fend for themselves in the streets. The movement received strong support from civil liberty groups. State governments were only too willing to unburden themselves of the financial responsibilities involved in institutional care. What seemed to be a humane approach only increased the number of homeless in society. Now efforts are being made by professionals to develop small housing facilities for their care. Some now recognize that continued structural support and care are still required.

Surgical Care

Massachusetts General Hospital in Boston was the first hospital to use general anesthesia in surgery. The first operation was performed in 1842 with anesthesia provided by Dr. Crawford Long. Soon chloroform and ether became standard anesthetic agents, which allowed for more frequent, less painful surgery.

Contemporary Medical Practices

"Miracle drugs" are a major part of the medical fabric of the twentieth century. Numerous researchers in universities, in pharmaceutical firms, and under government sponsorship have made and continue to make drug discoveries that stave off death and improve the quality of life.

Polio Vaccine

Poliomyelitis was a disease that, among others, crippled American President Franklin Roosevelt and killed and crippled many children. Eventually, two vaccines were developed: an injectable vaccine (by Jonas Salk, 1955) and an oral vaccine (by Albert Sabin, 1961). These vaccines have practically eliminated the disease commonly known as infantile paralysis.

Steptomycin

Selman Waksman (1888–1973) and his colleagues at Rutgers University in New Jersey began an intensive search to find another antibiotic to treat tuberculosis, known as the Great White Plague, which was then claiming numerous lives. Streptomycin, discovered in 1944, was the first antibiotic to be effective against tubercle bacillus, the infective agent in tuberculosis.

Whole hospital buildings were changed or eliminated as a result of new treatments. Tuberculosis sanatoriums and poliomyelitis facilities are examples of treatment centers outmoded by new therapy. The famed Willard Parker Hospital of New York was declared obsolete after drug and antibiotic treatments reduced contagion and the need for isolation in hospital buildings. More recently, ambulatory treatment of childhood disease has caused a dramatic reduction in the need for pediatric hospital beds.

Surgical Procedures

Technology continues at an accelerated pace, making real what only a few years ago appeared to be science fiction. New technology has resulted in shorter hospitalization and has given rise to home health care. For example, **cataract** surgery in the 1930s and 1940s was followed by a long postoperative recovery. The patient was housed in a darkened room and the head immobilized between sandbags. Now surgery is performed on an ambulatory basis with the patient going home the same day, once surgery is completed. Increasingly, diagnostic procedures and treatments are conducted in outpatient facilities.

Governmental Interventions in Medical Practice

Government pressures and controls have had their impact on the health care delivery system. Part of the impetus for ambulatory surgery has resulted from pressures by government, insurance companies, and the public at large to perform procedures quickly, eliminate hospital stay, and provide patients with the opportunity for recovery in their own home environment. Second options have helped to reassure patients that surgery is, in fact, necessary and justified. In many instances, insurance companies or employers require that prior approval be given for hospitalization if the company or employer is expected to be responsible for payment. Fewer needed beds have forced hospitals to close or merge. Hospital mergers reduce costs and provide greater economic efficiency.

Review of Therapeutic Advances Discovered in the Nineteenth and Twentieth Centuries

Drug Standards Set by Pharmacopoeias

The first U.S. Pharmacopoeia (U.S.P.) was published in Philadelphia in 1820 by the U.S. Pharmacopoeia Convention. This convention, founded on the American principle of representation, had **physician** representatives from all the existing states. The goal of the convention was to select the "official" drugs and to set up standards for their identity, purity, and assay methods. By 1850, pharmacists and physicians were members of the convention. The pharmacopoeia is revised every 10 years. The first pharmacist to be chairman of the convention was Charles Rice, superintendent of the General Drug Department at Bellevue Hospital in New York. He laid the foundation for the sixth edition of the U.S.P., published in 1882.

Biologicals

Serum therapy was initiated with the discovery of the germ theory by Robert Koch; the discovery of **vaccination** to provide **immunity** by Edward Jenner; and the discovery of antitoxins to neutralize microbial toxins by Emil von Behring. The vaccines, toxoids, and antitoxins were the first biologicals. Smallpox vaccine was introduced in the early 1900s, followed by vaccines for typhus, whooping cough, measles, mumps, rubella, diphtheria, tetanus, influenza, and polio. In 1987, a genetically engineered hepatitis B vaccine was marketed.

Hormones

Isolation of human hormones began in 1897 with adrenaline, followed by thyroxine (1916), insulin, cortisone, adrenocorticotropin (ACTH), estrone (1929), and testosterone (1935). These substances are important for replacement therapy and other therapeutic needs. Human insulin (humulin), a product of genetic engineering, was introduced in 1982.

Anti-infectives

Anti-infective therapy began with salvarsan (1907) and then prontosil (1935). A major breakthrough occurred with the discovery of penicillin (1928–1940). Other antibiotics soon followed: streptomycin (1944) and chloramphenicol (1947), known as the first broad-spectrum antibiotic.

Synthetics

Synthetic chemicals were rapidly developed, including phenobarbital (1912), Raudixin® (1953), Thorazine® (1954), Lithium (1960), and Valium® (1963).

Antihypertensives, antiarrhythmics, antianginals, vasodilators, and **beta blockers,** all improved cardiac and circulatory problems. Drugs were developed to meet problems in the major biologic systems.

Immunomodulators

The most recent category of drugs to be developed is the **immunomodulators.** Based on the theory of preserving the integrity of the immune system, immunostimulators are used when there is a deficiency, and immunosuppressants are used to prevent organ transplant rejection and to treat autoimmune diseases. These modulators preserve equilibrium in the second most complicated biologic system, the immune system. (The most complex is the nervous system.)

Drug Development

The use of medicinal substances is a part of every culture. Plants, minerals, and animal parts were the drug components until the early nineteenth century. The twentieth century has advanced drug therapy to a greater extent than the contributions of all ages past.

Hospital Development

Hospital care has moved within the evolution of the human race. The multifaceted health institutions of today, with all the advances of biomedical science, have retained the primary mission of hospitals. This mission is the humane, compassionate, contemporary, oriented goal to fight disease, control pain, and provide optimum quality of life through prevention, restoration, cure, or health maintenance. Human care remains a noble endeavor in which we, as health professionals, take our turns as consumer and provider.

Summary

Contemporary Health Care Issues

New delivery systems, such as **health maintenance organizations (HMOs),** emergicenters, and other facilities, have been developed to meet the public's desire for quick, early, and relatively inexpensive care. Much of the concern over the safety of performing surgery on an ambulatory basis has disappeared. Results of other health care delivery systems are being evaluated. Hospitals have been forced to find alternative means to bring in revenue to bolster flagging institutional finances. Some of the ideas have alarmed health care professionals. Advertising, television spots, candlelight dinners, exercise clubs, and day care centers are but few of the trendy ideas being utilized to bring the name of the local hospital to the attention of the public.

As the twentieth century draws to a close, the demand for service, the method of reimbursement for health care services, and the practice of medicine will greatly influence hospitals. Most assuredly, the awesome spector of AIDS will have a great impact in the remaining years of the century. Hospitals will continue to change and grow or diminish as medicine, **biotechnology,** science, politics, and public concerns assert their influence. As a result of these factors, hospitals will continue to develop their own special character.

Contemporary Pharmacy Concerns

Pharmacy practice in the latter part of the twentieth century in the United States has been, through many internal and external factors, reoriented from a product focus to a concern for the ways drugs are used by people. The incorporation of clinical studies in the pharmacy school curriculum; clinical drug research activities supported by the government, industry, and universities; and extensive drug information services are moving pharmacy into an esteemed health profession role in the twenty-first century.

Pharmacy Heritage

Recently there has been enthusiasm for tracing "roots." Knowledge of historical development provides a framework to clarify values, foster appreciation, and establish future focus. This chapter reviews the cultural, medical, pharmaceutical, and ethical dimensions of better care as documented in the history of the healing sciences. To fully appreciate this heritage as a member of a noble profession, it is important to relate to the major contributions that have been bequeathed to contemporaries in the service of the sick at various times in history.

ASSESSMENT

Multiple Choice Questions

1. Which of the following aspects of pharmacy are mentioned in the Old Testament?
   a. the role of the pharmacist
   b. professional norms of practice
   c. examples of healing herbs
   d. all of the above
   e. none of the above

2. The Edict of 1231, the Magna Carta of pharmacy, stated that
   a. pharmacists depend upon physicians to specify how prescriptions should be compounded
   b. no one has the right to inspect a pharmacy for standards
   c. drugs should be prepared in a reliable and uniform method
   d. all of the above
   e. none of the above

3. Pharmacopoeias contain
   a. herbal collections
   b. chemical drugs
   c. synthetic drugs
   d. official drug standards
   e. antidotes for herbal poisons

4. A famous rabbi-physician was
   a. Hippocrates
   b. Landry
   c. Mansur
   d. Maimonides
   e. Ezechiel

5. The town of Gheel is dedicated to the care of
   a. war veterans
   b. drug addicts
   c. the homeless
   d. psychiatric patients
   e. unwed mothers

6. Fabiola was a
   a. female physician
   b. Greek apothecary
   c. hospital benefactor
   d. mythical goddess of nursing
   e. Roman storyteller

7. The well-known military hospital in the town of Lititz was located in
   a. Pennsylvania
   b. New York
   c. Massachusetts
   d. Virginia
   e. New Amsterdam

8. The Pennsylvania Hospital was founded by
   a. George Washington
   b. Benjamin Franklin
   c. Abraham Lincoln
   d. Benjamin Rush
   e. William Penn

9. Deinstitutionalization has resulted in
   a. increased number of homeless
   b. bizarre street behaviors
   c. improved care for persons with emotional disorders
   d. empty institutions
   e. a, b, and d

10. The present health care system is being modified and refocused by
    a. economic pressures
    b. political influence
    c. scientific discoveries
    d. biotechnology
    e. all of the above

Matching

11. __b__ quinine

12. __c__ arsphenamine

13. __d__ streptomycin

14. __a__ digitalis

15. __e__ vaccination

a. heart problems

b. malaria

c. syphilis

d. tuberculosis

e. smallpox

True/False Questions

16. _____ Pharmacy has always been based on scientific findings.

17. _____ Galen and Paracelsus influenced the practice of medicine and pharmacy for hundreds of years.

18. _____ Garlic has been used since antiquity as a remedy for numerous health problems.

19. _____ Serum therapy uses only those herbs of therapeutic value.

20. _____ The early explorers who first came to American shores took some of the native American herbs back to Europe.

Bibliography

Cowen, D.L., & Helfand, W.H. (1990). *Pharmacy, an illustrated history.* New York: Harry N. Abrams, Inc.

Cowie, L. (1986). *Plague and fire.* London: Wayland Publishing.

Donahue, P. (1985). *Nursing, the finest art.* St. Louis: C.V. Mosby.

Dorland's illustrated medical dictionary (26th ed.). (1984). Philadelphia: W.B. Saunders Company.

Dubos, R. (1959). *Mirage of health.* New York: Harper and Row.

Garrison, F.H. (1929). *History of medicine.* Philadelphia: Saunders.

Ziegler, P. (1984). *The black death.* New York: Penguin Books.

2 Organizational Structure and Function of the Hospital

COMPETENCIES

After completion and review of this chapter, the student should be able to

1. Explain the primary function of a hospital.
2. List five functions related to patient "processing" activities.
3. Name four treatment modalities available in a hospital for patient care.
4. Explain the hospital's role in wellness programs.
5. Describe the roles of the hospital's governing board.
6. List the functions of the director of a medical department.
7. Mention the major diagnostic units in the hospital.

Introduction

Hospitals today are considered networks of health care services. These services focus on **diagnosis,** treatment, prevention, and health maintenance. This chapter will explore the organizational structure and functions that provide the care to maximize optimum therapeutic outcomes for the patients served.

When asked to explain what running a hospital was like, an experienced administrator once described it as running the largest hotel in town, the largest restaurant, the largest laundry, the largest laboratory, the largest employment office, the largest cleaning service, and so forth, all wrapped up in one. This scenario, although somewhat amusing, can be particularly helpful in understanding how patient care is delivered and how a hospital functions on a day-to-day basis. In this chapter we shall explore two concepts: (1) the functions of today's modern hospital and (2) how the hospital is organized to achieve those functions.

Hospital Functions

The primary functions of any hospital are to provide resources for and to assist the physician in (a) diagnosing the patient and (b) providing treatment for the patient. In carrying out these primary functions, a variety of secondary functions must also

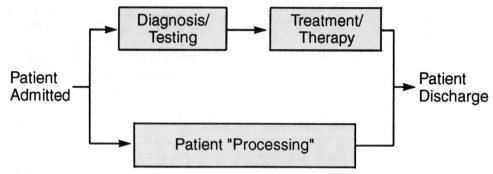

FIGURE 2–1 Simplified diagram of hospital functions

be performed (e.g., record keeping, billing, making plans for posthospital care.) This simple breakdown of functions is shown in **Figure 2–1.**

The "processing" of patients refers to all the functions and paperwork associated with a patient's stay in the hospital. These include the admission process, the medical records function, utilization review, billing, and **discharge planning,** to name a few.

The physician orders tests to confirm or identify the patient's diagnosis or medical condition. These tests are carried out in the various departments (e.g., radiology, medical laboratory, cardiopulmonary, and **neurosonology.**) Once the diagnosis has been determined, treatment or therapy may be appropriate, and may include surgery, physical therapy, respiratory therapy, or drug therapy. Each is carried out by the appropriate clinical service. Some departments, such as nursing, play an ongoing role in both the diagnosis and treatment functions.

The diagnosis and treatment of a patient is rarely a simple, straightforward process. Complications and unexpected ancillary test results can blur the distinction between diagnosis and treatment. It is not uncommon, for example, for one diagnosis to be treated only to have another health problem manifest itself. In today's aging society, older patients frequently present themselves at the hospital with multiple diagnoses and conditions, all interrelated to varying degrees, making the diagnosis/treatment functions quite complex. For purposes of understanding the hospital's overall functions, however, it is of importance to reorganize the sequence of diagnosis and treatment and the corresponding patient "processing" as being of primary significance to the structure and function of the hospital.

Another major function of hospitals that has gradually been developed over the past 10 to 15 years has been health education and promotion. Hospitals have taken on responsibility for not only helping patients recover good health, but also for helping them stay healthy. To this end, hospitals have sponsored smoking cessation programs, stress reduction classes, weight loss programs, and instructions in how to identify potential health problems, such as self-examination for breast cancer. Community screening efforts for blood pressure, mammography, cholesterol, and glucose levels are representative of similar efforts to uncover those people at risk of becoming ill before their health actually begins to deteriorate. In addition, hospitals have developed support groups for patients and families with such health problems as diabetes and cancer. Finally, hospitals have begun to play a coordinating role in helping whole groups of patients assess their health care needs and gain access to the appropriate health care providers. One group of patients for whom this function is prevalent is senior citizens.

If we are to superimpose these additional functions on Figure 2–1, it will now appear as shown in **Figure 2–2.**

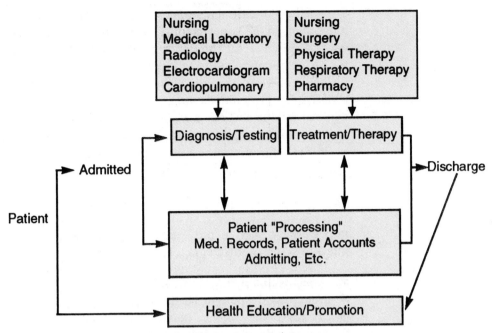

FIGURE 2–2 Expanded diagram of hospital functions

Anyone who has ever been in a hospital recognizes that there are a great many other things that go on that have not yet been addressed. Volunteers are available to answer questions or augment staff by assisting patients.

Dietary service counsels patients and prepares and serves patient and employee meals. Housekeeping keeps the hospital clean and plays an integral role in infection control. Plant engineering maintains the facility and provides the necessary heating or air-conditioning and other utilities. All of these activities, and others, are essential to the successful operation of a hospital.

Hospital Organization

Hospital organization and governance have traditionally been characterized as a three-legged stool: the governing body, the medical staff, and the hospital staff as led by the hospital's administration. It is a useful analogy since all three elements must be effectively integrated for a hospital to successfully support itself.

The governing body is usually called a **board of trustees** or **board of directors.** (In a governmental hospital these are sometimes known as a board of supervisors.) The board is charged with the ultimate responsibility of governing the hospital in the community's best interest. To this end, they are ethically, financially, and legally responsible for everything that goes on in the hospital. The board organizes itself into a variety of committees to perform the detailed activities required to govern the hospital. These committees encompass financial activities, community relations, planning, quality assurance, and personnel, as well as a variety of other areas of responsibility.

The medical staff consists of physicians, psychologists, podiatrists, dentists, and so forth, credentialled in their specialty or subspecialty to practice at the hospital. They are organized into departments such as medicine, surgery, family practice, ob/gyn, and pediatrics. The medical staff is sometimes further subdivided into subspecialty sections or groups such as cardiology, orthopedics, and neurology.

The medical departments have a department director or chair who oversees the functioning of the department. Typically these functions include establishing standards of practice for the department's specialty, providing continuing education for its members, monitoring individual physicians' performance, and providing a forum for the exchange of ideas and new techniques. The medical staff also organizes itself into multidisciplinary committees to perform specific activities that the medical staff as a whole is responsible for. These committee activities include reviewing pharmacy and therapeutics, **credentialling,** tissue review, quality assurance, and utilization review. Both the medical staff and the board of trustees also have executive committees that coordinate the work of all the other committees. They typically share sponsorship of a joint conference committee made up of representatives from both the board and the medical staff.

Like the medical staff, the hospital staff is organized around common functions separated into departments or services. Each department or service performs one or more of the following general categories of functions:

- Assist with the diagnosis via testing.
- Help treat the patient via therapy.
- "Process" the patient's paperwork or monitor the patient's treatment.
- Maintain the physical environment or support the patient's stay in the hospital.
- Support the functioning and management of the individual departments and/or hospital as a whole.

Diagnostic testing is carried out typically in the departments such as laboratory, radiology, nuclear medicine, and EKG. Therapy is provided in the departments of pharmacy, physical therapy, speech therapy, and radiation therapy. Some departments, such as nursing, psychiatry, and respiratory therapy, spend significant amounts of time both determining diagnoses and providing treatments.

Some departments perform "processing" functions that assist the patient throughout the stay without directly affecting diagnosis or treatment. Examples of these departments include **medical records,** admitting, patient accounts (billing), **utilization review,** and social services.

Another group of departments support the patient's stay either by contributing to the physical environment or by supporting the coordination of services to the patient. Included in this group would be communications, housekeeping, volunteers, laundry, plant engineering and maintenance, safety and security, and pastoral care. The dietary department, while providing support to the patient through ongoing nutrition, also can play a **therapeutic** role and a health teaching role.

Finally, a variety of departments and services are vital to the overall success of a hospital, but patients may never hear of them while around the hospital. These departments support the ongoing operation of the hospital and/or the individual services and include the departments of personnel, purchasing and general stores, **community relations and fund development,** planning, risk management, and accounting and finance. In addition, there are personnel who clerically support the activities of the medical staff.

Each hospital department/service is generally run by an administrative director or a section supervisor. These middle managers, in turn, report to representative members of the administration. These vice presidents report to either the executive vice president or directly to the president. Historically the departments were grouped according to common operating characteristics into four categories: nursing services, clinical services (testing and treatment departments), support services (support and facilities departments), and financial services (accounting, patient accounts, etc.). The organizational chart in **Figure 2–3** reflects this historical division of responsibility.

However, hospital organizational structure has changed dramatically over the years and is now tailored specifically to each hospital's activities and the capabilities of its department heads and administrative staff. Although some elements are common to all organizational charts, there is no longer one dominant organizational structure.

Matrix management and **product line management** are only two examples of organizational theory applied to the rapid technological and service delivery evolution that has taken place in health care. Matrix management structurally emphasizes the overlapping areas of responsibility among departments and the common areas of decision making. Product line management organizes the hospital not along the lines of comparable operating principles but by the end product or category of service being delivered.

It is not essential to fully understand organizational theory to appreciate how a hospital functions. What is important is to appreciate the great variety in the ways hospitals organize themselves and that, in each case, the communication and collaboration among departments are vital.

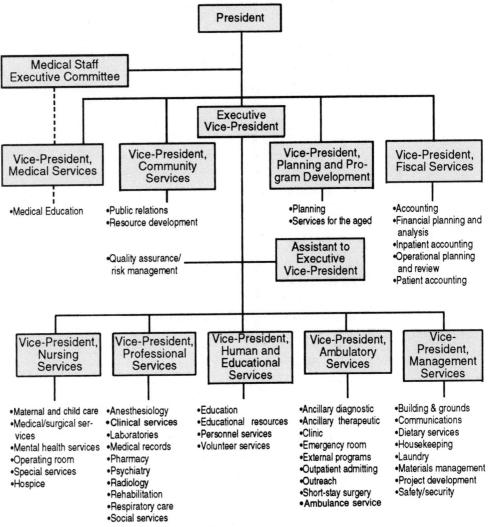

FIGURE 2–3   Hospital organization chart according to traditional divisions of responsibility

As a way of enhancing communications the hospital staff, such as the board of trustees and the medical staff, forms committees. Some committees are ongoing ones, such as safety and quality assurance committees. Many, however, are ad hoc working groups brought together to address a specific problem or concern. Once the desired resolution is achieved, these groups disband or form new committees to address different problems and issues. These ad hoc committees bring various departments together in a problem-solving situation without dramatically altering the organizational structure of the hospital or interfering with the reporting relationships carefully developed over time. As such they represent a flexible, informal organizational structure that allows the hospital to get its work done.

Summary

If there is one conclusion about hospital organizational structure and function that can be reached, it is that it will continuously change. New technologies are only now becoming available that will change whole departments or create new ones. New roles are continuously being proposed for the nation's hospitals and new organizational structures developed to meet the challenges that lie ahead. In short it is far from clear what hospitals will look like in the future or precisely how they will function. In light of the financial crisis hospitals are facing today, compounded by the technological revolution we are experiencing, we can be sure that hospitals will remain complex organizations that patients depend upon to adequately provide the quality care that is required. We can also be sure that proper and appropriate health care will continue to depend on accurate and precise communication of information and most importantly on the skill and dedication of those who staff our hospitals.

ASSESSMENT

Multiple Choice Questions

1. The primary functions of a hospital are to provide for which of the following:
   a. diagnosis
   b. treatment
   c. volunteer workers
   d. a and b
   e. a, b, and c

2. Patient "processing" activities include
   a. the admission process
   b. medical records function
   c. utilization reviews
   d. discharge planning
   e. all of the above

3. Most hospitals provide the following treatment modalities:
   a. surgery
   b. hypnosis
   c. acupuncture
   d. drug therapy
   e. a and d

4. Wellness programs in hospitals typically include
   a. smoking cessation programs
   b. handicap olympics
   c. strength training
   d. aerobics
   e. none of the above

5. The role of the hospital governing board includes responsibility for all the following except
   a. ethical concerns
   b. hiring of supervisory personnel
   c. legal and financial matters
   d. monthly on-site inspections of facility
   e. b and d

Matching

6. _____ maintains physical environment
7. _____ establishes medical standards of practice
8. _____ overall hospital governance
9. _____ social services
10. _____ monitors physicians' performance

a. board of trustees
b. medical staff
c. hospital staff

True/False Questions

11. _____ All hospitals conform to the same organizational structure.

12. _____ All hospitals function to provide required diagnostic and treatment services.

13. _____ Hospitals generally follow the patient into the community by discharge planning functions.

14. _____ Joint conference committees are made up of representatives from the board of directors and the medical staff.

15. _____ Clinical services include the testing and treatment departments.

Home Health Care

COMPETENCIES

Upon completion and review of this chapter, the student should be able to

1. Describe the evolution and future of the home health care industry, particularly related to home infusion therapy and home care pharmacy practice.

2. Explain the scope of services available to a patient requiring home health care.

3. Describe the five most common drug categories, medical indications for, and complications of home infusion therapy.

4. Describe the different types of infusion control devices used in home infusion therapy.

5. Describe the various roles for a pharmacy technician in a home infusion company.

Introduction

Home health care in the United States is a diverse and rapidly growing segment of the health care industry. It is rapidly becoming the predominant form of health care provision, replacing in-hospital care. Home health care, also called home care, can be defined as the provision of health care services to patients in their place of residence. The National Association for Home Care (NAHC) has identified a total of 17,561 home care agencies in the United States (NAHC, 1995). Home health care is as old as mankind; however, the first home health care agencies were established during the 1880s. On the basis of historical information obtained by NAHC, their numbers grew to 1100 by 1963 (NAHC, 1995). Pharmaceutical services were not a component of these early agencies, which consisted primarily of nurses, therapists, and home health aides. Retail pharmacies provided medications (primarily oral drugs) to patients in their home, through home deliveries by the pharmacy or the home health care nurse who picked up the medications for the patient. Pharmacy's role in home health care was then minor and indistinguishable from retail pharmacy practice. Indeed, home health care patients may have received less pharmaceutical care (i.e., clinical care) than their outpatient counterparts, because they rarely interacted with the pharmacist.

The first major boom in the number of home health care agencies occurred in 1965 with the enactment of Medicare. Medicare made home health care services available to the elderly, and beginning in 1973, to certain disabled younger Americans. Although the number of home health agencies doubled between 1967 and 1980 (NAHC, 1995), pharmacy's role in home health care had little increase because drugs were not a Medicare benefit. In 1983, Medicare initiated a prospective payment method of reimbursement for inpatient hospital care based on diagnosis-related groups (or DRGs) in an effort to reduce health care costs. This method of reimbursement provided economic incentives for hospitals to discharge patients as early as possible, reducing the length of a patient's stay in the hospital. This dramatically shifted patients from in-hospital care to the provision of care in the home setting. The number of home health care agencies doubled again between 1980 and 1985 (NAHC, 1995). Thus, in only 32 years, the number of home health care agencies grew from 1100 to over 17,000. The number of patients receiving home health care services grew to 7 million individuals. This time, however, pharmacy's role in home health care grew as well.

The role of pharmacy in the growth of home health care can be retraced to the birth of home infusion therapy during the early 1970s. Several university-based medical centers demonstrated the feasibility of providing nutritional support via the intravenous route, called total parenteral nutrition (TPN), in the home setting. This direct result of technological advances in infusion pumps allowed for smaller, yet more sophisticated pumps, and technological improvements in intravenous catheter materials and catheter placement techniques. These technological advances, with the implementation of the DRG-based method of hospital reimbursement and Medicare's willingness to pay for home TPN at one-third the inpatient rate, resulted in the birth of the home infusion therapy business. Once home TPN was established, other home infusion services were provided including home antibiotic therapy and pain management. Prior to this, TPN and drug infusion therapy were primarily hospital inpatient procedures. Now, there is almost no drug which cannot be administered safely in the home setting. Pharmacy's role in this field became prominent, and to this day, home infusion therapy remains pharmacy's predominant arena in home health care. In addition to hospitals as providers of home infusion therapy, the 1980s and 1990s saw entrepreneurial companies develop whose primary service was provision of home infusion therapy. During this time both the number of providers and the number of patients served grew. From 1982 through 1987, the compounded annual growth rate of the home infusion therapy industry was 58 percent (Conners & Winters, 1995). In 1987, it was estimated by the U.S. Office of Technology Assessment that 250,000 patients were receiving home infusion therapy (Conners & Winters, 1995).

Today the organizations and employers who pay for health care (including the U.S. government) are increasingly looking for ways to manage the cost of it. One predominant way of doing this in the 1990s is by managing the provision of care itself. This concept is called "managed care." Sometimes insurance companies, health maintenance organizations (HMOs), or employers directly provide this management of care. Other times they hire separate entities to manage the care for them. Under managed care, it has been increasingly realized that directing patients to the most appropriate and most cost-efficient health care setting at different cycles in their health care can reduce the cost of care without reducing (and sometimes increasing) the quality of care provided. Despite the tremendous growth of home health care in terms of number of patients and providers, the total cost of home health care is low. Annual expenditures for home health care in 1995 amounted to an estimated $27 billion (NAHC, 1995), which represents only 3 percent of the $1.069 trillion spent for personal health care in the United States in the same year. Compared with 42 percent for hospitals, home health care looks like a bargain. The numbers in **Table 3–1** further demonstrate this point. In addition, on the basis of satisfaction surveys, patients prefer home health care to hospital care, and one can see that the growth of home health care has not yet peaked. Even

TABLE 3–1

Comparison of Hospital, SNF, and Home Health Charges, 1992 and 1995 Estimates*

Charge per day	1992	1995
Hospital	$1459	$1810
Skilled nursing facility (nursing home)	264	293
Home health care	75	86

*Based on data provided by NAHC, 1995.

home infusion therapy, which has seen virtually no breakthroughs in technology and new therapies administered in the home in the past few years, is still experiencing a 13 percent annual compounded growth rate (Conners & Winters, 1995). The growth of pharmacy in home health care will continue into the next century. Many predict it will become the predominant health care setting for the provision of drug therapies and pharmacy practice.

Home Health Care Services

Home Health Services

Home health care consists of a wide diversity of health care services. The most frequently provided home care services are **home health services,** defined as the provision of health care services by a health care professional in the patient's place of residence, usually on a per visit basis. The predominant form of home health services is nursing. Other services include those of a dietitian, medical social worker, physical therapist, occupational therapist, and speech therapist. Some people also include respiratory therapists, dentists, and physicians in this group. Respiratory therapists are usually associated with the home medical equipment industry rather than with home health agencies. The provision of dental services in the home is relatively new, and extremely rare at present. Most people prefer to differentiate physician services in the home, referring to them as *home medical services.* Providers of home health services are called *home health agencies.* Home health agencies can be classified as public (governmental) agencies, nonprofit agencies, proprietary agencies, and hospital-based agencies. Most states require home health agencies to be licensed. Approximately 55 percent of home health agencies are Medicare certified (NAHC, 1995). To be Medicare certified, the organization must meet the Medicare Conditions of Participation and have a Medicare provider number. As part of the Conditions of Participation, the home health agency must provide nursing and one other home health service directly. Other services can be provided through a contracted provider. Nursing services can be high tech (e.g., infusion therapy) or low tech (e.g., diabetic teaching and monitoring) on an intermittent visit schedule or as 4- to 12-hour shifts called *private duty services.*

Personal Care and Support Services

The second most common form of home care services is **personal care and support services,** defined as the provision of nonprofessional services for patients in their place of residence. These services include homemaking, food preparation, personal care, and bathing. The individuals who provide these services are usually called **home health aides, homemakers,** or **personal care attendants.** Most personal care and support services are provided by home health agencies, although some companies (non-Medicare certified) specialize in this form of care exclusively.

Home Equipment Management Services

The third most prevalent form of home care services is **home equipment management services,** also referred to as **home medical equipment (HME)** services or **durable medical equipment (DME)** services. Home equipment management services can be defined as the selection, delivery, setup, and maintenance of equipment and the education of the patient in the use of the equipment—all performed in the patient's place of residence. Medical equipment includes wheelchairs, canes, walkers, beds, and commodes. It also includes higher technology items such as oxygen tanks, oxygen concentrators, ventilators, apnea monitors, phototherapy lights, infusion pumps, enteral pumps, and uterine monitors. Many providers include the sale of medical equipment and supplies (such as ostomy supplies) in this home care definition. However, the federal government and the Joint Commission on Accreditation of Healthcare Organizations (JCAHO), which accredits such providers, do not include the provision of products without services in their definition of home care. So such sales, without the corresponding services, would not be considered home care.

Home medical equipment providers are not required to be licensed in most states, although the U.S. Food and Drug Administration (FDA) and the Department of Transportation (DOT) require registration for distribution and transportation of oxygen. A large number of pharmacies are involved in the provision of home medical equipment services and sales which may be included in the definition of home care. Many HME organizations also provide clinical respiratory services, which include the professional services of a registered respiratory therapist for performing in-home assessments, monitoring of vital signs, oximetry testing, and/or administrating therapeutic treatments. Pharmacies are often involved in providing the respiratory drugs for these patients, either directly for the patient, or under contract from the HME provider.

Home Pharmaceutical Services

The last major form of home care service provided is **home pharmaceutical services,** usually defined as services provided to patients in their place of residence which procure, prepare, compound, dispense, and distribute pharmaceutical products and monitor patients' clinical status. To distinguish home care pharmacy services from other pharmacy services, including retail, two components to the services must be provided. First, the medications must be dispensed and delivered to patients in their home. Second, patients' clinical status must be monitored while they are in their home, and not through clinic visits and so forth. This can be done by evaluating physical assessment data from a nurse (or other professional) who visits patients in their home, monitoring lab data taken from patients in their home, calling patients at home on the telephone and evaluating their response to therapy, or using telemonitoring equipment set up in the home. In most cases when home pharmaceutical services are provided, home health services are provided as well, although not necessarily by the same company or organization.

Role of Pharmacy in Home Health Care

Although the predominant form of home pharmaceutical services provided is home infusion therapy (90 percent or greater), pharmacy practice in home care is not limited to a specific route of administration or dosage form (i.e., infusion). For example, patients who are homebound, who are required to be monitored and evaluated in the home, and who receive oral and topical therapies from a pharmacy are receiving home pharmaceutical services. A growing number of specialized mail-order pharmacies actually mail their drugs and employ pharmacists who monitor the patients' response to care between prescriptions, which is considered as providing home pharmaceutical services. The predominant specialty areas for such pharmacies include transplant/immunocompromised, cystic fibrosis, and hemophilia patients.

Home Infusion Therapy

According to the U.S. Office of Technology Assessment, home infusion therapy is described as a medical therapy that involves the prolonged (and usually repeated) injection of pharmaceutical products, most often delivered intravenously, but sometimes delivered via other routes (e.g., subcutaneously or epidurally) into patients in their home environment (Conners & Winters, 1995). Home infusion therapy is generally thought of as consisting of three services: pharmacy, nursing (home health), and equipment management services.

Pharmacy Services

Pharmacy services generally involve both compounding and dispensing the intravenous solutions into a ready-to-administer form. In many ways, this process is similar to the I.V. room of a hospital pharmacy. Preparation of sterile admixtures for home administration may require special techniques and more stringent environmental controls than a hospital I.V. admixture room. Unlike in a hospital where a medication is usually prepared within 24 to 48 hours of administration, home care may involve up to 1 month between preparation and administration, thus allowing a greater potential for microbial growth. More extensive quality control and end-product testing are also performed on the prepared products for the same reasons.

Another significant difference between home care and hospital pharmacy practice involves labeling of the admixture. Home care pharmacists have usually researched the stability of I.V. medications over longer periods of time; when research results indicate, they provide expiration dating much longer than manufacturers' recommendations. Prescription labels must conform to the requirements for the state pharmacy laws for retail pharmacies. The pharmacy is also responsible for the packaging and delivery of the prepared products to the patient's home. Delivery techniques vary from the use of one's own delivery vehicles and drivers, to the use of external contracted delivery services—both local and national (e.g., Federal Express), to having the nurse pick up and deliver the medications. Regardless of the delivery method, the pharmacy must always ensure that the product is packed to control the factors that affect the stability of the product (temperature, light, humidity, etc.) during delivery to the patient's residence.

The pharmacist working in home infusion is also responsible for the pharmaceutical care and clinical monitoring of the patient. The pharmacy monitors the drug therapy through evaluation of information received from the patient's nurse, the patient or family member or caregiver, the delivery driver, and the pharmacist's review of laboratory test results, which are often sent directly to the pharmacy. There is extensive communication regarding the care of patients with their physician and nurse, as well as other health care professionals involved and sometimes the patients themselves. The pharmacy maintains not only the normal prescription and dispensing records, but also a clinical record of the patients, called a *chart* or *home care record.* The home infusion pharmacy generally operates under outpatient or retail pharmacy laws, although many state boards of pharmacy have either additional or different regulations for home care pharmacies. The pharmacy is often involved in providing the nursing supplies, catheter care supplies, and the access device for the infusion therapy to patients. These infusion-related supplies and devices are sent with the medications to the patient, for use by the patient or nurse, in the patient's home.

Home Nursing Services

At least initially, most patients receiving home infusion therapy will also be receiving home nursing services. Nurses usually have considerable experience in handling I.V.s in an acute care setting before they care for home infusion patients. Major responsibilities of the home care nurse include educating the patient and/or family caregiver regarding administration of the infusion and care of the infusion site, performing dressing and infusion site changes, making in-home physical assessments, and monitoring the patient's health status. Nurses will also administer the medications initially, but the eventual goal is to train the patient or a family member to perform this task. Periodic visits are then made to monitor the patient's status and response to therapy. The nurse may also insert some types of I.V. access devices or catheters into the patient in the home. The choice of venous access device depends on the patient's condition, the length and type of infusion therapy, and the preferences of the patient, physician, and nurse. The selection of the access device can significantly affect the need for and quantity and type of supplies, nursing time and visits, and thus the overall cost. Certain devices also require more skill for insertion or placement than others. For instance, peripherally inserted central catheters (PICC), which are commonly used for 2- to 8-week home infusion therapy, are the most complicated venous access devices that can be inserted in the home. Insertion requires nurses who have undergone special training and are certified to perform this procedure. Sometimes nurses will also provide more traditional nursing home care to infusion patients (e.g., wound care), thus meeting all the patient's nursing care needs.

Equipment Management Services

Equipment management services include primarily the selection, delivery, and setup of an infusion control device (i.e., an infusion pump). These services are often performed by the pharmacy, but may also be performed by the home health agency or a separate HME provider. They also include the separation of clean (patient-ready) and dirty (returned) equipment, cleaning and disinfecting of equipment between patient use, and routine and preventative maintenance of the equipment including inspection, testing, and performing maintenance on the equipment. Equipment sent to patients also needs to be tracked and logged in compliance with the Safe Medical Devices Act (SMDA) of 1990. Backup equipment and/or services are needed for equipment malfunctions. As in a hospital or clinic setting, not all home infusion patients need an infusion pump. Gravity administration of the drug using the rate controller or clamp on the administration set or tubing can be safely used at home for some drugs and administration rates. Special infusion pumps and devices have been developed especially for the special needs of home infusion patients. Disposable administration devices and small lightweight pumps that do not require an I.V. pole are commonly used for home infusion therapy. When drug dilution is not required and the administration time is short, some patients may receive their medication as an I.V. push. Home care pharmacists must be able to decide whether an infusion device is required and what device or pump is appropriate for the patient, drug, and administration rate.

A home infusion provider may provide all three services (pharmacy, nursing, and equipment) to a patient together, separately, or in any combination. Some pharmacies are involved in the provision of home pharmacy services only, although the vast majority also provide infusion and enteral pumps. These pharmacies rely on the home health agency nurse to communicate patient assessment data in a timely manner and to coordinate care with the patient. Some insurers may want to pay only one provider. In this case, the pharmacy may contract with a home health agency, collect payment from the insurer, and pay the agency for the nursing services. This scenario may decrease the pharmacist's time required to obtain the assessment data from and coordinate care with the nurse, because the pharmacy controls the patient care and nursing service payment. The reverse scenario also occurs, however, in which the home health agency contracts with the pharmacy and the pharmacy receives payment from the home health agency. In this case, it is often difficult for the pharmacy to obtain the data needed in a timely manner. Decisions regarding the selection of a provider for a patient's home infusion therapy may be made by the insurers, patients, and physicians. Thus, some patients may receive pharmacy services only, whereas others will receive both nursing and pharmacy services from the organization. The trend to "one-stop shopping" by managed care providers, and increasing trend toward diversification by home care organizations, will result in many home infusion providers being part of a large organization that provides a vast array of home care services. Many home infusion therapy providers have also expanded into the long-term care market (as many providers of long-term care services are expanding into home care) to capture what is called the *post-acute* or *alternate site market*.

Types of Home Infusion Providers

Home pharmacy services, as part of home infusion therapy, usually can only be provided by a licensed pharmacy either alone or as part of a broader health care organization. The exception is physician practices, which can provide these services without a pharmacist or pharmacy out of their office under the auspices of their physician's license. This type is most commonly seen in oncology and infectious disease practices. Usually, physicians run an ambulatory infusion center as part of their office. Patients receive cancer chemotherapy, antibiotics, or any type of infusion while they are in the physician's office. Between physician visits, patients may return to the infusion center to receive their I.V. medications, or have them provided through home care. Even in cases when the patient predominately uses the infusion center, at times a nurse needs to visit the patient in the home (e.g., catheter problems in the middle of a weekend). Home care is usually provided by the nurses from the physicians' offices and is usually considered a sideline to their office-based practice. In these physician-based practices, nurses—not pharmacy technicians or pharmacists—are usually responsible for compounding and admixing the I.V. medications. Sometimes a local pharmacy is contracted to compound and deliver the medications to the physician's office, and occasionally a pharmacist is hired by the physician. Technicians are rarely used in this environment unless a pharmacist is present.

Other types of settings where home care pharmacy is practiced include retail or community pharmacies, institutional or long-term care pharmacies, hospital pharmacies, home health agencies, HME-based providers, infusion therapy specialty providers, and ambulatory infusion centers.

Retail or Community Pharmacies

Independent retail or community pharmacies are most likely to provide a variety of services including HME, ostomy care products, and diabetic care. Infusion therapy is usually a low-volume component. Pharmacists, and sometimes technicians, usually provide home infusion therapy services in addition to retail and other pharmacy duties. Most are "pharmacy-only" providers; however, a few pharmacies hire nurses to help coordinate home infusion therapy services and perhaps provide a limited amount of home health services. Delivery services are provided by nurses or the same delivery mechanism as the retail pharmacy/HME business. Some are part of a franchise in home infusion or participate in a home infusion network. Many are one-owner operations.

Institutional or Long-Term Care Pharmacies

Institutional or long-term care pharmacies primarily provide drug distribution services to a large number of nursing homes, prisons, and other institutional facilities, servicing an average 4000 patients daily. Although the primary business is oral therapies, many also provide I.V. therapies to long-term care facilities with subacute units. Home infusion therapy is usually a very-low-volume component. These organizations have extensive internal delivery systems (i.e., their own fleet of vans) and provide at least enteral and infusion pumps, though some may also supply other HME. Although these pharmacies may employ a nurse to assist with care coordination and education of the long-term care facility staff, home health services are rarely provided directly by these organizations, which tend to be pharmacy-only operations.

Hospital Pharmacies

Home infusion therapy is often provided by the hospital department of pharmacy in the inpatient I.V. admixture room or the outpatient pharmacy utilizing the existing staff. A pharmacist is assigned clinical responsibilities in home care and for interacting with the home health care team. The hospital usually provides a broad array of home health services, although these are operationally in a different department and may not even be on the hospital premises. Infusion pumps are either handled by the biomedical engineering department, the home health services department, materials management or the pharmacy department, or a combination of these. Delivery services are usually provided by the home care nurses, who pick up the medications from the pharmacy. Some hospitals have created a separate home infusion pharmacy independent of the inpatient pharmacy, especially when the volume remains high, which may be located on the campus of the hospital. Some hospitals have created a home infusion division (home health plus pharmacy) that resides off-campus, sometimes as a separate corporate entity, that looks and acts like an infusion therapy specialty provider.

Home Health Agencies

Home health agencies have purchased or implemented a pharmacy to supplement their home health services provision. These are usually large home health agencies that provide a wide array of home health services, and may have multiple home health offices. The pharmacy may service multiple home health branches, and usually looks and operates similar to an infusion therapy specialty provider.

HME-Based Providers

HME providers may also provide home infusion pharmacy services. Usually the primary role of pharmacies is to supply respiratory therapy medications which are needed for the home medical equipment and clinical respiratory needs of their patients. The home infusion pharmacy may operate similarly to a retail pharmacy-based infusion program or an infusion therapy specialty provider.

Infusion Therapy Specialty Providers

The infusion therapy speciality provider specializes only in the provision of home infusion therapy. Generally this organization provides home health services, although the nurses specialize in home infusion therapy only. Pharmacy occupies a prominent role in this type of organization. Infusion and enteral pumps are usually the only type of medical equipment provided by this company. Maintenance of the infusion and enteral pumps is usually performed by the company's employees. The infusion therapy specialty providers tend to have their own delivery staff and vans, depending on the size of the organization. This type of provider may service up to 1000 infusion patients per day. Smaller volume providers in this category also exist, however, and usually reside in suburban industrial office parks.

Ambulatory Infusion Centers

Ambulatory infusion centers consist of an office, usually in a doctor's office building. Patients are referred here to receive their infusions in a comfortable setting. The office consists of a series of rooms, each with a relaxing chair, infusion pump, and VCR. Nurses manage and run the office and administrate the drugs. The offices are generally licensed as pharmacies, and have a pharmacy and pharmacist present to prepare the I.V. admixtures for the nurses to administer. The nursing staff may provide limited home care services to patients treated by the center. As discussed, a nurse will need to visit the patient in the home and provide almost all deliveries. Many ambulatory infusion centers are owned by infusion therapy specialty providers and operate in a similar manner. Others are owned by physicians.

In all of the preceding cases, the provider can be independent or part of a regional or national chain. Some pharmacies serve patients seen by multiple home health agencies or home medical equipment providers, and service patients in multiple states whose geography is limited only by the areas serviced by overnight delivery services (such as Federal Express). Others are single-site providers that only serve their local community.

Types of Care and Therapies Provided

Although virtually any infusion can now be given safely to patients in their home, some forms of therapy have predominated, including antibiotic therapy, antiviral therapy, total parenteral nutrition, enteral nutrition, pain management, cancer chemotherapy, hydration, miscellaneous drugs, ancillary drugs, and preparing and dispensing medications for home care.

Antibiotic Therapy

Antibiotic therapy is by far the major form of home infusion therapy provided. Ceftriaxone (Rocephin™) and cefazolin, due to their long half-life and prolonged stability, account for about half of all home I.V. antibiotic use, with vancomycin following a close third. Other antibiotics used include amikacin, amphotericin B, ceftazidime, co-trimoxazole, clindamycin, ciprofloxacin, erythromycin, fluconazole, gentamicin, imipenem-cilastatin, metronidazole, nafcillin, penicillin G, piperacillin, and to-bramycin. Even drugs with short stabilities, such as ampicillin, are dispensed as vials for the patient to mix in the home.

A large percentage of all home infusion therapy patients receiving antibiotic therapy are AIDS patients (Conners & Winters, 1995). **Acquired immune deficiency syndrome (AIDS)** is a viral infection acquired *only* by transmission of bodily fluids. The virus involved is known as **human immunodeficiency virus (HIV).** Patients may acquire HIV, but not manifest AIDS for many years later. This disease, for which there is currently no cure, results in a breakdown of the patient's immune system, making the person susceptible to unusual infections (primarily unusual forms of pneumonia, tuberculosis, etc.), which ultimately lead to death. The most common causes of transmission of the virus are shared needles (in I.V. drug abuse situations) and sex. Health care staff who treat HIV-positive patients (patients with HIV infection) can only acquire the disease if stuck with a needle or object that has the patient's blood on it. Staff are usually trained in the appropriate precautions for handling products contaminated with patients' blood. Staff *cannot* acquire the disease through casual contact with the patient. In most cases, staff are more likely to give the patient an infection, or acquire other infections such as tuberculosis (TB) from the patient, hence the need for the strict use of infection control procedures in this population. These procedures commonly include hand washing, use of specially labeled containers for hazardous wastes, use of gloves, use of sharps containers for used needles/supplies, routine TB testing, and use of specially fitted TB masks. The procedures also require special training on the part of technicians and other staff in home care. Although some experimental treatments are being used to treat HIV infection, most antibiotic therapy is directed at prevention or treating these other infections the patient acquires. The course of AIDS is often prolonged, with the patient getting sicker and needing more medications over time. Because of this length of treatment needed and patients' desire for a decent lifestyle in their remaining days, home is the preferred site for care.

Other uses for antibiotics include other types of immunodeficient patients, such as transplant patients and cancer patients, whose immune systems are slowed by drugs that prevent transplant rejection or the chemotherapy used to treat cancer, respectively. Other common diseases treated by home antibiotics are osteomyelitis (bone infection), Lyme disease (a tick-borne infection that makes people weak and tired), cellulitis (an infection of the skin and surrounding tissues) common in diabetic patients, pneumonia and bronchitis (common respiratory diseases), pelvic inflammatory disease, urinary tract infections, endocarditis (infection of the heart), and cystic fibrosis (a childhood respiratory disorder that causes thick mucous secretions in the lung making the child susceptible to respiratory infections). Home antibiotic therapy is commonly used for such patients; however, many patients are being discharged home to finish their course of antibiotics started in the hospital. The diagnosis and reasons for the antibiotic use in such cases vary widely. Antibiotics may also be used to treat patients receiving other forms of home infusion therapy who develop catheter or line infections as a result of improper care or placement of their I.V. access site.

Antiviral Therapy

The predominant group of patients receiving antivirals are AIDS patients, although other immunosuppressed patients (e.g., cancer and transplant patients) may also receive this type of therapy. The predominant viral infections are cytomegalovirus, which affects the eyes, and herpes, which affects the skin and other tissues. The principal drugs in this group include acyclovir, ganciclovir, and foscarnet; however, new agents are constantly being introduced by the FDA or used on an experimental basis. Ganciclovir is the only agent in this group considered cytotoxic and requiring special handling, such as a cancer chemotherapy agent.

Total Parenteral Nutrition

Total parenteral nutrition (TPN) was the first type of home infusion therapy, but the number of patients receiving home TPN has decreased over the years. This therapy involves providing nutrient solutions containing amino acids—the building blocks of proteins, glucose, or sugar and fats, with electrolytes or salts, vitamins, and essential elements or minerals—directly into the right atrium of the heart. The purpose of TPN is to allow patients to receive all the nutrition/food they require to maintain normal body functions and survival. TPN should only be provided when patients cannot eat sufficient food or receive enteral solutions.

The primary reason for home TPN is that patients cannot absorb sufficient nutrients from their intestinal tract. The most common reason they receive home TPN is cancer. Cancer patients may have tumors which prevent nutrients from reaching their intestines and therefore cannot be absorbed or they may be too weak or emaciated (which is also seen with AIDS patients) to eat enough to survive. Other reasons for home TPN include Crohn's disease (an inflammatory disease of the gastrointestinal tract), surgical removal of the intestines, severe diarrhea from various causes, and hyperemesis gravidarum (severe vomiting during pregnancy). Some persons will require TPN for their entire life and some will receive home TPN only until whatever condition or disease has caused their inability to eat has been cured.

Peripheral parenteral nutrition (PPN) has a lower dextrose concentration than TPN, because TPN solutions are too concentrated to be infused into peripheral veins without causing severe pain and irritation and possible tissue damage. Because PPN is a short-term therapy which provides most but not all nutrients to sustain life, it is rarely used in home care. TPN products are prescription items that require a large amount of preparation time by the pharmacy technician. Because the solution is infused directly into the patient's heart, perfect aseptic technique is essential. TPN admixtures often require five to ten components and supplemental additives. To improve the accuracy of the compounding of TPN solutions and to decrease the potential of contamination which may lead to an infection in the patient, various compounding devices called *TPN compounders* have been developed. The Automix 3 + 3™ is a typical automated TPN compounder with a total nutrient admixture **(Figure 3–1)**. These TPN compounders generally involve a multichannel pump for the amino acids, dextrose, fats, and other additives connected to a personal computer. The personal computer helps with TPN admixture calculations and drives the pump. Microcompounding pumps have been developed for the electrolyte and other additives. Microcompounders are not commonly found in home infusion providers, although most of those providers who specialize in the provision of home TPN usually have a TPN compounder. Both of these compounding devices need to be calibrated and cleaned daily.

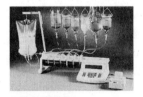

FIGURE 3–1
Automix 3 + 3™ and compounded TPN bag *(Courtesy of Secure™ Medical Products, Inc., Mundelein, IL)*

Enteral Nutrition

Enteral nutrition (EN) solutions are liquid nutrient solutions which are administered by mouth or through a feeding tube directly into the stomach or intestines. Enteral formulas such as TPN contain all the essential nutrients that a person needs for survival. *Home enteral nutrition (HEN)* is safer than TPN, because persons on HEN have fewer and less severe infections and complications than with home

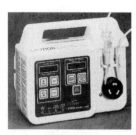

FIGURE 3–2
Enteral pump
(Courtesy of Nestle
Clinical Nutrition,
Deerfield, IL)

TPN. Care of the HEN patient is easier to learn for patients and their families and is less costly in the formulas and supplies and in the time required for the care. Enteral formulas are available in ready-to-use liquids or in powders that need to be reconstituted (usually in a blender). Powders are rarely compounded for the home care setting by the pharmacy, because they are usually stable only 24 to 48 hours. Hence, the patient is usually responsible for reconstitution. Changes in the types of enteral formulas a person receives are relatively infrequent so the pharmacy will deliver these solutions up to a month in advance. A few enteral nutrition products are prescription items, but most are nonprescription and can be acquired in community pharmacies and discount and grocery stores. The main role of the pharmacy for the HEN patient is the provision of an enteral pump, which is a special pump used to instill the enteral nutrition into the stomach or gut of the patient, at a controlled rate. An enteral pump, although similar to the infusion pumps used for intravenous solutions, is usually less costly, easier to operate, and requires less supplies **(Figure 3–2)**. The pharmacist may be responsible for monitoring the nutritional care of the patient, but sometimes the pharmacy is only a vendor for the products. Also, many patients on short-term TPN are transitioned from TPN to HEN before being allowed to return to a regular diet.

Pain Management

Many patients with cancer and AIDS have severe pain. Other patients may receive long-term pain therapy for nerve and muscle disorders, or short-term pain therapy following surgery. Although most patients are tried out on oral pain control, many do not respond because of the level of pain involved. After trying intramuscular or subcutaneous injections or transdermal (skin) patches, patients may receive continuous infusions of pain medications to achieve pain relief. Sometimes the infusions are continuous subcutaneous infusions, or continuous intravenous infusions. In severe cases, the pain medications are infused directly into the spinal cord fluid (epidural) or fluid surrounding the brain (intrathecal). In such cases, sterility and products without preservatives are important. Infusions of pain medications usually involve narcotic solutions. Most frequently, the narcotic infusion is administered by an infusion pump, known as a **patient-controlled analgesia (PCA) pump**, that provides a continuous flow of medication and also allows the patient to provide occasional boluses of pain medication when the continuous infusion does not provide sufficient relief. The pump controls the medication and bolus dose, the number of boluses, and the frequency that boluses may be given.

Cancer Chemotherapy

Almost any form of cancer chemotherapy can be given to patients at home, although predominantly they receive these products in the doctor's office or ambulatory infusion center. Almost all of these products are cytotoxic and require special labeling and precautions in handling. It is believed that prolonged and repeated exposure to these products may cause genetic defects and cancer. Special preparation techniques are used including special garments and attire. Preparation occurs in a class II biological containment hood, also called a **vertical hood.** This hood not only provides a sterile environment, but unlike other hoods, also protects the person working in the hood by containing any airborne product within the confines of the hood. These precautions prevent or minimize exposure to the cytotoxic agents by the technician or pharmacist who prepares them. Special spill kits are used to handle spills of these agents—again to minimize exposure. All staff and patients should be taught the special precautions for these agents. Please note that ganciclovir (an antiviral agent) shares these cytotoxic properties with cancer chemotherapy agents, and requires the same special precautions for handling. Even when cancer chemotherapy is not administered in the home, the ancillary treatment of cancer symptoms and the side effects of chemotherapy are administered there. Besides also receiving home pain medications, TPN, and antibiotics, as previously discussed, these patients may receive a number of other antinausea drugs, called antiemetic drugs (e.g., metoclopramide), blood products (e.g., erythropoietin, iron dextran, colony stimulation factor), and blood transfusions themselves.

Hydration

Basic I.V. solutions are sometimes provided to the patient (sterile water, normal saline, (or 5 percent dextrose in water [D5W]), or a combination of these. In some cases, these basic solutions are provided (with additional electrolytes or salts) not as ancillary medications, but as the primary therapy: hydration therapy. Hydration therapy is used for such problems as dehydration and hyperemesis (severe prolonged and repeated vomiting in some pregnant women). Regardless of whether it is used as the primary therapy or ancillary therapy, it is important to remember that these are prescription drugs. They must be dispensed and labeled as prescription drugs, rather than only supplies.

Miscellaneous Drugs

A variety of other drugs are dispensed to patients in the home care setting (see **Table 3–2**). Many of these products are newly developed through biotechnology—they are exact duplicates of products available in the body which are produced in laboratory by genetically engineered biological organisms, for instance bacteria such as *E. coli*. These are different than many drugs, which are chemically derived products, although they look or act like products in the body. Genetically engineered drugs tend to have less side effects than their chemical counterparts. Also,

TABLE 3–2   **Other Drugs Used in Home Infusion Therapy**

Drug	Indication
Methylprednisolone (Solu-Medrol™)	Immunosuppressed patients
OKT-3 (Orthoclone™)	Transplant patients
Deferoxamine	Hemophilia
Factors VIII, IX	Hemophilia
IV gammaglobulin	Immunosuppressed patients
Alpha-1-antitrypsin	Emphysema
Growth hormone	Growth deficiency in pediatrics
Beta-interferon	Multiple sclerosis
Erythropoietin	Red blood cell deficiency
Iron dextran	Iron deficiency
Colony stimulating factors (G-CSF, Gm-CSF)	White blood cell deficiency
Heparin	Thrombosis
Low molecular weight heparin	Thrombosis
Dobutamine	Severe congestive heart failure
Tocolytic therapy	Prolong or delay birth

because most products are exactly like their human body counterparts, they must be administered by injection and cannot be given orally. This attribute makes them excellent candidates for home infusion therapy. There is expected to be a major boon in new *biotech drugs* within the next few years, as a large number of companies are currently in the process of developing new biotech products.

Ancillary Drugs

The home infusion therapy nurse will provide a number of drugs to patients to assist in their main therapy. Most common are the line maintenance drugs—low dose heparin and saline—both of which are used to keep catheters from clogging due to blood clots. Low dose urokinase is also used for this purpose, but less frequently because of its higher costs. The pharmacy will also provide external products to clean catheter areas and prevent infections. Alcohol-based wipes and povidone-iodine products (gel, soap, etc.) are used in this capacity. Many nurses are given anaphylaxis kits, to have available in case a patient experiences an anaphylactic or severe allergic reaction to the drugs given. These kits will include epinephrine, diphenhydramine, methylprednisolone or another steroid, and other drugs to be given in an emergency based on a standard physician's order or protocol.

Preparing and Dispensing Medications for Home Care

The preparation and dispensing of medications in home infusion therapy requires specialized knowledge and skills. Both pharmacists and technicians from hospital pharmacy practice often take a year before they are comfortable with the nuances and differences of home care practice.

The pharmacist and technician must first be aware of the differences of outpatient versus hospital pharmacy law. In most states, home infusion therapy (even if dispensed by the hospital pharmacy) must adhere to outpatient pharmacy laws and/or special home care regulations, which are different from those of inpatient hospital pharmacy practice. For instance, inpatient pharmacists can often accept verbal orders relayed from a nurse on a floor. In outpatient pharmacy regulations, most states prohibit the pharmacist from accepting the verbal prescription from anyone but the physician directly (or the physician's employee agent), often resulting in the need to call the physician back to verify orders transmitted to the home care nurse. Outpatient prescription records and labeling requirements are different from those of the inpatient ones. Second, the pharmacist and technician must be aware of expanded stability and expiration dates of the products they prepare, beyond those used in hospital pharmacy, including special packaging requirements for delivery. Products must often be packed in coolers or Styrofoam-lined boxes for delivery in extremely hot or cold weather. Third, pharmacists and technicians need to be aware of special preparation techniques based on the infusion pump the patient will be using. For instance, the use of a fluid dispensing pump may be needed in preparing drugs in elastomeric devices, because of the tremendous pressure needed to fill them. Knowing that some pumps, such as the CADD pump, require that the drug be filled in a special cassette is an example of such expanded knowledge that is needed. Fourth, these patients (particularly those with HIV infections) have heightened needs for confidentiality, of which home infusion staff must be aware and thus show extra sensitivity. For example, staff should not leave supplies with a neighbor. Lastly, special preparation sterility techniques are required. The American Society of Health System Pharmacists (ASHP) has developed guidelines for the preparation of sterile drug products ("ASHP Technical Assistance Bulletin," 1993). Most hospitals prepare drugs at risk level I—the lowest risk level for potential transmission of infections by the prepared drug product; however, home care is at risk level II or III. Hence, special techniques and added precautions must be exercised. In addition to ASHP, the U.S. Pharmacopeia (USP) also has guidelines for the preparation and dispensing of sterile drugs used in the home ("Sterile Drug Products," 1993). In some states, adherence to these is required by law and regulation. Many state pharmacy laws also have special requirements for I.V.s prepared for home use.

Most of these guidelines center around the use of a *class 100 environment* (hood or room) for the preparation of sterile products, which indicates that the environment has less than 100 particles of dust and particulates per cubic meter of air. Sometimes *clean rooms* (specially filtered rooms to create a sterile environment) are required. In all cases, the sterile preparation area must be functionally separate from areas where nonsterile drugs are prepared. Traffic flow in and around the sterile preparation area should be minimized. The area should be free of clutter and particulate-generating materials (paper, boxes). Work surfaces and equipment should be cleaned daily with an appropriate antiseptic agent, and the floors (and the walls and ceiling if the paint and ceiling tiles are appropriately coated) should be cleaned monthly using a dilute bleach solution. The inside of the hoods should be free of papers and labels. Appropriate aseptic techniques must be used, final products should be visually inspected for particles or signs of deterioration, and more quantitative quality control techniques must be used, such as end-product testing.

Most importantly the timing of preparation and dispensing is critical in ensuring that the delivery of the product is coordinated with the needs of the patient, and nurse who may be administering the product. This is considerably more complex and difficult than meeting the delivery needs of inpatients.

Infusion Devices

Medications can be given by injection into the blood system by three different methods, each of which is determined by the volume to be injected and the time required for administration:

1. *Bolus* or *I.V. push* is the administration of a drug by directly pushing the barrel of a syringe to inject its contents directly into the vein. This approach is used for the rapid injection of drug into the vein and is reserved for situations when speed of response is key and when rate of administration or concentration of the drug will not negatively affect the patient.

2. *Intermittent injection* is the administration of the drug over 15 minutes to 4 hours (usually 0.5 to 1 hour), after which there is a period of no drug administration, followed by cycles of administration/no administration at intervals of 4, 6, 8, 12, 24, or more hours, hence the term "intermittent." Drugs administered by this technique are less concentrated than by I.V. push with a greater volume of fluid involved (usually 50–250 ml). Intermittent injection results in peak and valley effects in the level of drug in the blood.

3. *Continuous infusion* is the administration of the drug at a constant rate, and allows larger volumes of drug to be instilled over a longer period of time. Drugs administered by this technique are less concentrated than by intermittent infusion with a greater volume of fluid involved (usually 500–3000 ml). Continuous infusion results in a steady and continuous level of drug in the blood.

The preceding definitions assume that the drug is being administered into the blood. Each administration method, however, could be used for administering the drug *subcutaneously* (just under the skin), *intramuscularly* (into the muscle), *intrathecally* (into the brain's fluid), *intrasynovially* (into a joint's fluid), *epidurally* (into the spinal fluid), or into any body fluid or cavity. The volume, content, and concentration of the drug, however, may need to be varied. In addition, there are a variety of methods of accomplishing each approach. For instance, the I.V. push method can be administered manually (by hand), with the use of a syringe pump, or with the use of a bolus button on a PCA infusion pump. The intermittent and continuous infusions can be administered by a slow gravity drip method, by elevating the bag/bottle of drug above the access site (usually on an I.V. pole), or by using an infusion control device or pump when the accuracy of the infusion rate is important.

The function of an infusion control device, or *infusion pump,* is to regulate the rate of administration of a drug infusion. Following are several types of infusion control devices.

1. *Nonmechanical rate controller.* This type of device, sometimes called a "dial-calibrated gravity flow regulator," has no mechanical parts. It is not a pump, because the main force of the infusion remains gravity. However, the device accurately controls the infusion rate by controlling the size of the device's orifice, through which the drug travels. Examples of this type of device are the Dial-a-Flow® and the Rate Regulator®.

2. *Nonmechanical external pump.* This type of device also has no mechanical parts. The device exerts a positive infusion force and thus does not rely on gravity to work.

   a. The most common type of nonmechanical external pump is the *disposable elastomeric pump.* The drug is put inside a balloon reservoir (made of an elastomeric material), which expands within a hard plastic container. Because the pressure to expand the balloon is considerable, a special hand or mechanical pump must be used to fill the contents of this pump. The balloon provides the positive pressure. The diameter and length of a segment of the tubing controls the rate of infusion. These devices are available in various sizes and flow rates. A specific device is selected based on the medication and amount of fluid and rate at which the drug should be administered. These devices are small, extremely lightweight, and conveniently fit in the patient's pocket or in a small pouch. The convenience of a throwaway device and the freedom of movement during infusion makes these pumps preferred by most patients. Due to the disposable feature, the cost is often high and many payers will not reimburse for a device that is more costly than other infusion devices. Examples of this type of device **(Figure 3–3)** include the Intermate®, ReadyMED®, MedFlo II®, Eclipse®, and Homepump®.

   b. Another less common version of this pump is the *spring-controlled pump.* A plastic disc-shaped bag containing the drug is placed between two halves of the pump. A strong spring exerts pressure on a plate next to the bag to create the positive pressure. As in the elastomeric pump, the diameter and length of a segment of the tubing controls the rate of infusion. In this version, however, only the plastic bag containing the drug is disposable; the other components are reusable. An example of this type of pump is the Sidekick®.

3. *Mechanical peristaltic pump.* This type of pump is a mechanical device that delivers drug at a controlled rate by means of a system of rocking rollers or alternating motors. Many different manufacturers market these devices, which are useful for delivery of both large and small volumes of drug as either continuous or intermittent infusions or both continuous and intermittent admin-

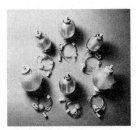

FIGURE 3–3

Elastomeric device
(Courtesy of Block Medical, Inc., San Diego, CA)

istration. Mechanical peristaltic pumps are available as pole-mounted pumps (common in many hospitals) or as portable or ambulatory pumps (commonly used in home care). Most of the pole mounts require electricity to operate, but have battery backup systems. The ambulatory pumps generally use 9-volt batteries, although some have special batteries and electrical charging units. Examples of these ambulatory pumps include the Verifuse®, CADD-Plus®, and Provider One Plus®. Some of the more portable versions (e.g., CADD Plus® and WalkMed 350®) require the drug be placed in a special plastic reservoir or cassette designed for the pump **(Figure 3–4)**. These devices usually are electronically controlled through visual displays and buttons. Multiple alarm systems prevent complications or alert the patient to pump failure problems. Most are programmed by the pharmacist or nurse before delivery to the patient, although others (e.g., Verifuse®) may be programmed remotely via computer commands given over the telephone line using a modem. Also, some versions have multiple channels acting as multiple pumps in one unit, and allowing up to four different drugs to be controlled by one pump. Examples of this type of pump include the Provider 6000®. Some models are specifically designed for PCA pain management, as they allow continuous flow plus bolus dosing and special programming and lockout features.

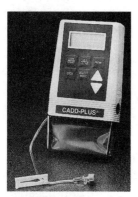

FIGURE 3–4
Mechanical peristaltic pump *(Courtesy of SIMS Deltec, Inc., St. Paul, MN)*

Another version of the mechanical peristaltic pump worth noting is the microinfusion pump. This pump allows extremely small volumes of drug to be continuously infused over long periods of time. Although the way the pump works is the same, the regular peristaltic pump would not be able to deliver this small a volume as slow as a microinfusion pump. This pump is important when highly concentrated solutions need to be administered very slowly to patients. Examples of this type of pump include the WalkMed 440 PIC®.

4. *Mechanical piston pump.* This pump is similar to the peristaltic pump except the basis of the pump is a double-acting piston that is electromagnetically operated by means of a battery. As the first system is activated, a magnetic field is created, moving the piston and forcing the drug from the piston cylinder. Simultaneously the second cylinder is recharged and the drug is infused during the next piston cycle. The advantage of this system is miniaturization, although several large, nonportable pumps are in this category. An example of this type of pump is the multichannel Lifecare Omniflow 4000®.

5. *Mechanical syringe pump.* This pump has been less popular in recent years, although it is extremely cost-effective. It uses regular syringes for the disposable reservoir and operates by several different mechanisms. One type uses an electromotor to drive the plunger at a slow rate. A screw assembly mechanism advances the plunger slowly, usually in pulses created by a motor drive variable. Examples of mechanical syringe pumps are the BARD Miniinfuser® and the MS-16®.

6. *Implantable pumps.* These pumps are surgically implanted just under the skin of the patient, with a catheter entering a vein or other cavity **(Figure 3–5)**. Implantable pumps usually work by a mechanical piston system or by means of gas pressure. In this latter type of system, pressure is created by a fluorocarbon vapor liquid mixture that forces against a collapsible diaphragm, discharging the drug through a flow-regulating tube. These pumps contain long lasting batteries and systems that keep the pump operating continuously for up to 10 years. Implantable pumps have either a fixed flow rate that is set by the manufacturer or the rate is externally programmed using an external electromagnetic wand. The advantage of implantable pumps is they are able to provide extremely small volumes of drug. Because many are implanted intrathecally, the risk of infection is less than other pumps as most require filling only once every 30 to 60 days. The

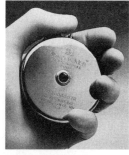

FIGURE 3–5
Implantable pump *(Courtesy of Medtronic, Inc., Minneapolis, MN)*

home care nurse fills the pump by injection into the pump chamber through the patient's skin. The disadvantages of these pumps are that they are extremely costly, they must be surgically implanted, and they cannot be shut off, so the internal reservoir must be continually filled with fluid or else serious complications can result. Implanted pumps include the Medtronic® and the Infusaid®.

Factors in the Selection of an Infusion Device or Pump

The selection of an appropriate infusion device or pump is complex. The pharmacy staff in cooperation with the home health nurse or agency, patient, payor, and others must consider what pump or device is appropriate for each patient. This decision includes factors related to the pump specifications such as flow range and volume; flow accuracy under optimal conditions; flow accuracy with temperature variations, low battery voltage, extended operation, back pressure and negative pressure; flow consistency; occlusion/flow restriction alarm and bolus volume after occlusion; and audible alarms and visual indicators. Other factors requiring consideration are equally important, such as quality of construction, design, ease of use, manufacturer support, operator's manual, and potential for *free flow* (a dangerous condition in which all of the infusion is accidentally administered in a short period of time). Practical considerations include the amount of time to train the patient, existing staff knowledge of pump operations, time of the infusion, patient's ability to ambulate, and the patient's home environment (e.g., stairs, carpeting).

A variety of devices are available for providing home infusion therapy. It was the advances in pump technology that led to the birth and growth of the home infusion therapy industry. Continuing advances to increase the features and reduce the size and expense of pumps will fuel the home infusion industry into the twenty-first century.

Equipment Management

A major role of the home infusion therapy company is the management of the infusion pumps and equipment provided to patients. This equipment may include I.V. poles, refrigerators, modems, and special telemonitoring devices (e.g., intrauterine monitors). If the organization is also a provider of home medical equipment, the range will expand even more. Home infusion companies have several responsibilities in this area. First, they are responsible for tracking each piece of equipment, whether it is with a particular patient, in the warehouse, or off-site for maintenance. In the event of a recall, the exact pump can be found. The FDA requires that home care companies accurately track the equipment they provide. Second, they are also responsible for ongoing routine and preventative maintenance of the equipment. Routine cleaning and maintenance should be performed in between each patient use, and at regular intervals (e.g., annually). Routine maintenance for infusion pumps should include, at a minimum:

1. A visual inspection of the structural integrity of the infusion pump casing and exposed operating parts (e.g., checking for cracks and broken external parts).
2. A check of the functionality of all buttons, switches, displays, and safety alarms. Alarms should be tested by simulating a malfunction to ensure that each alarm works.
3. A check of the battery charge, and recharging or replacing it.
4. Determination of the accuracy of the rate at which the pump delivers fluid, to ensure that it is within manufacturers' specifications.

5. Any other requirements or recommended procedures specified by the manufacturer in the operating manual for the pump.

A rate accuracy check (sometimes called a *volumetric check*) is important because it tests the basic function of the pump, which is to infuse solution at a controlled rate. As reimbursement policies limit the use of infusion pumps to drugs that require a controlled rate of infusion, the accuracy of that rate of infusion becomes more important. All maintenance should be documented. There should also be a mechanism for tracking equipment that requires ongoing routine and preventative maintenance (e.g., annually).

When equipment is received from patients, it should be identified and placed in an area designated for recovered equipment to be cleaned. It should never be mixed with clean patient-ready equipment. Also, obsolete equipment, or equipment that needs maintenance or repair, should be identified and separated from patient-ready and dirty equipment, including items not only in the warehouse but also in delivery vehicles. There should be appropriate systems for the delivery and setup of equipment in the patient's home. Finally, there should be a backup system for patients. Usually extra batteries are left with the patient or an extra pump. Extra backup pumps should be available. A 24-hour-a-day "on-call" system or the ability to replace the pump within a few hours, at any time, is also necessary.

Complications of Home Infusion Therapy

The complications of home infusion therapy are no different than hospital-based infusion therapy. Some believe the risk of infection by a serious, or resistant, organism is much less. Pharmacists and nurses often work together to monitor and prevent the complications of infusion therapy in home care. Complications that the provider may encounter include phlebitis, infiltration, sepsis, embolism, allergic reactions, and free flow.

Phlebitis

Phlebitis, the most frequently encountered complication of any infusion therapy, is inflammation at the site of the catheter insertion. If there is a blood clot involved, it is called *thrombophlebitis.* Depending on the situation, this complication has been estimated to occur in 3.5 to 7 percent of all patients receiving I.V. medications. Phlebitis can be caused by the drug, irritation by the catheter itself, or by an infection at the catheter site.

Infiltration

Infiltration occurs relatively frequently in patients with peripheral I.V.s, although it can occur with other types of venous access. The catheter is improperly placed or is dislodged from the vein and the drug is infused into the surrounding tissue rather than into the vein. This complication can be extremely painful, depending on the drug, and extremely serious in cases of infiltration by some cancer chemotherapeutic agents.

Sepsis

Sepsis is an infection in the blood which is a serious complication of infectious phlebitis left untreated. Sepsis is an overwhelming infection of the entire body and can be fatal. Each year it is estimated that 20,000 to 30,000 patients die from catheter-related sepsis.

Embolism

Embolism occurs when particulate matter, most commonly a blood clot, is introduced into the vein. This clot, or *emboli,* will travel through the bloodstream until it enters a blood vessel that is too small for it to flow through and then becomes lodged and eventually stops circulation. Because the tissue downstream of the embolism has its blood supply cut off, it will become oxygen starved and die, usually in the lung. The amount of damage varies but can include death. With the appropriate use of heparin or saline in catheter care, embolism from blood clots can be reduced. Air can also cause embolism. The delivery of air by the infusion pump is an issue that can be prevented.

Allergic Reactions

Allergic reactions may be the second most common cause of complication. The reaction may be mild, represented by a redness or rash, or it may be severe, represented by anaphylactic shock. The latter occludes the airway and results in death if not treated immediately. Patients are most commonly allergic to the drugs given (occurring in about 2 percent of patients), but more rarely are allergic to the plastic materials in the catheter or containers. Noting allergies in the medication history can often prevent disaster.

Free Flow

Free flow, as described, is a complication that results from the pump, due to a malfunction, causing the entire infusion to be delivered into the catheter in an extremely short period of time. Free flow can create a variety of problems depending on the drug and I.V. solution. For instance, if the product is TPN, the high glucose can cause a diabetic reaction, called *hyperglycemia,* and insulin may need to be given to the patient. Newer pumps are designed to prevent free flow.

Role of Technicians in Home Infusion Therapy

The role of the technician is more varied and more progressive in home infusion therapy than almost any type of pharmacy. The traditional and key role of the technician in home infusion therapy is in the preparation of sterile products in the I.V. room, under the supervision of a pharmacist. It is important to note that most states have more stringent requirements for technician supervision by a pharmacist in outpatient and home care settings (e.g., a pharmacist must be physically present within eyesight of the technician at all times). As previously discussed, this requires added knowledge and skills related to home care practice. In pharmacy environments that are more expanded, such as combined with a retail pharmacy, institutional pharmacy, or hospital pharmacy, the technician's role may be more varied and include duties and responsibilities in these other areas as well. Other roles for pharmacy technicians in home infusion therapy include:

- Driver or delivery representative or coordinator
- Warehouse supervisor
- Equipment management technician
- Patient service representative
- Purchasing agent or manager
- Billing clerk
- Case manager

Driver or Delivery Representative

The driver or delivery representative transports the products to the patient's home, and thus must be competent in infusion pump setup, troubleshooting, and the basics of equipment management; proper storage of the products in the home (i.e., which product must go in the refrigerator); infection control procedures; handling of hazardous materials and wastes; confidentiality; advanced directives and responding in emergency situations; identifying patients who may be abused or at nutritional risk; and so forth. It is important to remember that this individual may be the only employee of the home infusion provider who sees and talks to the patient directly. This individual may have to gather information, as well as provide information and care to the patient beyond routine delivery services.

Warehouse Supervisor/Technician

The warehouse supervisor/technician is responsible for the coordination and operation of the warehouse and may be responsible for coordinating deliveries, packing medications and supplies for delivery, controlling inventory of drug and supplies, handling returned hazardous materials and wastes, purchasing materials, and managing and maintaining equipment. Sometimes companies have a specially designated *equipment management technician* who handles the management and maintenance of the pumps, or it may be part of the overall responsibilities of the warehouse supervisor/technician.

Patient Service Representative

The patient service representative is responsible for contacting patients and making sure they have an appropriate inventory of ancillary supplies and medications—in essence helping the patients coordinate their home inventory of medications and supplies. This individual also serves as the major customer service representative to the patient and may assist in transmitting the patient's desires and requests to other staff in the organization. The patient service representative may also help coordinate deliveries with the warehouse supervisor/technician. This job is less "hands-on" and is generally more of a desk job.

Purchasing Manager

In large organizations, the purchasing manager is responsible for ordering drugs and supplies from wholesalers and manufacturers. This person may also be responsible for negotiating prices and purchasing contracts, and handling drug and product recalls. This responsibility may fall on the warehouse supervisor or pharmacist in smaller organizations.

Billing Clerk/Case Manager

The billing clerk/case manager is responsible for processing bills for home infusion therapy with insurance companies or Medicare carriers (the organizations responsible for paying the bills for Medicare patients). In addition, this individual may be responsible for negotiating prices with insurance company case managers, and for verifying a patient's insurance coverage and limits prior to providing care and getting authorization, if needed. This individual may also be responsible for getting initial information from the patient and referral source (physician, hospital, insurance company) to admit the patient to service.

The role of the technician in home infusion therapy can be challenging and varied compared with other practice settings. In addition, it often involves much latitude for job changes or advancement.

Summary

Home health care is a growing area for health care into the next millennium, and pharmacy practice in this environment is growing with it. Home infusion therapy predominates as a major service in home care that is pharmacy driven. The role of the pharmacist and pharmacy technician in home health care is rich and diverse. Knowledge of new biotech drug therapy, new pump technology, and vascular access devices (catheters) challenges the home infusion therapy practitioner and provides a rewarding career. The constant communication and teamwork involving the patient and health care team that is offered in home care is also professionally rewarding and enhancing. There is little doubt that many pharmacy practitioners will transition into home health care in the coming years, and that home health care will remain an important arena for pharmacy practice in the future.

ASSESSMENT

Multiple Choice Questions

1. Home health care as a site for the provision of health care has grown over seventeenfold in the past 32 years and provides services to over
   a. 1.3 million people
   b. 7 million people
   c. 10 million people
   d. 17 million people
   e. 31 million people

2. In 1993, home infusion therapy was growing at an annual compounded rate of
   a. 1.4 percent
   b. 7 percent
   c. 13 percent
   d. 38 percent
   e. 156 percent

3. Individuals who are called home health aides are involved in providing which of the following home care services:
   a. home health services
   b. home infusion therapy
   c. home medical equipment
   d. home pharmaceutical services
   e. personal care and support services

4. Home infusion therapy services involve the provision of home pharmaceutical services with
   a. home health services
   b. home medical equipment
   c. personal care and support services
   d. clinical respiratory services
   e. occupational therapy

5. The major form of equipment used in home infusion therapy is
   a. oxygen cylinders
   b. ventilators and concentrators
   c. pumps
   d. ostomy supplies
   e. blood glucose monitors

6. Home infusion therapy was made possible through technological improvements in
   a. drugs
   b. syringes
   c. catheters
   d. pumps
   e. sterile environments (e.g., hoods)

7. The types of pharmacies involved in the provision of home infusion therapy include
   a. retail pharmacies
   b. hospital pharmacies
   c. institutional or long-term care pharmacies
   d. HME providers
   e. all of the above

8. The most common form of home infusion therapy is
   a. antibiotics
   b. TPN
   c. pain management
   d. hydration
   e. cancer chemotherapy

9. The predominant diagnosis for patients receiving home antibiotic therapy is
   a. osteomyelitis
   b. Lyme disease
   c. AIDS/HIV infection
   d. staph infection
   e. sepsis

10. The most complex form of home infusion therapy to compound and admix is
    a. antibiotics
    b. TPN
    c. pain management
    d. hydration
    e. enteral therapy

11. The major differences between pharmaceutical services provided to home care patients and to hospital patients include the following EXCEPT
    a. different pharmacy laws
    b. lack of direct physician involvement
    c. packaging products properly for delivery
    d. expiration dating used
    e. level of sterile technique used

12. Drugs can be administered by continuous infusion using an infusion pump by any of the following routes of administration EXCEPT
    a. transdermally
    b. subcutaneously
    c. intravenously
    d. intramuscularly
    e. intrathecally

13. The method of pain management in which patients receive a continuous infusion of pain medication and are allowed to periodically bolus themselves on a limited basis is called
    a. pain relief control
    b. patient self-administered therapy
    c. cyclic pain therapy
    d. patient-controlled analgesia
    e. pain self-relief analgesia

14. An example of an elastomeric nonmechanical pump is
    a. Dial-a-Flow®
    b. Intermate®
    c. Infusaid®
    d. CADD-Plus®
    e. WalkMed 350®

Bibliography

ASHP technical assistance bulletin on quality assurance for pharmacy-prepared sterile products. (1993). *American Journal of Hospital Pharmacy, 50,* 2386–2398.

Catania, P.N., & Rosner, M.M. (Eds.). (1994). *Home health care practice* (2nd ed.). Palo Alto, CA: Markets Research.

Conners, R.B., & Winters, R.W. (Eds.). (1995). *Home infusion therapy: Current status and future trends.* Chicago: American Hospital Publishing.

Hicks, W.E. (Ed.). (1995). *Practice standards of ASHP, 1995–96.* Bethesda, MD: American Society of Health-System Pharmacists.

National Association for Home Care (NAHC). (1995). Internet site.

Sterile drug products for home use. (1993). *USP Pharmacopeial Forum, 19,* 6554–6584.

U.S. Congress, Office of Technology Assessment. *Home drug infusion therapy under Medicare* (OTA-H-509). Washington, D.C.

Long-Term Care

COMPETENCIES

Upon completion and review of this chapter, the student should be able to

1. Identify the three different types of long-term care facilities by sponsorship.
2. Identify the major source of funding for long-term care.
3. State why the rate structure of long-term care funding has such an important effect on services.
4. Identify the difference between a service pharmacist and a consultant pharmacist.
5. Describe the supportive role of the pharmacist and pharmacy technician.

Introduction

Society has long struggled with the obligation to care for those who can no longer care for themselves. Historically this obligation fell to immediate family members, or people of the same religion, tribe, or national background. The very earliest institutions had these religious or fraternal philosophies. Individuals not fortunate enough to be taken in by one of these charitable organizations were forced to live on the streets or to seek admission to institutions created by the governing entity, for example, the county poorhouse, the almshouse, or the local asylum.

In 1965 Congress passed two laws that would have a profound effect on this historical situation. The Medicare and Medicaid programs changed the way America provided for its frail and elderly population. Under Medicare, the elderly were guaranteed health care, and just as importantly, the children of the elderly were absolved of the legal responsibility of paying for care for their parents. The Medicaid legislation guaranteed payment for those deemed to be indigent. Thus, a new type of medical welfare was created. With these sound sources of income guaranteed, the growth of institutions willing to provide care mushroomed. Just as social security, a generation earlier, had guaranteed a source of income to the elderly and blind, these two pieces of legislation, commonly referred to as Articles 18 and 19, changed the way care was financed and who would ultimately pay the cost.

Types of Long-Term Care Facilities

The three types of nursing facilities are government sponsored, for-profit, and not-for-profit. The smallest percentage are those institutions run by the government at the federal, state, or county level. These may be veterans homes and hospitals or county-owned homes run for the benefit of its citizens or other similar grouping. These are the direct descendents of the poorhouses and almshouses. The second type of nursing home is referred to as a proprietary. This type of long-term care facility is by far the most numerous. These are owned by either one person, family, partnership, or corporation. They are run like a business and should make a profit for the investors. The most advanced type of this kind are the large corporations such as Beverly enterprises that are traded on the stock market. The last major type of long-term care facility is referred to as voluntary or not-for-profit. These facilities are the direct descendants of those charitable institutions that took care of their own particular followers. The term *voluntary* refers to the composition of the board of directors who serve without personal benefit or inurement, but do so from a wish to benefit society in some fashion. The second term, *not-for-profit,* defines what these institutions do with extra income. Instead of paying a profit or dividend to its shareholders like a for-profit institution rightly does, these facilities are obliged to reinvest the excess revenue back into programs or building improvements for the benefit of the population served. These facilities are not obligated to pay taxes and have the ability to raise funds for charitable purposes.

Regulation of Long-Term Care Facilities

All of these facilities are regulated by a complex system of laws, regulations, directives, and government oversight activity. Presently, this micromanagement of the industry shows no signs of lessening. Indeed, the Health Care Financing Administration (HCFA), a federal agency, has taken an extremely active role in driving the survey process which was formally a state function. Predictably, this strict oversight is directly connected to the large role in the funding from tax dollars necessary to fuel this large industry.

Income Sources

Funding for long-term care can be divided conveniently into three categories: tax dollars through Medicare and Medicaid, private pay, and third-party payers.

Medicare and Medicaid

The greatest amount comes from tax dollars through Medicare (physicians' visits, specialized supplies, limited skilled nursing services, etc.) and Medicaid, which is considered the payor of last resort. When all other sources of revenue are extinct, Medicaid pays for all legitimate costs associated with providing care.

Private Pay

Some revenues come from the private dollar. Basically, the revenue comes from individuals who have the assets (wealth) to pay for the care they receive until such time as their resources are low enough to be eligible for Medicaid.

Third-Party Payers

Third-party payers include insurance companies who have sold long-term care policies. Increasing in importance are the managed care companies that negotiate a price for those patients they are obligated to care for. It is most important to note that in the long-term care industry, payment for services is all-inclusive. The daily rate that is paid must cover all costs of providing adequate care. A large component of providing care is, of course, providing the drugs necessary for a quality life situation, which is why long-term care facilities have always been interested in cost containment. There is simply no mechanism for passing the cost of drugs along to the consumer. Because the drug bill is such an enormous figure, often equal to the entire annual food budget, long-term care administrators will search out those pharmacists and pharmacy technicians who are dedicated to obtaining the best product and providing the best services for the smallest dollar spent. Although the facility has little effective control over the physicians' prescribing habits, pharmacy professionals can often educate physicians about other cost-effective choices.

Population

Who lives in long-term care facilities? For the most part, residents are the elderly ill and frail individuals who will need increasing care for the rest of their lives. Some facilities specialize in care for children and specific medical conditions and diseases (such as AIDS and cancer). Rehabilitation facilities specialize in short-term stays for those individuals who have the ability to return to life in the larger community. For the most part, the challenge to those who operate these facilities is the need to balance between the rules, regulations, and efficient practice and the great need to recognize these residents as people who need to continue to participate in and enjoy what life has to offer them.

Because government policy and funding have created an impetus to admit skilled care patients, the population of today's long-term care facilities does not resemble that of 10 or 20 years ago. Today's facilities operate at much the same level of intensity as a small community hospital. Floor staffing in the modern long-term care facility is most commonly a charge nurse, possibly a second nurse on busy shifts, and several certified nursing assistants. Physicians, therapists, and consultants will all be present briefly at the facility to work with residents, but the great bulk of the work is carried out by the nursing staff. A model nursing unit will have forty to forty-five residents who will receive an average of seven prescriptions daily (with some drugs given several times a day). This brings the minimum number of total doses to about 300 doses daily that the charge nurses must administer.

The challenge for the pharmacist and pharmacy technician is to communicate the proper information so that each drug achieves the desired effect. Mindful that long-term care facilities care for residents 7 days a week, 24 hours a day, it is probable that many different individuals will perform the same function. The labeling must be clear to avoid misinterpretation by staff members. One popular medication system that is an effective aid for the charge nurse is the unit-dose system. In this system, individual pills are packaged in blister packs on a mock 30-day calendar card so that the nurse can check at any time to verify that the dosage has been given. Nurses are charged with the responsibility of properly administering medications to the resident. Nurses are taught the "five rights" of medication administration to ensure accuracy:

1. the right *patient*
2. the right *medication*
3. the right *dose*
4. the right *route*
5. the right *time*

Any procedure or helpful practice that enables the pharmacist or pharmacy technician to help the nurse reach that right person is of great value.

Pharmaceutical Personnel in Long-Term Care

Several types of arrangements exist by which long-term care facilities obtain the prescriptions for their residents. The larger facilities may have an in-house pharmacy staffed by pharmacists and pharmacy technicians. Most small to moderate size facilities, however, find it more sensible to obtain medications from a vendor or service pharmacy. Physicians' orders are transmitted to the off-site store and the filled prescriptions are delivered within a few hours. Drugs are then usually distributed to the units by the RN supervisor and become the responsibility of the charge nurse to properly store and eventually distribute.

The service pharmacies often provide an additional service by printing the medication administration record (MAR) for each resident, which saves the nurse some additional time. The service pharmacy also produces administrative reports as requested. Since prescriptions must be renewed every 30 days in a long-term setting, and since most of the prescriptions are for chronic ailments, it is possible for service pharmacies to forecast, to a large extent, what prescriptions will be repeated. The database maintained by these vendors is increasingly important as the government demands longitudinal quality assurance activities and accurate usage levels for reimbursement issues.

Consultant Pharmacist

The consultant pharmacist is also necessary to the long-term care facility. This person performs the mandated function of monthly reviews of the residents' drug regimes and will be watchful for unfavorable interactions or contraindications. This professional reports to the medical director, director of nursing services, administrator, and the attending physicians when a problem occurs. This consultant also participates on the various committees in the facility, such as quality assurance, medical board meetings, and so forth. Occasionally the consultant pharmacist is asked to provide in-service education for the nursing personnel. The consulting pharmacist is also available to guide the nursing personnel on the safe and legal disposition of unused prescriptions and proper survey preparation.

The Future of Pharmacy in Long-Term Care

Pharmacy was probably the first of the caring professions that became comfortable with the computer. Certainly the logic and structure of the apothecary arts are well suited to the strengths of the computer. In the future this natural linkage will become even stronger. With the advent of subacute care in long-term care facilities (with intravenous therapy and a completely new spectrum of high-tech drugs), the need for rational administration and continuous quality improvement will grow. As long-term care facilities increase their computer sophistication, information will be rapidly exchanged. On the other end of the spectrum, the healthier elderly who move to an assisted living environment will be responsible for taking their own medication. Direct professional supervision is lessened at a time when the person's ability to comprehend drug directions may be diminished. Hence, the challenge will be to package, label, and safeguard the product so that it will be used properly for maximum benefit.

Cost containment will increase in importance as the managed health care model becomes more popular. Some experts predict that the managed care model will depend more heavily on drug therapy as opposed to more expensive invasive procedures. Others maintain that more drugs will become over-the-counter items which always present a challenge for the dispensing pharmacist who must predict drug interactions with those prescriptions about which he has knowledge.

The controversy concerning the proper place of psychotropic drugs in the care of the elderly continues to drive the research for newer medications with known and unknown side effects. The pharmacist and allied technical support personnel will have to be committed to staying on the cutting edge of the information explosion to advise the medical community on these new products.

Summary

The pharmaceutical field, whether in a community store, institutional department, or as part of the growing pharmaceutical clearinghouses, will continue to be a vital service to the care and well-being of the growing elderly population. The challenge will be to make the product safe, convenient, and affordable for all.

ASSESSMENT

Multiple Choice Questions

1. Legislation that changed the way long-term care was financed is
   a. Medicare
   b. Medicaid
   c. better social security benefits
   d. both a and b

2. The newest type of long-term facility created by this legislation is
   a. voluntary, not-for-profit
   b. governmental
   c. proprietary
   d. community sponsored

3. The most important goal of pharmacy personnel in long-term care is to
   a. fill the prescription as per the physician's order
   b. write the directions so that no error can be made
   c. help the nursing personnel properly administer the medication by education and support
   d. all of the above

4. Drug regimen reviews on each patient are required
   a. upon admission
   b. upon change of orders
   c. monthly
   d. annually

5. The consultant pharmacist must report errors and discrepancies to the
   a. medical director
   b. director of nursing services
   c. administrator
   d. all of the above

6. Pharmacy technicians are most likely to be responsible for
   a. packaging the unit-dose cards
   b. providing credit on returned drugs
   c. administrative computer duties
   d. all of the above

7. Managed care companies will probably
    a. use more drug therapy than invasive procedures
    b. become more aggressive in the cost-cutting procedures
    c. exercise greater control over physicians' prescribing habits
    d. all of the above

8. Elderly populations are not only found in long-term care facilities, but also in
    a. assisted living arrangements
    b. subacute settings
    c. adult day care centers
    d. the community
    e. all of the above

9. To survive in the future, pharmacists and pharmacy technicians will have to become comfortable with
    a. quality assurance activities
    b. continuous monitoring/risk identification
    c. educational outreach
    d. computerization/information sharing
    e. all of the above

Completion

10. What are the "five rights" that nursing personnel must follow for proper administration of medications?

5 Regulatory Standards in Pharmacy Practice

COMPETENCIES

After completion and review of this chapter, the student should be able to

1. Describe the difference between statutes, rules, regulations, and quasi-legal standards.
2. Identify several federal and state regulatory agencies.
3. Explain the rules, regulations, and reasons for practice standards in health institutions.
4. State the need for the Food, Drug and Cosmetic Act.
5. Discuss quasi-legal standards that define accepted professional practice.
6. List several requirements of the Controlled Substance Act (CSA).
7. Recognize drugs that fall under regulation of the Controlled Substance Act.
8. State reasons for OSHA regulations.
9. Cite appropriate uses for tax-free alcohol.
10. State several basic components of the Patient's Bill of Rights.

Introduction

Rules and **regulations** are necessary to ensure the orderly and safe functioning of society while protecting and respecting individual prerogatives. No individual or enterprise is without regulation.

Regulations in health care provide for assurance of the safety and welfare of health care recipients, provide for the provision of "minimum standards" of a health care service, and provide standards by which to judge reasonable and prudent practice in a court of law. Additionally the implementation of new regulations overall have a very positive impact on the elevation and expansion of health care services and responsibilities.

Health care institutions are complex entities, providing services to every segment of our society. Because of the complexity of hospital services, every department in a health care institution is subject to regulation in some form. The profession of pharmacy—with its direct relationship to the public health, safety, and welfare—is, as such, under the watchful eye of regulatory agencies.

The objectives of this chapter are to give the technician an understanding of some federal and state regulatory agencies and the laws, rules, and practice standards affecting institutional pharmacy practice, and to provide an appreciation of the relationship of these regulatory standards to the specific activities of the pharmacist and the technician in a department of pharmacy.

Federal and State Statutes

Federal and **state statutes** enacted by a legislative body (Congress or state legislature) dictate the conduct of persons or organizations subject to the law. They also enable regulatory agencies to regulate a field pursuant to the mandate of the legislative body.

Two examples of statutes are the federal **Food, Drug and Cosmetic Act,** and the federal **Comprehensive Drug Abuse and Prevention Control Act.**

Rules and Regulations

Rules and regulations are promulgated by government agencies at the local, state, and federal levels. For example, regulatory agencies such as the **Food and Drug Administration (FDA)** and the Drug Enforcement Administration (DEA) can promulgate rules and regulations to enforce the Federal Food, Drug and Cosmetic Act and the Comprehensive Drug Abuse Act and Prevention Control Act respectively.

Quasi-Legal Standards

Quasi means "similar to." Accepted professional practice standards, standards set by the **Joint Commission on Accreditation of Healthcare Organizations (JCAHO),** and U.S. Pharmacopeia (U.S.P.) guidelines all appear to be "similar to" law although they are established by semigovernmental or private organizations. These are examples of **quasi-legal standards**—recognized by the federal government and many state governments. They have been sanctioned through statutes and regulations.

Regulatory Agencies

The discussion that follows will illustrate the regulatory agencies affecting health care institutions. In addition, quasi-legal standards and professional practice standards as outlined in the JCAHO and **American Society of Health System Pharmacists (ASHP)** practice standards will be outlined. To represent the state level, New York regulatory agencies are used as an example.

Federal versus State Drug-Control Laws

Because federal laws and regulations vary from those of particular states, practicing pharmacists and technicians must learn certain basic rules in order to know where they stand in complying with the law. These rules can be summarized as follows:

1. The pharmacist is equally responsible for compliance with both federal and state laws and respective regulations governing his or her pharmacy practice.
2. If the federal law or regulation is more stringent than the comparable state law or regulation, or vice versa, the more stringent law or regulation must be followed. In many cases the state law or regulation is more stringent than its federal counterpart.

State Regulatory Agencies

Every state will have its own unique structure for the regulation of the education, licensing, and discipline of the profession of pharmacy. It should be noted that laws change from state board to state board. For example, some allow technicians to compound I.V.s, but others do not. The following outlines professional regulation in New York State.

Professional Regulation in New York State

In the state of New York, the board of regents issues licenses to practice under Title VIII of the Education Law in thirty-one fields, comprising virtually all of the areas of practice traditionally called professions.

The New York system of professional regulation is unique in that it places a citizen body, the board of regents, in charge of the education, licensing, and discipline of the professions. It is also unique in providing for boards to advise the commissioner of education and the board of regents on all matters relating to licensure and discipline. The boards, each aided by an executive secretary (appointed by the board of regents), provide communication links to the professions and the public. The boards make recommendations on policy and on disciplinary issues and provide advice to the department of education and the board of regents.

State Board of Pharmacy

In most states, responsibilities of the **state board of pharmacy** are to ensure that (1) the public is well served professionally by pharmacists, and (2) the drugs distributed and dispensed within each state meet standards for purity and potency and are properly labeled.

Other responsibilities include but are not limited to

- licensure and registration of pharmacies
- dealing with complaints of professional misconduct
- disciplinary proceedings
- regulations relating to filling and refilling prescriptions (oral and written)
- substitution (generic and therapeutic)
- labeling
- inspections
- poison schedules

Long-Term Care Facilities

A **long-term care facility (LTCF)** is a facility that is planned, staffed, and equipped to accommodate individuals who do not require hospital care, but who are in need of a wide range of medical, nursing, and related health and social services. These services are prescribed by or performed under the supervision of persons licensed to provide such services or care in accordance with the laws of the state in which the facility is located.

The establishment, maintenance, and operation of long-term care facilities are regulated by the states. The majority of the states vest regulatory power in the state health department, although a few states vest power in the state welfare department. Laws and regulations vary from state to state; however, minimum federal standards have been established that must be met in each state. For a long-term care facility to participate in Medicare (Title XVIII) or Medicaid (Title XIX) programs, the facility must comply with the federal Conditions of Participation—Pharmaceutical Services. These regulations are enforced through appropriate state agencies.

The rules governing the handling of pharmaceuticals in long-term care facilities are contained in certain federal laws, the pharmacy practice statutes of the state, and other food and drug statutes and regulations of the state. The following is a brief review of the rules and regulations applicable to pharmaceutical services in long-term care facilities.

Conditions of Participation—Pharmaceutical Services

The long-term care facility provides appropriate methods and procedures for dispensing and administering drugs and biologicals. Whether drugs and biologicals are obtained from community or institutional pharmacies or stocked by the facility, the facility is responsible for providing such drugs and biologicals for its patients. The facility must also ensure that pharmaceutical services are provided in accordance with accepted professional principles and appropriate federal and state laws.

Standard: Supervision of services

The pharmaceutical services are under the general supervision of a qualified pharmacist who is responsible to the administrative staff for developing, coordinating, and supervising all pharmaceutical services. The pharmacist (if not a full-time employee) devotes a sufficient number of hours, based on the needs of the facility, during regularly scheduled visits to carry out these responsibilities. The pharmacist reviews the drug regimen of each patient at least monthly, and reports any irregularities to the medical director and/or director of nursing services. The pharmacist submits a written report at least quarterly on the status of the facility's pharmaceutical service and staff performance, and participates in the facility's quality assurance committee.

Standard: Control and accountability

The pharmaceutical service has procedures for control and accountability of all drugs and biologicals throughout the facility from the point of initiation of a drug order to its administration to the resident/patient and reconciliation of doses administered. This includes procedures for procurement of pharmaceuticals, storage, administration, and their ultimate destruction and/or return to the provider pharmacy.

The scope of pharmaceutical services of long-term care facilities includes

- review of patient records
- review of medication orders
- review of "Stop Order" policies
- monitoring the drug therapy regimen
- review of procurement, labeling, and dispensing of medications
- review of storage of medications

- review of distribution, administration, and charting of drugs
- review of emergency medication supply
- review and development of pharmaceutical policy and procedures
- participation in committees and quality assurance activities
- participation in in-service education and training
- review of physical facilities and equipment

Federal Regulatory Agencies

An example of a federal regulatory agency is the Department of the Treasury—Bureau of Alcohol, Tobacco and Firearms.

Tax-Free Alcohol

In hospitals that use large amounts of **tax-free alcohol,** the hospital pharmacy is normally responsible for the procurement, dispensing, storage, and accountability of tax-free alcohol.

The federal government's philosophy with respect to the use of tax-free ethyl alcohol is that the alcohol will be used only for specific purposes: It will not be used for beverage purposes, is not for resale, and is used in accordance with uses stated on the alcohol permit. If not used according to stated purposes, a tax will be levied for its procurement and subsequent use. In pursuit of this goal, the federal government has devised a number of regulations that mandate specific federal forms to be completed by users of tax-free alcohol.

The federal regulatory agency responsible for controlling tax-free alcohol is the Bureau of Alcohol, Tobacco and Firearms (ATF), Department of the Treasury.

Title 27 of the Code of Federal Regulations (CFR) outlines the procedures and the persons eligible for the procurement, dispensing, storing, and recovering of tax-free alcohol. Tax-free alcohol may be used by hospitals, clinics, blood banks, and sanatoriums for specific research, analysis, or testing.

Tax-free alcohol may be stocked by hospital pharmacies pursuant to applicable federal regulations. These regulations prohibit the selling or distribution of tax-free alcohol to any person off the premises.

To obtain a permit to purchase and use tax-free alcohol, one must first submit to the regional ATF director an "Application for Permit to Use Alcohol Free of Tax." The permit serves as authorization to withdraw tax-free alcohol from a distillery. Permits are issued to cover only those acts included on the application. Actual uses of tax-free alcohol include but are not limited to mouthwash, pharmaceutical floor stock, sterilizing solutions, preparations of laboratory stains and reagents, and tincture of iodine.

There must be adequate storage facilities available for the prevention of unauthorized access to tax-free alcohol. These facilities are to be large enough to hold the maximum quantity of tax-free alcohol that will be on hand at any one time as allowed by the permit.

A bond is required for persons who withdraw more than 1500 proof gallons of tax-free alcohol per year.

When tax-free alcohol is received, the permittee must account for any loss of contents made in transit. The tax-free alcohol may not be removed from its original packaging unless required by city or state fire code.

Accurate detailed records of all receipts, shipments, usage, destructions, and claims to the withdrawal and use of tax-free alcohol must be kept for easy access by ATF officers. Records must be kept on file for 3 years after the date of transaction. All records must be kept at the permit premises.

A physical inventory must be made of the tax-free alcohol on a semiannual basis. If a loss is incurred, a claim for allowances must be filed with the regional director.

Taxable Alcohol

Pharmacy departments may have to compound pharmaceutical preparations and/or fill outpatient prescriptions requiring the use of alcohol, both of which will be used for resale off hospital premises. The alcohol purchased for use in these or similar instances must be alcohol for which appropriate federal and state taxes have been paid. Similarly, alcohol used for beverage purposes within the institution must comply with state law in this regard.

Federal Food, Drug and Cosmetic Act

The Federal Food, Drug and Cosmetic Act is the federal law (statute) through which the Food and Drug Administration promulgates its rules and regulations. In 1938, Congress enacted the Food, Drug and Cosmetic Act as an improvement over the initial federal drug control law, the 1906 Pure Food and Drug Act.

The Federal Food, Drug and Cosmetic Act provides for the following:

- It protects the public health by requiring that only safe, effective, and properly labeled drugs are introduced in commerce.
- It protects the public health by requiring the food or cosmetic preparations subject to the act to be safe and properly labeled.
- It protects the public health by requiring that drugs and/or medical devices for human use be safe and effective. It requires that drugs and devices conform to government standards or that premarketing government approval for **investigational drugs** or devices be obtained.
- It provides that the manufacture, processing, packaging, or holding of drugs comply with "good manufacturing standards" set by the FDA.
- It is enforced by the federal Food and Drug Administration (FDA), which promulgates regulations implementing the act.
- It requires that over-the-counter (nonprescription) drugs be labeled for safe use by consumers in self-medication.

Durham-Humphrey Amendments

The Durham-Humphrey Amendments (enacted in 1951) provided for additional safeguards for prescriptions and over-the-counter drugs.

- They require that prescription drugs (legend drugs) be dispensed to the patient only, pursuant to a practitioner's prescription or directly dispensed by the practitioner.
- They provide that the prescription shall ONLY be refilled as authorized by the practitioner.
- They require that oral prescriptions be reduced in writing and filled by the pharmacist.
- They require particular labeling for both prescription drugs and nonprescription drugs.
- They provide that dispensing (or distributing) a drug in violation of labeling requirements shall be deemed "misbranding" of the drug.
- They provide that a drug containing any filthy, putrid, or decomposed substances or packed or held under unsanitary conditions shall be deemed "adulterated."

- They provide for FDA seizure of drugs misbranded or adulterated.
- They give the FDA broad inspection powers over factories, warehouses, or establishments where drugs, food, devices, or cosmetics are made or processed.
- They provide for limited FDA inspection of pharmacies.
- They provide for the reporting, collection, and evaluation of **adverse drug reactions.**
- They provide for the coordination of **drug recalls** with pharmaceutical manufacturers.
- They provide for the coordination of the FDA's Drug Quality Reporting System (DQRS).

An FDA Regulation

Patient package inserts

FDA regulations require the distribution of **patient package inserts (PPIs)** to each female patient who receives estrogenic or progestational drugs. The PPI, an informational leaflet written for the lay public describing the benefits and risks of each medication, should not be confused with the manufacturer's product insert.

The requirements of the regulation are met if the PPI is provided to the patient before administration of the first dose of the drug and every 30 days thereafter as long as therapy continues. The physician or nurse is responsible for distributing the PPI to inpatients. The pharmacist is responsible for distributing the PPI to outpatients.

Adverse Drug Reactions

A definition of an adverse drug reaction is any unexpected, obvious change in a patient's condition that a physician suspects may be due to a drug, that occurs at doses normally used in humans, and that (1) requires treatment, (2) indicates decrease or cessation of therapy with the drug, or (3) suggests that future therapy with the drug carries an unusual risk in this patient.

Most hospitals have a policy that all suspected adverse reactions to drugs will be brought to the attention of the physician, investigated, documented in the patient's chart, and reported to the FDA when necessary.

Upon suspecting that an adverse drug reaction has occurred, the nurse should follow hospital procedure.

1. Alert the prescribing physician that an adverse drug reaction may have occurred and initiate appropriate treatment, if necessary.
2. Record the suspected adverse drug reaction on the patient's chart.
3. Using the hospital's procedures established for reporting an adverse drug reaction, notify the pharmacy of the suspected reaction. If appropriate and agreed upon by the physician, pertinent data will be supplied to the Food and Drug Administration on their "MedWatch Form" (Form FDA 3500), as shown in **Figure 5–1.**
4. The back of the form contains advice about voluntary reporting, including important phone numbers, and also functions as a "self-mailer" to the FDA.

Drug Recalls

All drug recalls are voluntary, either manufacturer initiated or FDA requested, and the result of reports from the manufacturer or health professionals.

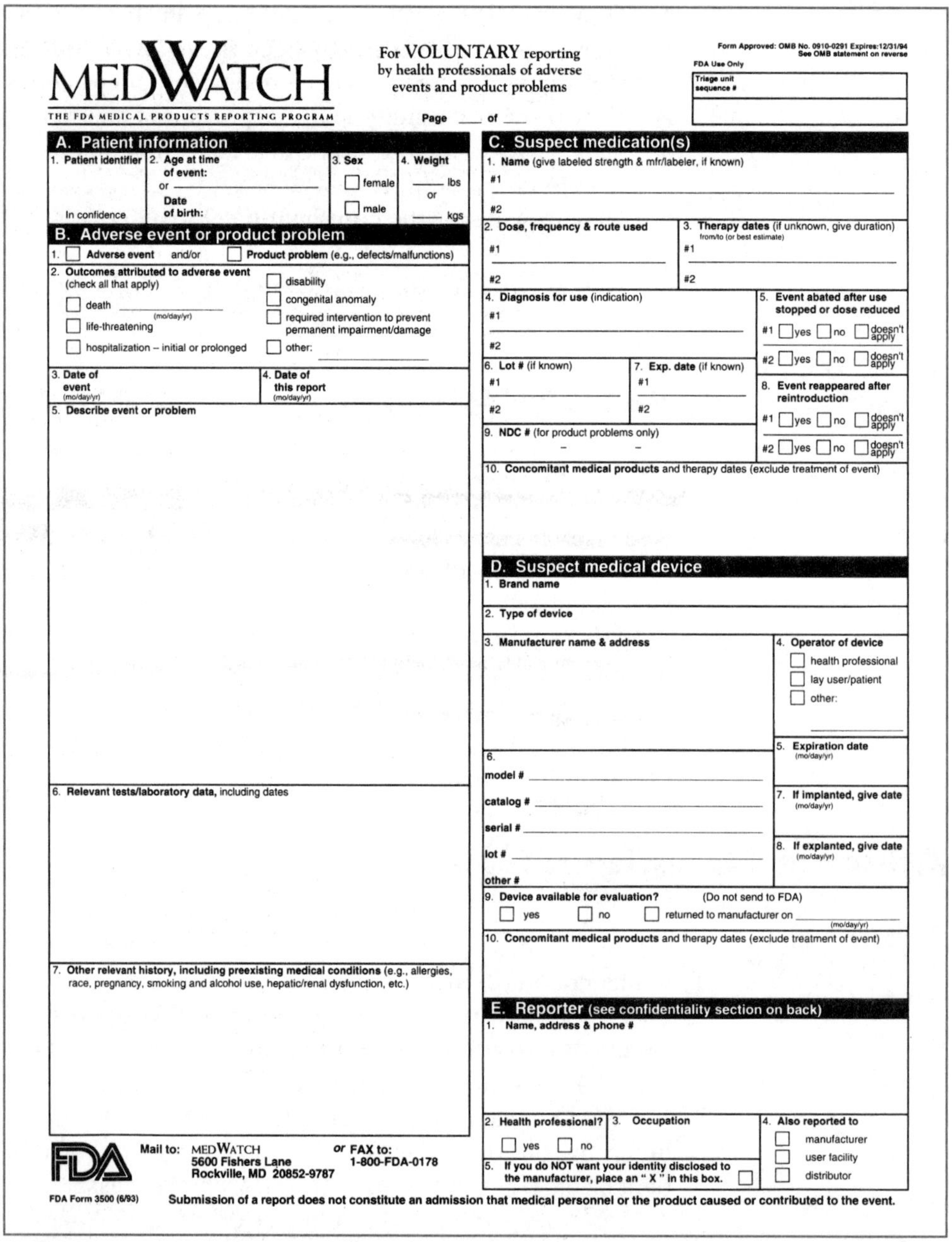
MEDWATCH
THE FDA MEDICAL PRODUCTS REPORTING PROGRAM

For VOLUNTARY reporting by health professionals of adverse events and product problems

Form Approved: OMB No. 0910-0291 Expires: 12/31/94 See OMB statement on reverse
FDA Use Only
Triage unit sequence #

Page ___ of ___

A. Patient information
1. Patient identifier — In confidence
2. Age at time of event: or Date of birth:
3. Sex ☐ female ☐ male
4. Weight ___ lbs or ___ kgs

B. Adverse event or product problem
1. ☐ Adverse event and/or ☐ Product problem (e.g., defects/malfunctions)
2. Outcomes attributed to adverse event (check all that apply)
☐ death ___ (mo/day/yr)
☐ life-threatening
☐ hospitalization – initial or prolonged
☐ disability
☐ congenital anomaly
☐ required intervention to prevent permanent impairment/damage
☐ other: ___
3. Date of event (mo/day/yr)
4. Date of this report (mo/day/yr)
5. Describe event or problem
6. Relevant tests/laboratory data, including dates
7. Other relevant history, including preexisting medical conditions (e.g., allergies, race, pregnancy, smoking and alcohol use, hepatic/renal dysfunction, etc.)

C. Suspect medication(s)
1. Name (give labeled strength & mfr/labeler, if known) #1 #2
2. Dose, frequency & route used #1 #2
3. Therapy dates (if unknown, give duration) from/to (or best estimate) #1 #2
4. Diagnosis for use (indication) #1 #2
5. Event abated after use stopped or dose reduced #1 ☐ yes ☐ no ☐ doesn't apply #2 ☐ yes ☐ no ☐ doesn't apply
6. Lot # (if known) #1 #2
7. Exp. date (if known) #1 #2
8. Event reappeared after reintroduction #1 ☐ yes ☐ no ☐ doesn't apply #2 ☐ yes ☐ no ☐ doesn't apply
9. NDC # (for product problems only) – –
10. Concomitant medical products and therapy dates (exclude treatment of event)

D. Suspect medical device
1. Brand name
2. Type of device
3. Manufacturer name & address
4. Operator of device ☐ health professional ☐ lay user/patient ☐ other:
5. Expiration date (mo/day/yr)
6. model # catalog # serial # lot # other #
7. If implanted, give date (mo/day/yr)
8. If explanted, give date (mo/day/yr)
9. Device available for evaluation? (Do not send to FDA) ☐ yes ☐ no ☐ returned to manufacturer on ___ (mo/day/yr)
10. Concomitant medical products and therapy dates (exclude treatment of event)

E. Reporter (see confidentiality section on back)
1. Name, address & phone #
2. Health professional? ☐ yes ☐ no
3. Occupation
4. Also reported to ☐ manufacturer ☐ user facility ☐ distributor
5. If you do NOT want your identity disclosed to the manufacturer, place an " X " in this box. ☐

FDA Mail to: MEDWATCH 5600 Fishers Lane Rockville, MD 20852-9787 or FAX to: 1-800-FDA-0178

FDA Form 3500 (6/93) Submission of a report does not constitute an admission that medical personnel or the product caused or contributed to the event.

FIGURE 5–1 MedWatch form for voluntary reporting by health professionals of adverse events and product problems *(Courtesy of the Food and Drug Administration)* *(continues)*

Classes of Recalls

The FDA medical staff determines the health hazard potential of a product (e.g., sub-potent labeling errors, adverse drug reactions) and assigns a drug recall classification.

1. *CLASS I*—A situation in which there is a reasonable probability that the use or exposure to a violative product will cause severe adverse health consequences or death.
2. *CLASS II*—A situation in which the use or exposure to a violative product may cause temporary or medically reversible adverse health consequences.

ADVICE ABOUT VOLUNTARY REPORTING

Report experiences with:
- medications (drugs or biologics)
- medical devices (including in-vitro diagnostics)
- special nutritional products (dietary supplements, medical foods, infant formulas)
- other products regulated by FDA

Report SERIOUS adverse events. An event is serious when the patient outcome is:
- death
- life-threatening (real risk of dying)
- hospitalization (initial or prolonged)
- disability (significant, persistent or permanent)
- congenital anomaly
- required intervention to prevent permanent impairment or damage

Report even if:
- you're not certain the product caused the event
- you don't have all the details

Report product problems – quality, performance or safety concerns such as:
- suspected contamination
- questionable stability
- defective components
- poor packaging or labeling

How to report:
- just fill in the sections that apply to your report
- use section C for all products except medical devices
- attach additional blank pages if needed
- use a separate form for each patient
- report either to FDA or the manufacturer (or both)

Important numbers:
- 1-800-FDA-0178   to FAX report
- 1-800-FDA-7737   to report by modem
- 1-800-FDA-1088   for more information or to report quality problems
- 1-800-822-7967   for a VAERS form for vaccines

If your report involves a serious adverse event with a device and it occurred in a facility outside a doctor's office, that facility may be legally required to report to FDA and/or the manufacturer. Please notify the person in that facility who would handle such reporting.

Confidentiality: The patient's identity is held in strict confidence by FDA and protected to the fullest extent of the law. The reporter's identity may be shared with the manufacturer unless requested otherwise. However, FDA will not disclose the reporter's identity in response to a request from the public, pursuant to the Freedom of Information Act.

The public reporting burden for this collection of information has been estimated to average 30 minutes per response, including the time for reviewing instructions, searching existing data sources, gathering and maintaining the data needed, and completing and reviewing the collection of information. Send your comments regarding this burden estimate or any other aspect of this collection of information, including suggestions for reducing this burden to:

Reports Clearance Officer, PHS
Hubert H. Humphrey Building,
Room 721-B
200 Independence Avenue, S.W.
Washington, DC 20201
ATTN: PRA

and to:
Office of Management and
Budget
Paperwork Reduction Project
(0910-0230)
Washington, DC 20503

Please do NOT
return this form
to either of these
addresses.

FDA Form 3500-back   **Please Use Address Provided Below – Just Fold In Thirds, Tape and Mail**

**Department of
Health and Human Services**
Public Health Service
Food and Drug Administration
Rockville, MD 20857

NO POSTAGE
NECESSARY
IF MAILED
IN THE
UNITED STATES
OR APO/FPO

Official Business
Penalty for Private Use $300

BUSINESS REPLY MAIL
FIRST CLASS MAIL   PERMIT NO. 946   ROCKVILLE, MD

POSTAGE WILL BE PAID BY FOOD AND DRUG ADMINISTRATION

MED**WATCH**
The FDA Medical Products Reporting Program
**Food and Drug Administration
5600 Fishers Lane
Rockville, MD 20852-9787**

FIGURE 5–1 MedWatch form for voluntary reporting by health professionals of adverse events and product problems *(continued)*

3. *CLASS III*—A situation in which the use or exposure to a violative product is not likely to cause adverse health consequences.

FDA field checks

A post recall audit is done by the FDA to verify that manufacturers, wholesalers, pharmacists, or customers have received notification about the recall and have taken appropriate action.

Repackaging of Drugs

Repackaging of drugs in a pharmacy requires the use of a repackaging record. A repackaging record must be maintained including the name, strength, lot number, quantity, name of the manufacturer and/or distributor, the date of repacking, the number of packages prepared, the number of dosage units in each package, the signature of the person performing the repacking operation, the signature of the pharmacist supervising the repacking, and such other identifying marks added by the pharmacy for internal record-keeping purposes. Drugs repacked for in-house use only must have an expiration date 12 months or 50 percent of the time remaining to the manufacturer's expiration date—whichever is less—from the date of repacking.

Investigational Drugs

Drugs marketed in this country for either human or animal use must receive the approval of the appropriate bureau of the Food and Drug Administration (FDA). This approval is sought by submission of a New Drug Application (NDA). FDA regulations in effect since 1962 state that to receive approval, the drug must be shown to be both safe and efficacious for the use intended. Since a body of evidence supporting safety and efficacy must be included, sometime prior to this approval the drug must have been actually used by physicians for the conditions named in the application. It is, therefore, during this period of preapproval use that a drug is considered to be investigational. Individuals or pharmaceutical companies desiring to ship or receive drugs that are not covered by an approved NDA must notify the FDA of their intent. This takes the form of an exemption from approved status and is commonly referred to as an investigational new drug (IND) exemption.

Preclinical Studies

Administration of biologically active substances to humans carries unavoidable risk. This risk can be identified through adequate preclinical research. Such research uses animal subjects and establishes the drug's basic biological and toxicological characteristics.

After a new drug's chemical properties and structure are established, biochemical studies are conducted to determine its absorption, distribution, metabolism, and elimination. This information facilitates extrapolation of animal data to humans and provides the basis for establishing suitable dosage regimens.

Clinical Studies

Phase I studies

Phase I clinical studies represent the first time a new drug is introduced into human beings. Emphasis is now placed on elucidating the safety of the new agent by defining the pharmacokinetic, toxicological, and pharmacological parameters associated with its use in humans. Such studies should be performed with its use in humans.

Five to twenty participants, with a few serving as a control (placebo) group, are utilized for Phase I clinical trials. Studies with a control group usually are performed double blind [i.e., both the investigator and the subjects are unaware of which drug (active versus placebo) is being administered].

The starting dose of the drug administered to the subjects is less than that expected to show clinical activity; it is also a level considerably below that associated with adverse effects in animals.

In some Phase I studies, drugs known to have high risks associated with their use (e.g., cancer chemotherapeutic agents) are not given to normal subjects but rather to patients who have failed all known effective treatment for the disease.

Phase II studies

Phase II clinical studies are a continuation and expansion of the activities initiated during Phase I trials. Considerable pharmacokinetic and pharmacological data about a drug are generated during Phase I studies, and the relative degree of safety for human use is determined. In Phase II studies, the emphasis shifts toward establishing the activity of the new drug in actual clinical situations.

Phase II studies should be conducted by experts in management of the disease state being treated who can proficiently evaluate the response of the disease process to the drug. Protocols are developed that specifically address the goals and objectives of the research, the controls and treatments used, the parameters assessed, and the personnel involved.

Upon completion of Phase II studies, the sponsor reaches a critical crossroad in the life of a new drug. To proceed, evidence of safety and efficacy must be established. Unfavorable outcomes may lead to the abandonment of further research with the drug or to additional preclinical and Phase I work. Favorable results determine whether broad clinical trials are warranted. If an affirmative decision is reached, Phase III studies are initiated.

Phase III studies

The decision to initiate Phase III clinical trials follows a comprehensive review of the preclinical and Phase I and II clinical study results. The need to provide substantial proof of efficacy based on "adequate and well controlled clinical investigations" is the primary emphasis of Phase III clinical studies. Phase III studies establish the acceptable use of the drug.

Due to the scope of this phase of clinical research, many hundreds of patients may need to be evaluated before meaningful results can be obtained. Therefore, the same study could be conducted in many research centers.

As the clinical exposure to an investigational agent increases, the likelihood of idiosyncratic and allergic reactions, as well as previously undocumented side effects, increases.

Approval for marketing can be sought only upon completion of all the aforementioned research. To obtain marketing approval, a completed NDA form and other materials (such as proposed labeling, case report tabulations, and drug samples) must be sent to the FDA for review. The response to the NDA submission may be "approved," "approvable" (if certain specified data are provided), or "not approved." The drug may be marketed only upon issuance of an approval letter.

Handling

The procedures for handling investigational drugs are an important part of hospital drug distribution systems. These procedures will naturally reflect the extent to which an institution is involved with research, the resources available, and the particular needs of the hospital. For most community hospitals, the main activities related to investigational drugs will most likely involve the storage, distribution, and control of investigational drugs. In a large teaching hospital, investigational-drug use may result in numerous services and responsibilities.

The basic responsibilities of a hospital pharmacy handling investigational drugs are as follows:

- *distribution and control of investigational drugs,* including drug procurement, storage, inventory management, packaging, labeling, distribution, and disposition of unused drugs
- *clinical services,* such as patient education, staff in-service training, and the monitoring and reporting of adverse drug reactions

- *research activities,* such as participating in the preparation and/or review of research proposals and protocols, assisting in data collection and analysis, serving on the institutional review board (IRB), and conducting pharmaceutical research
- *clinical study management,* which might involve working on study reports to the research sponsor and coordination of study personnel activities

Investigational Use of Marketed Products

Physicians often use a marketed drug for an indication or in a manner not in the approved product labeling. In doing so, the physician must have sound evidence or a firm scientific rationale that justifies the intended use. Use of drugs in this fashion is not subject to FDA regulation, nor is it subject to review unless so required by institutional policy as established by a committee within the hospital known as the institutional review board.

Institutional Review Board

The institutional review board (IRB) is a board, committee, or other group formally designated by an institution to review, to approve the initiation of, and to conduct continuing review of biomedical research involving human subjects in accordance with FDA regulations. The purpose of IRB review is to ensure that

- risks to subjects are minimized;
- risks to subjects are reasonable in relation to anticipated benefits;
- informed consent will be sought and documented from each prospective subject or the subject's legally authorized representative;
- where appropriate, the research plan makes adequate provision for monitoring the data collected to ensure the safety of subjects;
- there are adequate provisions to protect the privacy of subjects and to maintain the confidentiality of data.

Orphan Drugs

The Orphan Drug Act was enacted into law January 1983. The law provides incentives to drug manufacturers to develop and market drugs (**orphan drugs**) for the diagnosis, treatment, or prevention of rare diseases or conditions. A rare disease is one that affects less than 200,000 persons in the United States or one that affects more than 200,000 persons but for which there is no reasonable expectation that the cost of developing the drug and making it available will be recovered from the sales of the drug. Examples include Aminopyridine for the relief of symptoms of multiple sclerosis and Amsacrine for acute adult leukemia.

The Controlled Substances Act

The Controlled Substances Act (CSA) of 1970 (effective May 1, 1971) is the major federal law regulating the manufacture, distribution, and sale (dispensing/administration) of certain drugs or substances that are subject to or have a potential for abuse or physical or psychological dependence. These drugs or substances are designated as "controlled substances." The law provides a "closed" system for legitimate handlers of these drugs, which should help reduce the widespread diversion of these drugs into the illicit market.

The Drug Enforcement Administration (DEA) is the lead federal law-enforcement agency charged with the responsibility for combating controlled substance abuse. The DEA was established July 1, 1973. It resulted from the merger of the Bureau of Narcotics and Dangerous Drugs, the Office for Drug Abuse Law Enforcement, and other drug enforcement agencies. The DEA was established to more effectively combat narcotic and dangerous drug abuse through enforcement and prevention. In carrying out its mission, the DEA cooperates with other federal agencies, foreign as well as state and local governments, private industry, and other organizations.

Schedules of Controlled Drugs

Controlled substances are classified into five schedules.

Schedule I
The controlled substances in Schedule I include drugs having no accepted medical use in the United States and have a high abuse potential. Some of the drugs or substances in Schedule I are heroin, marijuana, LSD, peyote, mescaline, psilocybin, and hallucinogenic substances.

Schedule II
The controlled substances in Schedule II include drugs having a high abuse potential with severe psychic or physical dependence liability. Some drugs in Schedule II are opium, morphine, codeine, hydromorphone (Dilaudid), Pantopon, methadone hydrochloride (Dolophine), meperidine hydrochloride (Demerol), cocaine, oxycodone hydrochloride (Percodan), and oxymorphone (Numorphan). Also included are amphetamines such as Dexedrine, Desoxyn, Preludin, and Ritalin, and certain other drugs such as amobarbital (Amytal), pentobarbital (Nembutal), and secobarbital (Seconal). Some drugs included in Schedule II are also found in other schedules when combined with other drugs.

Schedule III
The controlled substances in Schedule III include drugs having an abuse potential less than those in Schedule I and Schedule II. Some drugs in Schedule III are compounds containing limited quantities of certain narcotic drugs and nonnarcotic drugs (e.g., Tylenol with codeine). Also included in this schedule are barbiturates not listed in another schedule and certain depressants such as glutethimide (Doriden), methyprylon (Noludar), nalorphine (Nalline), and paregoric.

Schedule IV
The controlled substances in Schedule IV include drugs having an abuse potential less than those listed in Schedule III. Some drugs in Schedule IV are barbital, phenobarbital (Luminal), chloral hydrate (Noctec), ethchlorvynol (Placidyl), meprobamate (Equanil, Miltown), paraldehyde, methohexital, chlordiazepoxide (Librium), diazepam (Valium), oxazepam (Serax), clonazepam (Clonopin), lorazepam (Ativan), and propoxyphene hydrochloride (Darvon Compound).

Schedule V
The controlled substances in Schedule V include drugs having an abuse potential less than those listed in Schedule IV. Drugs in Schedule V consist mainly of preparations containing limited quantities of certain narcotic drugs generally for antitussive and antidiarrheal indications.

Some of the drugs in this schedule are Lomotil, Actifed C Expectorant, Phenergan Expectorant with Codeine, and Robitussin A-C syrup.

Symbols

Each commercial container of a controlled substance is required to have on its label a symbol designating the schedule to which it belongs. The symbols for controlled substances are: (I) or C-I; (II) or C-II; (III) or C-III; (IV) or C-IV; and (V) or C-V.

Records and Reports

Hospitals and other health care facilities authorized to purchase, possess, and use controlled substances must keep a number of records both within the pharmacy and at the individual nursing units to ensure appropriate use and control of the controlled substances. These records and reports may include the following:

- an order signed by a person authorized to prescribe, specifying the controlled substance medication for a specifically indicated person
- a separate record at the main point of supply for controlled substances (This shows the type and strength of each drug in the form of a running inventory. The inventory indicates the dates and amounts of such drugs compounded at that site or received from other persons, and their distribution or use.)
- a record of authorized requisitions for such drugs for distribution to the nursing units (Such records must indicate receipt at the nursing unit by the signature of a person authorized to control the nursing unit.)

With each substock of controlled substances an administration sheet must be furnished. The administration sheet lists the type of controlled substance, dose, and number of doses furnished to the nursing unit. The sheet also indicates

- name of patient
- name of prescribing physician or practitioner
- date and hour of administration
- quantity of administration
- balance on hand after each administration
- signature of administering nurse

An entry must be made in the patient's chart to indicate administration of the controlled substance. The entry includes the name of the administering nurse and the date and hour of administration.

Order Forms

A triplicate order form is necessary for the transfer of controlled substances in Schedules I and II. Under the Controlled Substances Act, the use of the order forms will be for Schedules I and II only. No charge is made for order forms.

Registration

The Controlled Substances Act exerts its control by way of federal registration of all persons (except the ultimate user or patient) in the legitimate chain of procurement to distribution or dispensing of controlled drugs. Every person or firm who manufactures, distributes, conducts instructional activities with, conducts chemical analysis with, conducts research with, exports, imports, prescribes, administers, or dispenses controlled substances or who proposes to engage in the same must register with the federal Drug Enforcement Administration (DEA) of the U.S. Department of Justice.

Classification of registrants

Registrants are divided into groups by activities. Hospital pharmacies register as dispensers of nonnarcotic and narcotic Schedule II–V drugs. In many cases state law is much more stringent than federal law and therefore will not allow things that would be authorized under federal law. To illustrate, New York State's rules and regulations on controlled substances have several significant differences with federal law and are also stricter than the federal law. For example, all benzodiazepines are classified and handled as Schedule II controlled substances in New York State to curb abuse of these drugs. In addition all Schedule II controlled substances in New York State require an official NYS triplicate prescription. When a practitioner writes a prescription for a Schedule II controlled substance, a triplicate prescription must be used. These are purchased from the state of New York.

The medical practitioner retains the first copy of the triplicate for 5 years. The patient receives both the original and the second copy of the triplicate once the prescription is written by the practitioner. The pharmacist filling the prescription retains the original copy for 5 years and sends the second copy to NYS Bureau of Controlled Substances, which maintains a computerized record of physician prescribing of Schedule II controlled substances.

Additionally, the dispensing of Schedule II controlled substances requires affixing an orange label containing a NYS caution statement, "Controlled substance, dangerous unless used as directed," and the federal transfer warning statement, "Caution: Federal law prohibits the transfer of this drug to any person other than the patient for whom it was prescribed."

Lost or Stolen Order Forms

Both federal and state laws have requirements for drug security and regulations for reporting lost or stolen order forms (and in New York State, lost or stolen triplicate prescriptions), drug theft, inventory discrepancies, and so forth.

Inventory Requirements

The Controlled Substances Act requires each registrant to make a complete and accurate record of all stocks of controlled substances on hand every 2 years. The biennial inventory date of May 1 may be changed by the registrant to fit the regular general physical inventory date, so long as the date is no more than 6 months from the biennial date that would otherwise apply. The inventory must be maintained at the location appearing on the registration certificate for at least 2 years.

Most pharmacy departments take a physical inventory of their controlled drugs much more frequently than required by federal law. Some departments take controlled drug inventories on a daily basis to ensure appropriate accountability and reconciliation.

Destruction of Controlled Substances

To dispose of any excess or undesired stocks of controlled substances, a pharmacy is required to contact the state Bureau of Controlled Substances and/or the DEA office for disposal instructions and to request the necessary form(s) from each. The state bureau and/or the DEA office will advise the registrant of the procedures to be followed.

Federal Hazardous Substances Act

The Federal Hazardous Substances Act was enacted in 1960. The Consumer Product Safety Commission enforces this act.

Poison Prevention Packaging Act

The **Poison Prevention Packaging Act** of 1970 is an amendment to the Hazardous Substances Act. It regulates certain substances defined as household substances. It requires that these substances be packaged for consumer use in "special packaging" that will make it significantly difficult for children under the age of 5 to open, but not difficult for adults to open.

The "special packaging" is often referred to as "child-resistant containers." One of the main purposes of the act is to extend the special packaging requirements to both prescription and nonprescription drugs.

Special exemptions

Drugs dispensed on prescription or on a medical practitioner's order are exempt from the special packaging requirement if the prescribing doctor specifies a non-complying container in the order or prescription or if the patient or customer receiving the drug requests a noncomplying container. Another exemption is made for OTC items for elderly or handicapped persons. This exemption allows the manufacturer to market one size of commercial consumer container with noncomplying packaging; but for the exemption to apply, such noncomplying packaging must contain the printed statement, "This package for households without young children." The manufacturer must also market popular sizes of the products in the special packaging as required.

Here is a brief list of substances that are currently required to be sold or dispensed to consumers in the "special packaging."

1. Aspirin-containing preparations must be sold or dispensed to consumers in the special packaging or child-resistant containers.
2. Controlled substances must be dispensed to consumers only in the special packaging or child-resistant containers.
3. Prescription only (legend) drugs for oral human use must be dispensed to the consumer only in child-resistant containers, unless the patient or guardian requests a non-child-resistant container and signs a release to this effect. Exempt from the special packaging requirement for legend drugs is the dispensing of sublingual nitroglycerin preparations and the sublingual and chewable isosorbide dinitrate (Isordil) preparations. These drugs are prescribed for angina pectoris sufferers who must be able to quickly get at their medication.

Occupational and Safety Act

The Occupational and Safety Act of 1970 was passed to assure every working man and woman in the nation safe and healthful working conditions. Under the Occupational and Safety Act, the Occupational Safety and Health Administration (OSHA) was created to decrease hazards in the workplace, to maintain a reporting system for monitoring job-related injuries and illness, and to develop mandatory job safety and health standards.

OSHA is authorized to conduct workplace inspections to determine whether employers are complying with standards issued by the agency for safe and healthful workplaces. Workplace inspections are performed by OSHA compliance safety and health officers. Similarly, states with their own occupational safety and health programs conduct inspections using qualified state compliance safety and health officers.

Several OSHA standards and guidelines apply to all departments in health care institutions. Several standards that would relate most specifically to the department of pharmacy and some other departments are discussed next.

Air Contaminants

Employees are to be protected from air contaminants and chemicals that could cause injury or illness with regard to potential carcinogenic agents. OSHA published *Guidelines for Cytotoxic (Antineoplastic) Drugs* as a meaningful tool for pharmacy employers and employees handling chemotherapy drugs. The publication provides information regarding personal protective equipment, monitoring, training, and so forth.

Flammable and Combustible Liquids

Appropriate storage containers (vault, cabinet, etc.) must be provided for pharmaceuticals such as alcohol, acetone, and flexible collodion.

Portable fire extinguisher

A sufficient number of portable fire extinguishers of the appropriate type, depending on the hazards in the department, must be available and immediately accessible.

Eye and Face Protection

Employees performing functions where there are hazards of flying objects (glass), liquids, and so forth, such as in the prepackaging area of the pharmacy, are to be provided with appropriate eye and/or face protection.

General Concerns about Hazardous Materials

Bulk storage and receiving areas, such as the pharmacy storeroom, must have unobstructed aisles, shelving must be secured to prevent accidental falling, and the area must be kept clean and dry.

Hazardous Drugs and Chemicals

An OSHA regulation that became effective May 23, 1988, requires that employees know about the hazards of all chemicals to which they are exposed.

Hazard Communication Standard

The Hazard Communication Standard (HCS) is based on the simple concept that employees have both a need and a right to know the hazards and identities of the chemicals to which they are exposed when working. They also need to know what protective measures are available to prevent adverse affects.

The purpose of this standard is to ensure that the hazards of all chemicals are evaluated and that information concerning these hazards is transmitted to affected employees. This transmission of information is to be accomplished by a comprehensive hazard communication program that includes container labeling and other forms of warning, material safety data sheets (MSDS), and employee training.

1. **Written hazard communication program**
   Employers must develop and implement a written hazard communications program that includes a list of the hazardous chemicals known to be present by obtaining the appropriate Material Safety Data Sheets (MSDS) for all toxic/hazardous substances in every department.

2. **Material Safety Data Sheets (MSDS)**

MSDS must be provided by the manufacturer, importer, or distributor for each hazardous chemical used in a workplace. The MSDS must be in English and must contain the following information:

- chemical and common names
- if a mixture, chemical and common names of ingredients
- physical and chemical characteristics, such as flash point and vapor pressure
- physical hazards, including potential for fire, explosion, and reactivity
- health hazards, including signs and symptoms of exposure (Both acute and chronic effects should be included.)
- routes of entry into the body
- OSHA permissible exposure limit (PEL)
- precautions for safe handling and use, including hygienic practices and protective measures during repair or maintenance
- procedures for cleanup of spills and leaks
- emergency and first aid procedures
- date of preparation of MSDS and/or date of latest revision
- name, address, and telephone number of manufacturer, importer, or distributor.

The employer must maintain copies of the required MSDS for each hazardous chemical in the workplace and ensure that they are readily accessible to employees during each work shift. See Appendix A–1 for further information.

Omnibus Budget Reconciliation Act

In adopting the federal Omnibus Budget Reconciliation Act (OBRA) of 1990, Congress recognized the escalating pressure to expand social programs, particularly those that impact on the increasingly larger and more politically active older citizens. Senator David Pryor of Arkansas, the principal author and sponsor of OBRA 90, was convinced that the pharmacist could play a key role in improving the effectiveness of drug therapy and reduce the overall costs.

OBRA 90 mandated three main provisions that affect the profession of pharmacy. First, manufacturers are required to provide their best (i.e., lowest) prices, which they offer to any customer, to Medicaid patients by rebating to each state Medicaid agency the differences between their average price and their "best" price. Second, drug-use review and patient counseling is now mandated. Third, the act authorizes government-sponsored demonstration projects relating to the provision of pharmaceutical services. The last two provisions of the law are discussed here and are the impetus for new state regulations.

OBRA 90 requires states to implement regulations consistent with the objectives of the federal law prior to January 1, 1993. In New York State, these regulations took effect on December 4, 1992. States are required to mandate prospective drug-use review, establish programs for retrospective drug-use review, and implement educational programs to rectify problems uncovered as a result of the aforementioned drug-use review programs. Although the original federal regulations mandate such programs for Medicaid patients only, virtually every state has implemented the new regulations for all patients to assure all patients a high level of professional service.

In New York State, pharmacists are now required to maintain individual patient medication profiles which are expected to contain, in addition to patient demographic information such as the name, address, telephone number, gender, and date of birth, additional information including:

- known allergies and drug reactions
- chronic diseases
- a comprehensive list of medications and medical devices and other information appropriate for counseling about the use of prescription and over-the-counter drugs

Utilizing this patient medication profile, pharmacists are expected to conduct a "prospective drug review" before dispensing or delivering a prescription to a patient, or the patient's caregiver, which would include screening for the following:

- therapeutic duplication
- drug-drug interactions, including serious interactions with the over-the-counter drugs
- incorrect drug dosage or duration of treatment
- drug-allergy interactions
- clinical abuse or misuse

After a prospective drug review, regulations require that counseling be provided to each patient and must include all "matters which in the pharmacist's professional judgement, the pharmacist deems significant," including:

- the name and description of the medication
- the dosage form, dosage, route of administration, and duration of drug therapy
- special directions and precautions for preparation, administration, and use by the patient
- common severe side effects or adverse effects or interactions that may be encountered, including their avoidance and action required if they occur
- techniques for self-monitoring drug therapy
- proper storage
- prescription refill information
- action to be taken in the event of a missed dose

For mail-order pharmacies, counseling and patient profile information may be conveyed by toll-free long-distance telephone and are usually patient initiated.

Although any qualified employee of a pharmacy may initiate the offer to have the pharmacist counsel a patient (e.g. technicians), only a pharmacist or a pharmacy intern can provide the actual counseling. The objective of the counseling to the patient or the patient's caregiver is to improve patient medication compliance, to avoid medication misadventures, and to improve drug therapy outcome.

Pharmacists should note that if a patient refuses to supply information necessary for maintenance of a patient profile, or refuses counseling, the pharmacist may fill a prescription as presented, provided the patient's refusal is documented in the records of the pharmacy. The law, however, expects pharmacists to make a reasonable effort to obtain, record, and maintain the required information. The federal and state regulations use terms such as "counseling," "offer to discuss," and "reasonable effort." These terms mandate that the distribution of printed material and the posting of a sign, alone, do not meet the spirit or letter of the law. Pharmacists are also advised to ensure that physical barriers and other impediments do not exist to discourage patients from receiving professional counseling.

If these new regulations are viewed in a positive manner, and as an opportunity to expand and develop a true professional role for pharmacists within the community, the viability of pharmacy practice will be enhanced. The public has need for a readily available professional who will assist them in improving their health care outcomes.

Quasi-Legal Standards

Practice Standards, Guidelines, and Statements

The American Society of Health System Pharmacists (ASHP) has developed an extensive series of practice standards covering numerous aspects of hospital pharmacy practice. Practice standards provide a basis for evaluation, review, and goal-setting for the hospital pharmacy director. In a court of law the practice standards define accepted professional practice and assume quasi-legal status. The system of law in the United States relating to the practice of medicine, pharmacy, and other health professions is based on "reasonable and prudent" practice. Practice standards define reasonable and prudent practice. A practitioner who fails to meet these standards may be found negligent by the courts.

Joint Commission on Accreditation of Healthcare Organizations

The Joint Commission on Accreditation of Healthcare Organizations (JCAHO) is a not-for-profit, nongovernmental corporation whose member organizations are the American College of Physicians, the American College of Surgeons, the American Hospital Association, and the American Medical Association. These organizations, through the JCAHO, have established optimal standards for the operation of hospitals. Compliance with JCAHO standards is voluntary. Any hospital may request a survey to determine if it is compliant.

JCAHO Accreditation

Noncompliance with a JCAHO standard results in a "recommendation." The JCAHO will not accredit a hospital with excessive recommendations or one that fails to meet certain essential recommendations. The JCAHO issues a certificate of accreditation to hospitals that substantially comply with its standards. Accreditation is currently for 3 years. To continue its accreditation beyond this period, a hospital must be resurveyed.

Failure to meet the JCAHO standards or the loss of JCAHO accreditation can severely affect a hospital's prestige. The hospital may find it difficult to attract qualified physicians and the adverse publicity may cause patients to seek admission elsewhere. Furthermore, JCAHO-accredited hospitals can automatically participate in the Medicare program. Without this accreditation, a hospital has to pass an annual Medicare survey.

Legal Status of JCAHO Standards

The JCAHO provides uniform nationally recognized standards that define quality patient care. Many hospitals (accredited and nonaccredited) base their policies, procedures, and quality assurance (QA) criteria on commission standards. Because these standards are widely accepted, the courts have used them in lieu of local or community practice norms. In some instances they have become the expected legal standard of care. Therefore, failure to meet JCAHO standards may open the hospital and the pharmacy to legal difficulties.

Comprehensive Accreditation Manual for Hospitals

With the publication of the 1995 Comprehensive Accreditation Manual for Hospitals (CAMH), the JCAHO moves the Agenda for Change from the abstract to reality and provides hospitals with a critical tool for the establishment of an integrated care assessment process focused on the patient and the effects of care.

In the past, standards and the survey evaluation were designed around departments such as nursing, pharmacy, laboratory, or dietary; in contrast, the current standards are designed around functions performed within the organization and involving many departments working together.

The central core of the CAMH contains three major sections of performance-focused standards. Each section encompasses a group of functions, or structures with functions, that enable hospitals to provide patient care. The standards themselves provide a framework to ask and answer the following questions: Are we doing the right thing? Are we doing the right things well? Is performance being improved within major functions?

To fulfill and improve the processes that define patient care, collaboration is critical. The design of the CAMH and the related survey process allow for effective assessment of the presence or absence of that collaboration among caregivers.

The components of the survey process

The survey team consists of, at least, a physician, an administrator, and a nurse. It reviews presurvey management reports to provide an orientation to an organization. The survey team will depend on interview observation and documentation review techniques to understand the organization and its performance of patient care and management responsibilities.

1. **Opening conference**

   The survey begins with a brief opening conference, which includes an overview presentation of performance improvement activities by the organization's leadership. This conference is an opportunity for "show and tell."

2. **Document review**

   Document review is intended to familiarize the survey team with the organization. Bylaws, policies and procedures, rules and regulations, and other documents are requested in advance to work a preliminary indication of performance and standards of compliance and to set the stage for the interactive survey components that follow.

3. **Patient care unit visits**

   The patient care unit visit is the interactive component of the survey team interviews with managers, direct care providers, hospital staff, and patients. The team will spend as much as half its time in the organization visiting patient care settings to access consistency of performance in executing the expectations established by the organization's leadership and articulated in the policies and procedures. All of the surveyors will visit patient care areas separately.

Staff should be prepared to articulate policy and procedure for patient care activities in which they play a role, and the relationship of these policies to the performance of their daily responsibilities. They may be asked to illustrate that role or comment on the care in a specific patient case.

A typical inpatient visit is scheduled in advance, allowing the hospital the opportunity to prepare for the interviews, and normally includes the following:

- The surveyor(s) meets with key individuals who are elected by the hospital, including a physician, nurse, pharmacist, dietician, and other caregivers typically involved with patient care on that particular unit.
- A tour of the unit provides the surveyor with an opportunity to review and observe the overall operation of the unit, including activities such as the storage of medications and the availability, placement, and function of life safety equipment.

■ Selected patient records evaluated in open case review ensure that documentation in the patient record reflects the established policy and procedures. Open case review involves interviews or discussions with caregivers, including pharmacists with the objective of ensuring that caregivers
- ■ are aware of, and familiar with, established policies and procedures;
- ■ can articulate how those policies and procedures are implemented; and
- ■ can relate their execution of the policies and procedures to care of individual patients and performance improvement.

■ Together the surveyor and the unit manager will select a patient or patients to be interviewed, including a patient who is being discharged. Patients will be asked how they felt about their care and their caregivers and may be asked specific questions about whether the care they received reflected the intent of the established policies and procedures.
- ■ For example, a diabetic patient with a complex medication regimen might be interviewed regarding the patient education provided during the inpatient stay and in preparation for discharge.
- ■ Instructions for medication use continue to be a major focus of attention, ensuring that patients understand their condition and treatment while in the hospital, as well as what will happen after discharge.

4. **Function interviews**

Surveyors will devote a portion of their visit to 1-hour multidisciplinary interviews with selected caregivers and administrative staff. One function for this portion of the survey is medication use and nutrition care.

5. **Leadership interviews**

Senior leaders in the organization, including administrators, medical staff leaders, nursing leadership, and department heads, will participate in this survey segment. It will focus on planning, integration, and communication among leaders and with the overall organization and the community.

6. **Competence assessment systems**

Throughout the CAMH are standards supporting the belief that every patient who comes to an accredited organization has the right to expect clinicians, administrators, and support staff capable of doing their jobs and doing them well to meet patient needs.

7. **Other survey activities**

While most pharmacy-related survey issues have been incorporated into the patient care area surveys and the medication use interview, a dedicated pharmacy services visit is scheduled with the primary purpose of reviewing medication storage and control systems.

Patient's Bill of Rights

Many states have established a **patient's bill of rights** for hospital and health care institutions. This bill of rights ensures that all patients—inpatients, outpatients, and emergency service patients—are afforded their rights. The hospital's responsibility for assuring patients' rights includes both providing patients with a copy of these rights and providing assistance to patients to understand and exercise their rights.

For the purposes of illustration, the following is an example of the New York State Hospital Patient's Bill of Rights.

PATIENTS' RIGHTS

As a patient in a hospital in New York State, you have the right, consistent with the law, to

- Understand and use these rights. If for any reason you do not understand or you need help, the hospital must provide assistance, including an interpreter.
- Receive treatments without discrimination as to race, color, religion, sex, national origin, disability, sexual orientation, or source of payment.
- Receive considerate and respectful care in a clean and safe environment free of unnecessary restraints.
- Receive emergency care if you need it.
- Be informed of the name and position of the doctor who will be in charge of your care in the hospital.
- Know the names, positions and functions of any hospital staff involved in your care and refuse their treatment, examination or observation.
- A no smoking room.
- Receive complete information about your diagnosis, treatment and prognosis.
- Receive all the information that you need to give informed consent for any proposed procedure or treatment. This information shall include the possible risks and benefits of the procedure or treatment.
- Receive all the information you need to give informed consent for an order not to resuscitate. You also have the right to designate an individual to give this consent for you if you are too ill to do so. If you would like additional information, please ask for a copy of the pamphlet "Do Not Resuscitate Orders—A Guide for Patients and Families."
- Refuse treatment and be told what effect this may have on your health.
- Refuse to take part in research. In deciding whether or not to participate, you have the right to a full explanation.
- Privacy while in the hospital and confidentiality of all information and records regarding your care.
- Participate in all decisions about your treatment and discharge from the hospital. The hospital must provide you with a written discharge plan and written description of how you can appeal your discharge.
- Review your medical record without charge. Obtain a copy of your medical record for which the hospital can charge a reasonable fee. You cannot be denied a copy solely because you cannot afford to pay.
- Receive an itemized bill and explanation of all charges.
- Complain without fear of reprisals about the care and services you are receiving and to have the hospital respond to you and if you request it, a written response. If you are not satisfied with the hospital's response, you can complain to the New York State Health Department. The hospital must provide you with the Health Department telephone number.
- Authorize those family members and other adults who will be given priority to visit consistent with your ability to receive visitors.
- Make known your wishes in regard to anatomical gifts. You may document your wishes in your health care proxy or on a donor card, available from the hospital.

It is incumbent upon health care workers to be familiar with the bill of rights and to ensure compliance with it.

Summary

There are numerous statutes, rules, regulations, and quasi-legal standards of practice that regulate the pharmacy profession in institutional settings. In many instances they are minimum standards and requirements that have been established to protect the patient and to ensure safe and effective drug therapy. Pharmacists and technicians should be familiar with and ensure compliance to these standards in their daily activities and responsibilities.

ASSESSMENT

Multiple Choice Questions

1. A patient package insert is required to be given to all patients who are taking
   a. steroids
   b. analgesics
   c. estrogenic drugs
   d. vaccines
   e. all of the above

2. Which of the following is considered a controlled substance?
   a. Demerol
   b. morphine
   c. Valium
   d. Phenergan expectorant with codeine
   e. all of the above

3. Regulations affecting pharmacy practice encompass
   a. federal and state statutes
   b. state rules and regulations
   c. CSA regulations
   d. JCAHO standards
   e. all of the above

4. Which of the following is not an approved use of tax-free alcohol?
   a. educational organizations for scientific use
   b. hospitals for medical use
   c. laboratory use for scientific research
   d. beverage purposes
   e. all of the above

5. The Food, Drug and Cosmetic Act encompasses which of the following?
   a. protection of public health
   b. refill authorization of prescription drugs
   c. collection of adverse drug reaction reports
   d. over-the-counter drugs' labeling requirements for safe consumer use
   e. all of the above

6. Controlled substances are required by federal law to have appropriate safeguards with their use. Which of the following is not an issue?
   a. inventory requirements
   b. dispensing records and reports
   c. administration of records and reports
   d. storage
   e. patient consent

7. Adverse drug reactions should be reported to the FDA for
   a. documentation
   b. revision of prescribing information
   c. possible drug recall
   d. a possible warning statement
   e. all of the above *(circled)*

8. A class I recall does not include
   a. voluntary manufacturer initiation
   b. possibility of severe health consequences
   c. FDA initiation *(circled)*
   d. assignment of the drug recall classification by the FDA
   e. any of the above

9. The intent of the Occupational Safety and Health Administration (OSHA) is
   a. to monitor job-related injuries
   b. to develop job safety and health standards
   c. to conduct workplace inspections
   d. to ensure a safe and healthful workplace
   e. all of the above *(circled)*

10. Pharmacy practice standards, guidelines, and statements
    a. define reasonable and prudent practice *(circled)*
    b. establish minimum standards for the profession
    c. are established to protect the patient
    d. ensure safe and effective drug therapy
    e. accomplish all of the above

True/False Questions

11. __F__ Regulatory agencies stipulate similar goals for pharmaceutical services of both long-term care facilities and hospitals.

12. __T__ The Poison Prevention Packaging Act of 1970 requires certain substances to be packaged for consumer use in "child-resistant containers."

13. __F__ The pharmacy standards of the Joint Commission on Accreditation of Healthcare Organizations (JCAHO) provide a quasi-legal standard of practice for the profession. *(handwritten: Hospitals)*

Bibliography

American Pharmaceutical Association, American Society of Consulting Pharmacists, American Society of Hospital Pharmacists. (1986). *Pharmaceutical services in the long-term care facility.* Washington, D.C.

American Society of Health System Pharmacists. (1998). *Practice standards of the American Society of Hospital Pharmacists, 1997–1998.* Bethesda, MD.

Code of Federal Regulations (27 parts, 1–199). (1985). Part 22, pp. 507–530. Washington, DC: Federal Register National Archives and Records Administration, revised April 1, 1988.

Fink, J.L. III. (1989). *Pharmacy law digest.* Media, PA: Harwal Publishing Co., DC-86.

Investigators Handbook (a manual for participants in clinical trials of investigational agents, sponsored by the division of cancer treatment, National Cancer Institute). Bethesda, MD.

Joint Commission of Accreditation of Healthcare Organizations. (1995). *Comprehensive accreditation manual for hospitals.* Oakbrook Terrace, IL: Joint Commission on Accreditation of Healthcare Organizations.

McNeill, L., & Talley, J.R. (1986). Tax-free alcohol. *Hospital Pharmacy, 21,* 335–37.

N.Y.S. Department of Health. Vol. A., chap. III, "Administrative Rules and Regulations," subchapter J, "Controlled Substances," part 80, "Rules and Regulations on Controlled Substances."

United States Department of Justice, Drug Enforcement Administration. *Pharmacist's manual. An informational outline of the Controlled Substances Act of 1970.*

United States Department of Labor, Occupational Safety and Health Administration. *OSHA inspections.* OSHA-2098.

University of the State of New York, The State Education Department, State Board of Pharmacy. *Pharmacy Handbook.* Albany, NY.

PART II

The Profession of Pharmacy

6

An Ethical Pharmacy Concern: The Informed Drug Consent

COMPETENCIES

Upon completion and review of this chapter, the student should be able to

1. Describe the ethical foundation that requires a patient to be informed concerning the risk and benefits involved in taking potent medications.
2. List the objections to providing information regarding the risks (side effects) that can be anticipated with the therapy.
3. Explain the requirements for good communication skills to inform a patient of possible serious side effects.
4. Mention five factors that could modify the patient's fundamental right to know the risks involved in a particular drug regimen.

Introduction

This chapter deals with an important aspect of pharmacotherapy: the patient's right to know the benefits and the risks involved in the medications that the prescribing physician decides are in the patient's best interest, for healing, alleviating symptoms, or long-term replacement therapy.

Modern medication treatment has moved from botanical products to gene therapy. The benefits are great, but so are the risks. Some serious, even life-threatening, risks can be anticipated; many risks cannot be predetermined. However, the question is, "What information regarding medication risk information should be made available to the patient?"

Today's pharmacy technician is viewed as an integral member of the health team generally and the pharmacy team specifically. This ongoing professional concern about medication risk disclosure is a topic with which the pharmacy technician should be familiar.

The Consumer and Drug Risk Information

Few things carry more weight than writing, filling, and taking a physician's prescription. Every prescription has one or more substances that, in some persons, may have serious unwanted effects as well as desired effects. This fact is the ineradicable part of pharmacotherapeutics—to gain the benefit, the risk must be run.

Regardless, patients eager for relief or cure rarely know or even ask about the risks. Physicians eager for therapeutic success may minimize those risks, mention them only in passing, or not know them as well as they should. However, if consent to the choice of a drug and management of the risks of taking it are to be morally valid, patients need information and the time to understand those risks.

Providing appropriate risk information is an essential ethical obligation of physicians, pharmacists, and nurses. In a way appropriate to each role, each shares in this responsibility and is a moral accomplice if harm comes to the patient through neglect of this obligation.

To clarify what this obligation entails, four basic questions need to be addressed.

1. What is the ethical foundation for, and the content of, the obligation to inform patients about medication risks?
2. What are the objections to providing such information?
3. Is it ever justifiable to withhold or distort information for the good of the patient?
4. To what degree do the patient's age, mental competence, emotional state, and education modify the fundamental obligation?

This discussion covers the *therapeutic* rather than the experimental use of drugs, the *particularized assessments* in individual patients rather than the general issue of risk assessments in policy formulation, and *ethical* rather than legal aspects.

What Is the Moral Foundation for the Obligation of Providing Information about Risk?

The ethical roots of the obligation of providing information about risk are embedded in human nature, the principles of autonomy, and the ends and purposes of the therapeutic relationship.

By nature, human beings have the capacity to make rational decisions and choices about how to live their lives based on their own values and purposes. It is this capacity that grounds the principle of autonomy—the principle that requires each of us to behave toward others in such a way as not to inhibit, indeed, to enhance, their capacity for self-governing decision and action.

The end and purpose of the therapeutic relationship is the good of the patient. That good has two components—medical and personal—expressed in the patient's value sets. To act for the good of the patient requires, at a minimum, protection of the patient from physical harm; but this is not sufficient. It would be equally harmful to violate the humanity of the patient by usurping his or her capacity for reasoned decision even for a good purpose (e.g., making sure he or she agrees with the "right" drug regimen).

Respect for both human nature and the capacity for self-governing decisions is actualized in the doctrine of informed consent. This doctrine requires that patients have the information they need to make a reasoned choice and to ensure that the choice is free of coercion. For the healing professional, respect for persons must be more than mere acquiescence to the principle of autonomy. It also carries the beneficent responsibility to help patients make their own choices and to enhance their capacity to do so.

The obligation to inform patients of the risks of treatment is grounded, therefore, in the most fundamental sources of general and medical morality. The patient who faces the decision to take a potent medication must be provided with the information without which choice can be neither free nor informed. Only the patient can decide whether the magnitude and probability of benefit outweigh the magnitude and probability of harm. Further, without a knowledge of side effects, patients cannot do their part in risk management (i.e., to recognize and report side effects and prevent further harm to themselves).

What Are the Objections to this Obligation?

Recognition of the fundamental right of patients to make their own decisions is now well accepted among bioethicists and increasingly among clinicians. Nevertheless, specific objections are still raised to disclosure of risk information in drug therapy.

A very old objection is that the decision to undertake a drug regimen is so complex that the patient could not possibly make an "informed" decision. It would be wrong, therefore, to place this burden on the patient. This is a spurious objection. First, it is a disservice to the increasing number of educated patients who want to know and can grasp the facts. Moreover, patients do not need to understand every facet of clinical pharmacology, only the analysis of costs and benefits as viewed from the perspective of their own values, the kind of life they want to lead, and the risks they consider worth running. It is the physician's responsibility to give the patient the opportunity for choice and to enhance the autonomy of that choice. Almost all patients, with sufficient effort, can be helped to comprehend the nature and severity of risks to their health.

Another objection is that the knowledge of side effects will frighten the patient away from beneficial treatment or affect compliance negatively; but this is just as likely to happen without knowledge as with it. Patients often listen to friends or misinterpret symptoms as danger signs and discontinue a drug on their own. Discussing risk at the start of treatment and assuring patients of surveillance will put fears in a more realistic light and enable patients to evaluate symptoms. Finally, increasing numbers of patients are aware of the problems of drug side effects and will worry as much about not being told.

Some physicians say consent cannot be "free" because the patient is anxious, wants to be cured, and will accept whatever the doctor recommends. This may be so, but the only antidote is to disclose risks so that anxiety can be addressed. As anxiety wanes, the patient can more realistically evaluate the results and side effects of the recommended drug.

Finally, some physicians think informed consent is a sham because doctors can get any choice they want by the way they present the data and whether they put stress on the advantages or the dangers. This is true, but it is all the more reason for the physician to enhance the patient's autonomy.

How Is the Obligation Fulfilled in Practice?

In the clinical situation, fulfillment of the obligation centers on obtaining a morally valid consent for initiation of a drug regimen. This is more than a legally valid consent, which requires signature, witnesses, and a one-time explanation of what is to be done: A morally valid consent must have four characteristics—it must be competent, informed, reasoned, and free of coercion.

Only fully *competent patients* can give morally valid consent. Clearly, if a patient is not competent mentally for any reason—as a result of a psychiatric disorder, chronological immaturity, or cerebral dysfunction, whether physiological or organic—he or she cannot make a reasoned decision.

To fulfill the ethical obligations of *informed consent,* the physician's duties are several. First, the physician must possess and transmit the relevant information. It must be up-to-date, accurate, and honestly presented with uncertainties clearly defined.

Unfortunately, adequate information about risks is often not available. The physician must apprise the patient of this fact so uncertainty can be factored into the assessment. Clearly this is an area in which physicians should enlist every source available, especially clinical pharmacologists and clinical pharmacists in risk management.

Risk identification, determination of risk probability, risk assessment, and risk management must be recognized as distinct processes, each of which requires specific knowledge and attention. Simply to identify a risk is not sufficient. The risk must be personalized by relation to the patient's age and susceptibility (genetic, ethnic, etc.), and to the presence of other disorders and other medications, all of which can modify risk probability and magnitude.

Much argument is expended in defining "how much" to tell. There is no formula that will satisfy everyone. Some suggest the physician should supply what a reasonable person would want in order to make a decision. In general, the patient needs to know most about the most serious effects with high probability and probably less about side effects with very low probability and minor or negligible harm. Low-probability, high-magnitude risks (e.g., fatal reactions to anesthesia or urographic contrast material) should be made known. For example, in the case of urographic contrast, patients should know that risk of fatal reactions is reduced by use of low osmolality contrast material, which is more expensive but reduces the incidence of fatal reactions from 1 in 30,000 to 1 in 250,000. On the whole, if errors are to be made, they should be on the side of disclosure.

A valid decision must also be a *reasoned* one. Whether the decision is considered right or wrong by the physician is not the question. The test of a reasoned decision is whether it follows logically on the patient's values in relationship to the risk data. The logic of assent is as important as the assent or dissent itself. Patients can make the right decision for the wrong reasons and vice versa.

The decision must be *free of coercion.* Coercion can occur in subtle ways (e.g., by withholding all or part of the information or by disproportionate emphasis on the dangers or the benefits of a particular treatment). Some may justify these ethical infractions in the name of helping patients or guarding them against their own poor judgment. This is morally indefensible, and does not mean that physicians should refrain from saying what they believe is in the patient's interests or from trying to persuade the patient when they believe the patient's decision is grievously in error. The lines between overt coercion, deception, manipulation, and persuasion are difficult ones to draw; however, the difficulty does not justify abandoning the effort. Much depends here on the character and ethical sensitivity of the physician.

Finally, the patient must *understand* the information presented. Simply presenting the information, however honestly, is not sufficient. The physician must take pains to see that it is understood and that new information is added as it appears in the literature. Patients should also be monitored as the drug is being taken for their comprehension of the risks and for signs of harm.

Obtaining valid consent is not a one-time affair. The physician should periodically check the patient's comprehension of risk. A period without incident can lull doctor and patient into a false sense of security. Obviously, if autonomy is to be respected, the patient can withdraw consent at any time and must be given this opportunity.

The physician has the duty to enhance the patient's decision-making capacity when possible. This requires treating reversible physiological disturbances of sensorial state that result from fever, infection, and toxic and metabolic states. Treatment might be started before the patient is competent to consent to restoration of the capacity, but when decision-making capacity is restored the patient must again become part of the decision-making process so far as risk evaluation is concerned.

When risks are very high and benefits marginal, physicians should be free not to run those risks even with a competent patient who is willing to run any risks. With incompetent patients, surrogates are under obligation to limit harms. The physician may refuse an eager surrogate when the physician believes the risks are too high. The right of a competent patient or surrogate to refuse a drug regimen does not become a right to demand any drugs he or she might want.

Pharmacists and nurses also share in these responsibilities, each in the way that relates to the profession. Pharmacists are responsible primarily for risk management but also, as occasions require, for risk identification and assessment of risk probability. Nurses are responsible primarily for education and monitoring relating to risk management.

These responsibilities cannot be neatly compartmentalized. Pharmacists' and nurses' duties overlap with those of physicians. They are obliged to work cooperatively with each other and the physician to protect the patient's interests. Any member of the therapeutic team who is aware that patients are endangered due to lack of proper risk information must take appropriate action to avoid that harm. None of this is a threat to the physician-patient relationship. It merely recognizes the ethical responsibility and moral complicity of all team members. Even if such action were a threat, the nurse or pharmacist would not be relieved of duty to protect the patient. All of this being so, the obligation to share information and plans for a drug regimen among team members is obvious.

Is It Ever Justifiable to Intentionally Withhold Information?

Traditional medicine sometimes has justified withholding information from a patient to avoid precipitating depression, loss of hope, or suicide. This has been called the "therapeutic privilege." It is accepted by some bioethicists today as a rare but legitimate reason for bypassing informed consent. This is a privilege that should be used with the utmost caution, if ever. It would be valid only if the physician had very weighty evidence and serious harm could occur if the patient knew all the side effects of the drugs he or she was taking.

The problem is usually not the information provided but the way it is provided. Far too often, the process is seen as data transmittal and not genuine communication on a continuing basis with another human being. Any anxiety or depression produced is more often the result of the physician's attitudes and personality than of the information itself. No sure formula is available to prevent harm when providing information. However, some general requirements for effective communication can be listed: The information must be adjusted to the patient's age, educational level, and cultural, social, and linguistic group, as well as to the patient's personality. This is not something the physician needs to do alone. Indeed, it may be that other health care professionals are more skilled in this area. The physician is then obliged to involve them in the process, especially when patients' competence and capacity for decision making are marginal or lost entirely.

Educational and Cultural Differences

Educational and cultural differences between patients and health professionals need special consideration. Educational differences require that the major issues be made as clear and simple as possible. If language differences exist, proper interpretation is necessary so that patients and surrogates can comprehend the nature and gravity of the decisions.

Finally, in our culturally diverse nation, cultural differences are of increasing importance. As it has been developed thus far, medical ethics is Anglo-American in its bias, but there are cultures in which individualism and autonomy are not prime ethical imperatives. Patients from those cultures expect their families to share in the decision or even make the decision for them. In some cultures, only the father or tribal chief makes decisions. These cultural differences should be respected short of inflicting serious physical damage to patients.

Summary

Providing information about risks of drug regimens is an ethical responsibility of physicians, pharmacists, and nurses. It is grounded in the principle of respect for the distinctive capacity of humans to make their own choices about their own lives. It is expressed in the principle of autonomy and actualized in informed consent.

This chapter outlines the specific obligations of health professionals that arise from the principle of respect for persons, both for those who have the capacity to make their own decisions and for those who do not.

Although the writing and filling of prescriptions are everyday occurrences, the decisions involved in this process are far from trivial ethically. Indeed the frequency with which medicines are prescribed and the commonplace, or unexceptional, aspect of the process, in addition to the vulnerability of those for whom medications are ordered, impose heavy responsibilities on physicians, nurses, and pharmacists to conduct all aspects of a drug regimen with the utmost sensitivity to the welfare of their patients.

ASSESSMENT

Multiple Choice Questions

1. The primary responsibility to discuss the possible harmful effects of a prescribed drug rests upon the
   a. physician
   b. pharmacist
   c. nurse
   d. laboratory technician
   e. pharmacy technician

2. A reason why physicians may put more stress on the benefits rather than the risks is
   a. to satisfy the patient
   b. to expedite the prescribing process
   c. for the desire for therapeutic success
   d. for the lack of adverse reaction knowledge
   e. all of the above

3. The end and purpose of the therapeutic relationship between members of the health care team and the patient is
   a. medical, to improve health and prevent therapeutic harm
   b. personal, to respect the person's autonomy in self-determination
   c. both a and b

4. The doctrine of informed consent requires that
   a. the patient has the information necessary to make an informed consent
   b. the patient's choice be free of coercion by the physician, pharmacist, or family
   c. a health professional—physician, pharmacist, or nurse—be available to answer any further questions the patient may have regarding the risks and benefits of the drug
   d. all of the above

5. The obligation to inform a patient of the risks and benefits of a potent drug is fundamentally based on
   a. medical morality
   b. patient concern
   c. malpractice issues
   d. all of the above
   e. none of the above

6. A positive effect of the patient's knowledge of the possible adverse or side effects of a medication is
   a. the patient may reject the drug
   b. the patient may become anxious and nervous
   c. the patient may recognize and report early indications of an adverse effect

7. A moral valid consent to take a potent drug requires the following characteristic:
   a. The patient is competent to make a decision.
   b. The patient is informed of both the benefit and the risk.
   c. The patient has the ability to make a reasoned choice and is able to weigh the benefits while, at the same time, consider the adverse effects.
   d. The choice must be free of coercion.
   e. All of the above

8. Patient incompetency can include
   a. psychiatric disorder
   b. illiteracy
   c. chronologic immaturity
   d. cerebral dysfunction
   e. a, c, and d

9. Information presented to the patient should
   a. emphasize the facts that will encourage the patient to consent to the drug regimen
   b. be up-to-date, accurate, and honestly presented

10. Drug risk information should be personalized for the individual patient because
    a. persons react differently psychologically
    b. genetic makeup of individuals differs
    c. patient's state of health is a factor
    d. other drugs or diseases can modify reactions
    e. all of the above

Bibliography

Pellegrino, E.D. (1995). Medication risks: The ethics of informed consent in pharmacotherapy. In *Communicating Risk to Patients* (pp. 23–27). Rockville, MD: The United States Pharmacopeial Convention, Inc.

Drug-Use Control: The Foundation of Pharmaceutical Care

COMPETENCIES

Upon completion and review of this chapter, the student should be able to

1. State the mission of pharmacy practice.

2. Explain pharmaceutical care.

3. Describe the drug-use process.

4. Explain the importance of control in the drug-use process.

5. Explain the role of the pharmacist versus the role of the technician in the drug-use process.

6. Discuss trends in the drug-use process and how these may affect the roles of the pharmacist and technician.

Introduction

After a brief introduction, you will learn about the **drug-use process** and its connection to **pharmacy practice.** You will also learn about **control** of this process and how control is measured and enforced. You will have a clear understanding of the role of the pharmacist versus the role of the technician. The future of drug-use control will be discussed and how it may affect the pharmacist and technician.

It is critical that you thoroughly understand the basic principles of pharmacy practice and the drug-use process. This is where pharmacy technicians spend most of their time and put forth most of their effort.

Profession of Pharmacy

History

The preparation of medicines started in ancient civilizations; however, it was the Greeks and Romans who made pharmacy a true profession. The emergence of the pharmacist and pharmacy shop came about in Baghdad in 762, then spread to western Europe. American pharmacy mostly grew from the British colonies in the New World. However, there was some Spanish-American influence as well. During the early 1900s pharmacy grew from an art to a science. In earlier days pharmacists mostly prepared medicines from natural sources. Later pharmacists started to understand how medicines worked and embraced the role of safeguarding the patient from harm. Today the pharmacist is a highly respected professional in the United States.

Purpose

The societal purpose of **pharmacy** is to help patients make the best use of their medications. Pharmacists do this by discovering, preparing, and dispensing medication. They also provide information about medicine, protecting the public from harm, and teach students in the art and science of pharmacy. The profession is made up of three basic parts: research, education, and practice.

Practice of Pharmacy

Mission

The **pharmacy mission** is to help people make the best use of medication. Pharmacy practice has several traditional functions: the procurement, storage, preparation, **dispensing,** and distribution of medication. A newer dimension is a more clinical or patient-oriented role. In this role, the pharmacist provides information about drugs and the effects (good or bad) of drugs on the care of patients. Pharmacists distribute this **drug information** to requesting physicians, nurses, other health professionals, patients, or the public. Most recently, pharmacists are providing unrequested drug information when it is in the best interest of the patient.

Pharmaceutical Care

Pharmaceutical care is the application of pharmacy practice to the patient. Pharmaceutical care is the responsible provision of drug therapy to achieve definite outcomes that improve a patient's quality of life. Pharmaceutical care blends traditional practice (i.e., drug preparation and dispensing) and **clinical pharmacy practice.**

In delivering pharmaceutical care, the pharmacist is responsible for (1) accepting responsibility for the patient; (2) directly interacting with the patient; (3) exhibiting a caring attitude and caring actions; (4) establishing a definite outcome for each drug used; (5) trying to improve a patient's quality of life; and (6) identifying, resolving, and preventing medication-related problems.

Medication-related problems prevent the achievement of a positive or improved patient outcome. There are eight medication-related problems: (1) having an untreated condition; (2) receiving a drug for which there is no indication; (3) an underdose; (4) an overdose; (5) a drug interaction (one drug interferes with the actions of another drug); (6) an adverse drug reaction; (7) wrong drug prescribed; and (8) not receiving a prescribed drug.

Pharmacists often use **pharmaceutical care plans** (see **Figure 7–1**) to help track patient's progress, the medication-related problems, their recommendations, changes in therapy, and progress toward the therapeutic goals established through the pharmaceutical care process.

Practice Sites

Pharmacy is practiced in many different sites, such as community pharmacies, chain drug stores, and hospitals. Pharmacists also provide service to nursing homes, managed care facilities, etc. Thus, models for delivering pharmaceutical care may differ. What does not change is the goal of achieving **ideal drug therapy** (**Figure 7–2**).

PHARMACEUTICAL CARE PLAN

Pharmacist Name: _____

Patient Identifier

Vital Statistics and History

Age _____ Race _____ Sex _____ Ht _____ Actual Wt _____ IBW _____ Adj. BW _____ ClCr _____ BP _____ HR _____ R _____ Temp _____

CC _____   Date of Admission _____

HPI _____

PMH _____

Drug History PTA (i.e. Rx: scheduled, prn; OTC; ETOH; Tob; Drugs)

Active Problem List Supporting Labs

1. _____
2. _____
3. _____
4. _____
5. _____
6. _____

Date Start	Date D/C	Drug/Dose/Interval	Monitoring Parameters/Precautions	Desired Outcome	Therapeutic Outcome Achieved	A	B

A. Medication Related Problems: 1. Untreated Indication 2. Improper drug selection 3. Subtherapeutics dosage 4. Failure to receive drug 5. Overdosage (toxic) 6. Adverse Drug Reactions/SE 7. Drug Int./Drug-Food Int. 8. Drug use without indication 9. Other (explain) 10. None Identified   B Recommendations: 1 = Followed 2 = Partially Followed 3 = Not Followed 4 = Information Only 5 = None

FIGURE 7–1 Pharmaceutical care plan

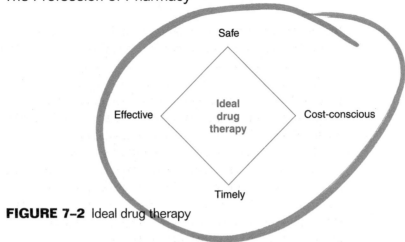

FIGURE 7–2 Ideal drug therapy

Pharmacy is a time-honored profession. Pharmacists are licensed by society to help people make the best use of medication. Pharmacy technicians work under the direct control of pharmacists. They help pharmacists fulfill their societal duty.

The Drug-Use Process

Definition

The drug-use process is the series of steps necessary to move a drug product from purchase to patient use. The drug-use process includes the identification of a need for a drug and the purchase, storage, manufacture, or preparation of the drug. It also includes the prescribing, labeling, dispensing or distribution, and administration of a drug and monitoring its effect(s).

Traditional elements of the drug-use process include purchasing and distribution. A newer dimension, often termed clinical pharmacy practice, includes an assessment of the need for the drug and whether the preferred drug is being used. It also includes monitoring the drug's effectiveness or unwanted effects. Blending the traditional and clinical parts of pharmacy produces pharmaceutical care for the patient.

The goal of the drug-use process is to produce safe, timely, effective, and cost-conscious therapy for the patient. During this process, the needs and feelings of the patient must always be kept in mind. All patients should be treated with respect, kindness, and compassion. This is the trademark of the health care worker. Nurses, physicians, and other health care workers are customers of the pharmacy service. They also should receive respect. Meeting the needs of our patients and customers accurately, on time, every time, provides quality care.

The pharmacy technician is an important part of the drug-use process. What does it take to be successful? The technician must understand the importance of getting the right drug, to the right patient, at the right time, with respect and compassion.

Control of the Drug-Use Process

Control

At the heart of the drug-use process is control. Control is any method used to eliminate or reduce the potential harm of the medication distributed. The provision of pharmacy service is a series of clinically related control functions. **Drug-use con-**

trol is "that system of knowledge, understanding, judgments, skills, controls, and ethics that assures optimal safety in distribution and use of medication" (Brodie, 1967).

The importance of drug-use control is to protect the health and safety of the patient. It is the foundation and mainstream of pharmaceutical care. Drug-use control is a chain of events that protects the patient from harm. Each link in the chain must follow the other, be strong individually, and together provide control. If a break occurs, safety may be lost and the patient may be harmed.

Patients suffer from the unwanted effects of drugs. Such events are called **medication misadventures.** Medication misadventuring is what can go wrong in the "therapeutic adventure" of using a medication—errors in prescribing judgment, system errors in the process of bringing drug products to the ultimate users, and idiosyncratic responses to medications.

Types of medication misadventures include medication errors, adverse reactions, allergic reactions, and unwanted drug interactions. The severity of these problems can range from mild discomfort to death.

A recent study showed that 3.7 percent of patients suffered disabling injuries while hospitalized. Of these, the highest number of disabling events was due to drugs (19 percent). The drugs causing the most adverse effects were antibiotics (16.2 percent), antitumor drugs (15.5 percent), and anticoagulants (11.2 percent). Antibiotics kill germs, antitumor drugs are for cancer, and anticoagulants keep the blood from clotting too much.

An example of a chain of control events and procedures in hospital pharmacy practice includes the selection of qualified pharmacy personnel, proper work flow, specifications for drug procurement and storage, systems for product preparation, and the interpretation and verification of drug orders. It would also include the checking of drug preparation, the distribution of medication to patient care units, drug storage throughout the hospital, and verifying that medication has been administered as ordered. These areas and others need constant monitoring to ensure proper control.

Pharmacists and pharmacy technicians work together to provide a system of checks and balances called drug-use control. This helps ensure patient safety. Drug-use control is the most important part of delivering pharmaceutical care. Society depends on the pharmacy profession to protect it from the potential harm of medication.

The pharmacy profession has various methods to provide control in the drug-use process, including laws, standards of practice, guidelines, documents, initialing, and monitoring.

Laws

Laws, rules, and regulations are intended to protect the public from harm. Pharmacists need to pass an examination and are licensed "to first, do no harm." Society trusts the pharmacist to protect it from drug misadventures. There are many laws that pharmacists must follow. They are responsible to various agencies to make sure that all laws are obeyed. These agencies include the state board of pharmacy, the state health department, the drug enforcement agencies, and others.

What the technician does in the pharmacy varies from state to state. As long as the technician is working under the supervision ("within sight and sound" in most states) of the pharmacist, there should be no legal problems. All drug labeling and preparation should be actively and carefully checked by the pharmacist.

American Pharmaceutical Association

2215 Constitution Avenue, NW
Washington, DC 20037-2985
(202) 628-4410 Fax (202) 783-2351
http://www.aphanet.org

The National Professional Society of Pharmacists

CODE OF ETHICS FOR PHARMACISTS

PREAMBLE

Pharmacists are health professionals who assist individuals in making the best use of medications. This Code, prepared and supported by pharmacists, is intended to state publicly the principles that form the fundamental basis of the roles and responsibilities of pharmacists. These principles, based on moral obligations and virtues, are established to guide pharmacists in relationships with patients, health professionals, and society.

I. **A pharmacist respects the covenantal relationship between the patient and pharmacist.**

Considering the patient-pharmacist relationship as a covenant means that a pharmacist has moral obligations in response to the gift of trust received from society. In return for this gift, a pharmacist promises to help individuals achieve optimum benefit from their medications, to be committed to their welfare, and to maintain their trust.

II. **A pharmacist promotes the good of every patient in a caring, compassionate, and confidential manner.**

A pharmacist places concern for the well-being of the patient at the center of professional practice. In doing so, a pharmacist considers needs stated by the patient as well as those defined by health science. A pharmacist is dedicated to protecting the dignity of the patient. With a caring attitude and a compassionate spirit, a pharmacist focuses on serving the patient in a private and confidential manner.

III. **A pharmacist respects the autonomy and dignity of each patient.**

A pharmacist promotes the right of self-determination and recognizes individual self-worth by encouraging patients to participate in decisions about their health. A pharmacist communicates with patients in terms that are understandable. In all cases, a pharmacist respects personal and cultural differences among patients.

IV. **A pharmacist acts with honesty and integrity in professional relationships.**

A pharmacist has a duty to tell the truth and to act with conviction of conscience. A pharmacist avoids discriminatory practices, behavior or work conditions that impair professional judgment, and actions that compromise dedication to the best interests of patients.

V. **A pharmacist maintains professional competence.**

A pharmacist has a duty to maintain knowledge and abilities as new medications, devices, and technologies become available and as health information advances.

VI. **A pharmacist respects the values and abilities of colleagues and other health professionals.**

When appropriate, a pharmacist asks for the consultation of colleagues or other health professionals or refers the patient. A pharmacist acknowledges that colleagues and other health professionals may differ in the beliefs and values they apply to the care of the patient.

FIGURE 7–3 Pharmacy code of ethics *(adopted by the membership of the American Pharmaceutical Association, October 27, 1994) (continues)*

VII.   **A pharmacist serves individual, community, and societal needs.**

The primary obligation of a pharmacist is to individual patients. However, the obligations of a pharmacist may at times extend beyond the individual to the community and society. In these situations, the pharmacist recognizes the responsibilities that accompany these obligations and acts accordingly.

VIII.   **A pharmacist seeks justice in the distribution of health resources.**

When health resources are allocated, a pharmacist is fair and equitable, balancing the needs of patients and society.

FIGURE 7–3 Pharmacy code of ethics *(continued)*

Standards of practice

The pharmacy profession has set up its own rules. These rules, which pharmacists hold each other to follow, are called **standards of practice.** Although these rules are not laws, breaking a standard of practice can be serious. Standards of practice allow pharmacists to apply peer pressure to self-police the profession.

An example of standards of practice is the pharmacy code of ethics (**Figure 7–3**). Following the code of ethics and other standards of practice helps provide control to the drug-use process.

Guidelines

There are also other guidelines, such as site-specific policies. These guide pharmacy personnel on what is required by the employer or the director or manager of the department. Policies are not to be broken, except in unusual situations, such as emergencies or for patient safety reasons as determined by the pharmacist.

Procedures are guidelines on the preferred way to perform a certain function. They often follow a policy statement. Procedures guide how to perform the function to follow the policy. Procedures may be set up by the employer (company, hospital, etc.), department, store, or committee. Unlike policies, procedures are true guidelines. They may sometimes be bent or broken for good reason to serve a higher purpose, such as patient benefit. However, before bending or breaking a procedure, the technician should always check with the pharmacist.

A **job description** is also a guideline. Like policies, these add control to the work process. A job description defines the knowledge (education, skill, and experience), problem solving, and responsibility needed to do a job. It also outlines the boundaries and expectations of a specific job.

A **drug formulary,** used in most hospitals, is also a type of guideline used for control. A drug formulary is a group of medicinal agents selected by the medical staff with the help of the pharmacy. A formulary represents the ideal drugs, or **drugs of choice,** for the patients served by the hospital. The medical staff, when obtaining privileges to practice at the hospital, agree to follow the formulary as much as possible. In this manner, there is some control, by helping avoid less desirable therapeutic agents.

Documents

One of the major methods of helping ensure control in the drug-use process is the use of **control documents.** Control documents come in many forms, such as records, sheets, logs, and checklists. To reduce paperwork, more and more of these documents are being computerized.

TABLE 7–1

Types of Control Documents and Their Purpose

Document Type	Purpose	Example
Purchasing/Inventory	To have an adequate supply of medication that is fresh	Master Emergency Drug Box Sheet
Workload		
Amount	To maintain proper staffing	Orders processed/Day Log
Reminders	To remind what needs to be done	Daily I.V. Proof Cleaning Sheet
What's done/not done	To ensure completeness of a function	Monthly Nursing Unit Inspection Sheet
Accuracy*	To prevent errors in preparation, packaging, and labeling	Master Formula Sheet
Accountability*	To document who did what	Unit-Dose Cartfill Sheet (Figure 7–5)
Variance	To see where standards are not being met	Missing-Dose Log
Performance	To track individual performance of workers	Unit-Dose Cartfill Sheet (Figure 7–5)
Drug tracking controlled substances*	To track the movement of drugs and to prevent loss	Narcotic and Controlled Substance Record
Repackaged and relabeled*	To track lot numbers and expiration dates	Manufacturing Log (Figure 7–4)

*A legal requirement in most states.

Control documents monitor various parts of the drug-use process. **Table 7–1** provides examples of the various types of control documents and their purpose. Documents with the specific purpose of documenting the manufacture, repackaging, or relabeling of drugs are required by law. For protection, it is also a standard practice to document who did what to a manufactured or prepackaged **prescription** or **drug order.** The manufacturing log outlines these activities (**Figure 7–4**). Prescriptions for medication are written by physicians in their office. Drug orders for medication are written on the patient's charts in the hospital. Prescriptions slightly differ from drug orders.

Pharmacists are required by law to ensure the accuracy of all drugs dispensed to a patient. All drug carts are checked by pharmacists and any problems so noted (**Figure 7–5**). They are also responsible for the **controlled substances** (drugs of abuse) ordered, stored, and used at their practice site. The use of other control documents is at the discretion of the pharmacist in charge, but often is the standard of practice.

Initialing

Having technicians' initials on their pharmacy work is very important. For legal reasons, certain procedures in the drug-use process must be initialed by the pharmacist, and oftentimes by the technician. Although the pharmacist is always responsible for what the technician does, it is important that they initial their own work. In this way, they will not get blamed for something they did not do. Each practice site will differ on what needs to be initialed; therefore the technician will need to ask.

DRUG/STRENGTH.DILUENT/VOLUME	LOT #	MANUFACTURER/LOT # EXP. DATE	# ITEMS PREPACKED	TECH	R.PH	EXP. DATE

FIGURE 7–4 The manufacturing drug log documents personnel and activities involved in manufactured or prepackaged prescriptions or drug orders

Monitoring

Perhaps the most important part of the control process is continual monitoring. Monitoring is used by pharmacists and technicians to prevent harm to patients. This is done before the drug leaves the pharmacy.

Pharmacists have at least 5 or 6 years of intense education about drugs, disease, and patient care. When a drug is ordered, their first function is to assess the appropriateness of therapy for the patient. Physicians may not always be correct in what they order, due to a variety of reasons. Pharmacists work cooperatively with physicians and are the check and balance to help protect patients. If the drug is correct, the pharmacist then checks the **dose,** other medication used, and so on. Even if the drug prescribed is safe and effective, the pharmacist will check one more item. Is there an alternative drug that is equally effective and safe, but less expensive?

Pharmacists will also be working to make sure their patients receive the **first dose** of medication quickly and safely. The goal is to achieve ideal drug therapy. If, during the monitoring process, pharmacists spot an error or potential problem, they contact the physician and make the necessary changes or adjustments.

Pharmacists will also be monitoring and checking the work of the technician. Monitoring is for accuracy and speed in getting the medication order or prescription dispensed to the patient.

It is very important for technicians to monitor their own work. The goal is to catch errors before the pharmacist does. In this way errors are reduced and the technician becomes a valuable part of the pharmacy team. When checking work, the **rule of three** applies:

1. Check the drug label when taking it from the shelf.
2. Check the label after counting or removing the drug.
3. Check the label after returning the drug to stock.

Unit _____   Filled by _____

Wing/Team _____   Checked by _____

Date Filled _____   Checked with _____ RPH

No. of drawers filled _____ Adverse Drug RX _____ PT _____

Room No./ Name	Problem	Solution	If Filling Error

FIGURE 7–5 Unit-dose cartfill sheet

Surprisingly, the label may often change in this process. The pharmacist must always check and initial the technician's work.

It is also important to be watchful for errors being created by fellow workers, including technicians and pharmacists. It is the technician's duty to speak up and not let patients be harmed. Check with the supervisor about the company's policy. Each pharmacy differs on how this situation is handled.

What will happen if you, the technician, make a critical error that gets through the system and harms a patient? This is locally determined. Legally the pharmacist is always responsible; however, you may be severely counseled or dismissed. In most situations your employer is legally responsible for your actions and will be maintaining adequate malpractice insurance to protect you financially in lawsuits. However, you should always check this out with your employer before starting your job.

Pharmacist and technician monitoring happens throughout the drug-use process. This helps prevent errors from occurring that may harm the patient. Quality assurance programs monitor what took place versus what should have taken place. A **quality standard** is set up, such as "we will have 'first doses' of medication available for the nurse to **administer** (give the drug) within 30 minutes of receiving the order." Added to this is a **compliance rate,** such as 95 percent, which means that the standard will be met 95 of 100 times measured. Then every so often, (e.g., once a month), a sample of orders is measured to see how often the standard is met. If the standard is not met, the situation is investigated to see why, and a change is made to correct the situation.

A pharmacy service may have several quality standards and measurement systems in place to check the quality of its service. In general, ideal standards are those that directly measure the outcome of pharmacy service on patients. Another example of a quality standard is "no medication, dispensed in error, will reach the patient."

Enforcement

Another method of control in the drug-use process is **enforcement.** Enforcement in following policies and procedures is usually accomplished through supervisory monitoring. Pharmacy workers who do not follow policies or procedures may need to be counseled by the supervisor. The results may be a verbal warning, a written warning, suspension (with or without pay), or termination. Suspensions and terminations usually involve serious or repeated violations of important policies or procedures.

Another method of achieving control of the drug-use process through enforcement are **employee performance evaluations.** Routinely, usually once a year, the supervisor meets with the employee and evaluates the employee's performance. How well an employee has worked is compared with what is expected. The expected is usually explained in an **action plan** and/or job description. Evaluations provide feedback to employees on how they are doing and how they can improve. This feedback provides added control and continuous improvement to the drug-use process.

Control is critical in ensuring that everything goes right in the drug-use process. Without it patients can be seriously harmed from the drugs. Various processes are in place to work together to ensure that drug-use control is working. Technicians, working under the direct supervision of the pharmacist, are an important part of controlling the drug-use process.

Emerging Practice Patterns

As the pharmaceutical care model develops into its full potential, the roles of the pharmacist and the technician will change dramatically. The pharmacist, based on increased education and training, will be used more directly in patient care. The physician will rely much more on the pharmacist. The pharmacist will advise on the preferred medication to use and the preferred way to monitor its effects. The pharmacist will become responsible to the patient for therapeutic outcome or failure. To do this, the pharmacist will more and more practice outside the pharmacy, closer to physicians, nurses, and patients. The patient will rely more on the pharmacist for advice on drugs and protection from medication misadventures.

The pharmacist will need increased education to move into the more clinical, patient-oriented role. Such education is provided through the doctor of pharmacy degree (Pharm.D.), the recognized clinical practice degree in pharmacy. After graduation additional training may also be needed, which is often obtained through a 1- or 2-year residency training program. Pharmacy residents learn to provide pharmaceutical care and to effectively communicate and interact with physicians and nurses.

Pharmacists will also need to be less tied to the drug distribution system to apply their clinical skills. How to do this without adding significant expense to the health care system is critical. In doing so, the profession will use more automation. Computers will be used extensively to track the medications prescribed and when they are needed. Furthermore these computers will be connected to automated dispensing machines. Such machines will package, correctly label, and bar-code custom-made doses of medication for specific patients.

In hospitals each patient's I.V. solution and medication drawer will be prepared correctly every time. This will be done by robots, robotic arms, or devices that are directed by computers and guided by bar coding. Pharmacists will no longer be tied to the distribution system. Very little checking will be needed, only occasional monitoring.

Nurses, when giving patient's medication, will use portable bar code readers. They will scan their name badge and the patient's wristband with the bar code reader. This will tell the computer who is doing what to whom. (The "what" is what drug is being given.) The nurse will scan the bar coding of the medication dose with the portable bar code reader. Information will travel via microwaves to a computer receiver in the patient's room. The computer will turn on a green light on the bar code reader if the medication is correct. The nurse will push a button on the bar code reader to indicate that the medication has been given. The computer will automatically record the medication as given and charge for it.

Such a system is close at hand. It will significantly liberate the pharmacist from the drug distribution system. Some pharmacists will still be needed to oversee the automated process, but these pharmacists will have additional specialized training in automation and drug safety.

What about the role of technicians in this future picture? Technicians will exist, although in less numbers. They will be better trained and do many of the functions now performed by pharmacists. The pharmacy technician of the future will do higher-level functions, run automated drug distribution and preparation equipment, and interact with computers. Thus, the technician will need some formal education and certification.

Summary

A career in pharmacy is a time-honored profession. Its purpose is to discover, prepare, dispense, and provide information about medicine, and to safeguard the public from medicinal errors. It also teaches students in the art and science of pharmacy.

The mission of pharmacy practice is to help people make the best use of medication. The pharmaceutical care model integrates the traditional and clinical parts of pharmacy practice.

The foundation of pharmaceutical care is control of the drug-use process. Various processes work together to control that process, which protects patients from drug misadventures. Pharmacists are sanctioned by society to help protect patients from the harmful effects of drugs. Pharmacy technicians, working under the direct control of the pharmacist, help the pharmacist control the drug-use process.

In the future, pharmacists will be active in assisting physicians and patients use medication wisely. Automation and better trained pharmacy technicians will help liberate the pharmacist for this more clinical role.

ASSESSMENT

Multiple Choice Questions

1. The societal purpose of pharmacy practice is to
   a. dispense medication
   b. provide drug information
   c. help people make the best use of medication
   d. prepare drugs

2. The drug-use process is
   a. when people abuse drugs
   b. methods used to prepare drugs
   c. steps involved in moving a drug from identification of need to use
   d. how drugs are administered

3. What is drug-use control?
   a. any method used to reduce harm from medication
   b. federal drug enforcement regulations
   c. a method to accurately measure who uses drugs
   d. FDA manufacturing rules

4. Why is control needed in the drug-use process?
   a. to protect patients from harm
   b. to satisfy FDA requirements
   c. to keep drugs from being illegally diverted
   d. to satisfy quality assurance requirements

5. Which of the following is not a drug-use control method?
   a. formulary
   b. laws, rules, and regulations
   c. prescriptions
   d. policies and procedures

6. What is a medication misadventure?
   a. errors
   b. adverse reactions
   c. side effects
   d. all of the above

7. What major duty do pharmacists perform for society?
   a. prepare medication
   b. protect patients from medication harm
   c. supply drugs
   d. keep drugs from being illegally diverted

8. Pharmacy technicians will legally perform their duties as long as they
   a. check everything they do
   b. read all labels three times
   c. have all labels and products checked by the pharmacist
   d. are certified

9. A major change that will soon dramatically change the pharmacy practice is
   a. the use of automation, such as robots
   b. more direct patient contact by the pharmacist
   c. a higher level of attention to drug safety, effectiveness, and cost
   d. all of the above

10. How will the change(s) in question 9 affect technicians?
    a. They will be more involved in running machines.
    b. They will be doing higher-level functions.
    c. They will need more education.
    d. all of the above

Bibliography

ASHP guidelines on a standardized method of pharmaceutical care. (1996). *American Journal of Health System Pharmacists, 54,* 1713–1716.

Brodie, D.C. (1967). Drug-use control: Keystone to pharmaceutical service. *Drug Intelligence and Clinical Pharmacy, 1,* 63–65.

Cowen, D.L., & Helfand, W.H. (1990). *Pharmacy: An illustrated history.* New York: Harry A. Abrams, Inc.

Hepler, C.D. (1985). Pharmacy as a clinical profession. *American Journal of Hospital Pharmacists, 42,* 1298–1306.

Hooks, M.A., & Maddox, R.R. (1998). Implementation of pharmaceutical care—A process for professional transformation. *Southern Journal of Health System Pharmacists, 3,* 5–12.

Manasse, H.R. (1989). Medication use in an imperfect world: Drug misadventuring as an issue of public policy, part 1. *American Journal of Hospital Pharmacists, 46,* 929–944.

Manasse, H.R. (1989). Medication use in an imperfect world: Drug misadventuring as an issue of public policy, part 2. *American Journal of Hospital Pharmacists, 46,* 1141–1152.

Drug Information Service

COMPETENCIES

After completion and review of this chapter, the student should be able to

1. Define *pharmaceutical care* and relate it to drug information.
2. List five purposes of a drug information center.
3. Describe the responsibilities of a drug information specialist.
4. List 20 items of knowledge that can be identified for a particular drug.
5. Discuss the ASHP guidelines related to medication information activities.
6. Describe the major duties of a pharmacy technician in drug information services.

Introduction

The traditional role of the hospital pharmacist has been closely associated with drug compounding and dispensing services. Over the past several years, this phase of practice has been changing with the additional mission of providing pharmaceutical care. **Pharmaceutical care** is the direct, responsible provision of medication-related care for the purpose of achieving definite outcomes that improve a patient's quality of life.

The pharmacist as a provider of drug information, in the generic sense, is nothing new. It is probably safe to say that pharmacists have been dispensing information and drugs as part of their responsibilities since the beginning of the profession. Traditionally, this information has been confined to the physical or chemical properties, dosages, sources, formulations, and so on. What is new is the development of the concept of the pharmacist as a provider of clinically useful drug information that can be applied to the therapeutic management of patients. The evolution of this concept resulted in the formation of organized, centralized drug information services. Just as the efficient delivery of health care to increasing patient populations has led to the centralization of these services, the dissemination of drug information by pharmacists has had to be organized in a similar manner. In this fashion, the greatest possible utility of drug information centers is achieved.

Today we are faced with a highly complex society. Despite our technological achievements, we are still plagued with disease, poverty, and insufficient education. These are problems that have been part of the human condition for centuries, but the time has come when we should begin to apply our knowledge to provide people with a more efficient system of health care. One way to accomplish this goal is through the formation of drug information services.

Drug Information Service

The purposes of a drug information service are

1. to deal with problems encountered with all modes of drug therapy;
2. to develop optimal therapeutic regimens;
3. to keep abreast of new medical discoveries;
4. to inform all health care personnel of these discoveries; and
5. to answer any other questions that may arise in regard to any other aspects of medicine and drug therapy.

Reading this brief synopsis one may ask, "Is this not one of the duties of a physician, to keep informed about new medical discoveries?" The answer to the question is, of course, yes. One must keep in mind, however, that in the United States, there is one physician for approximately every 600 people, and that every month there are hundreds of new medical findings that are published in thousands of books, journals, and newsletters, which makes it virtually impossible for every physician to be completely up-to-date on all the new literature. A major function of a drug information service is to obtain and evaluate information from the literature on the important new discoveries and to make this information known to the health care professionals that the center serves.

Another important service that such a center can provide is in the field of drug interactions. Many patients are on multidrug therapies, and a drug information service can provide the physician with all pertinent information about interactions and possible side effects that may be encountered. Thus, the physician saves the time otherwise needed for individual research of these problems.

The system of medical care that results when drug information services are utilized allows for much greater efficiency of professional functions by pharmacists, and provides up-to-date information to health care professionals and better patient care.

Drug Information

The term *drug information* is fast becoming a cliché, but what is it exactly? The term, as used in "drug information center," "drug information service," or "drug information specialist," should not be construed to mean simply basic factual information that can be gleaned from the literature. Rather, it should imply the ability to communicate to the practitioner the clinically relevant information that can be used to facilitate the practice of rational therapeutics that results in positive patient outcomes. However, one should not be deceived by this seemingly simple definition. The complexity of the drug literature creates enormous problems for the pharmacist in filling this need. Some of the problems in providing drug information services deal essentially with how to best communicate existing information.

The activities of a drug information service are characterized as being primarily communicative in nature. These communication activities are essentially divided into three broad categories—the collection, evaluation, and dissemination of drug information. The net result of these activities should be improved patient care through more rational drug therapy as influenced by the efforts of the drug information service.

Definition of Drug Information

A drug information service exists as a source of information. Drug information includes, but is not necessarily limited to, such particular items of knowledge as chemical names, structures and properties, identification, diagnostic or therapeutic indications, mechanisms of action, recommended doses and dosage schedules, administration, absorption, metabolism, detoxification, excretion, side effects, adverse reactions, contraindications, interactions, chemical and therapeutic incompatibilities, costs, advantages, signs and symptoms, treatment of toxicities, clinical efficacy, comparative data, clinical data, drug use data, and any other information useful in the diagnosis and treatment of patients with drugs. Drug information does not include advertising material, drug detailing, clinical impressions, "testimonial" type reporting, inventory control, or purchasing information.

Drug Information Specialist

The objective of a drug information service is to exist as a resource for information on all aspects of drugs and drug therapy for health professionals. Its primary purpose is to provide clinically relevant drug information in response to patient-specific and general requests from health care practitioners in hospitals, skilled care facilities, and the community at large. The goal of this effort is to promote the effective and safe use of drugs in the diagnosis and treatment of disease through selection, evaluation, and dissemination of the drug literature.

Drug information services include, but are not limited to, gathering, reviewing, evaluating, organizing, summarizing, and distributing information on drugs by various methods to other health care providers and health care consumers. The pharmacist responsible for the drug information service is the drug information specialist, and this specialty can be divided into (1) the drug literature specialist, and (2) the clinical drug communication specialist.

The drug literature specialist (drug documentation specialist) has the principal functions of accumulating, organizing, and expediting access to the documents that constitute the published record of clinical drug research. This specialist provides on-demand literature searches, bibliographic compilations, computer-processed information retrieval services, and other medical librarian functions.

The drug information specialist (clinical drug communication specialist) provides close and continuing support to the clinician, increasing the latter's efficiency and effectiveness in patient care by supplying selected literature evidence in justification of specific drug usage practices. This specialist must be able to discriminate among the literature sources used to convey specific concepts or conclusions concerning a particular drug or patient-specific problem. Because of the expertise in the critical analysis of the current drug literature, this pharmacist is able to direct the clinician to the minimum amount of material necessary to reach an intelligent, informed, independent conclusion concerning a particular question relating to drug therapy.

The drug information specialist has at his or her disposal books, journals, computer data bases, retrieval systems, and literature files from which to search in depth for information not readily available. This person then evaluates and interprets the literature, from which comes a comprehensive answer to the inquirer. This last statement, "evaluates and interprets the literature," differentiates the drug information pharmacist from a medical librarian who also has access to books, journals, and files.

The drug information service can be considered a specialized "library" with emphasis placed mainly on the pharmacological properties of drugs and drug therapy.

It is easy to see how the specialty of clinical pharmacy relates to the drug information service. One definition of the clinical practice of pharmacy is the communication of drug information which relates to the promotion of safe and rational drug therapy that achieves positive patient outcomes. The drug information service pharmacist is a specialist acting as a fact-finding clearinghouse, capable of gathering and analyzing drug data, and communicating in-depth drug information when requested. When defining the clinical pharmacy specialist, we refer to a person whose main responsibility in the clinical area is to monitor the drug therapy of particular patients. Therefore, both pharmacists are specialists in drugs—one in the centralized area and the other in the clinical environment. Without the benefit of a central drug information service, clinical pharmacists would have to provide their own mechanism for retrieval and dissemination. It is too cumbersome and time consuming for clinical pharmacists to conduct in-depth literature searches, since it is a full-time job for them to monitor patients receiving drugs on the nursing units. This information support should be provided by the centralized drug information service.

The physician, as one of the primary users of drug information, should have at his or her disposal a good source of information within the hospital setting. The drug information pharmacist has the responsibility of, and the time to devote to, researching the answers to hundreds of questions in reference to patient care, medical education, and drug research activities. The information cycle can be considered to include the following:

1. **Investigation** by research, experimentation, and clinical and preclinical drug studies
2. **Publication** in representative journals of medicine, nursing, and pharmacy
3. **Identification and evaluation** of scientific papers and articles
4. **Recording** of papers for filing, microfilming, dating, and numbering
5. **Organization** for filing systems and classifying (National Library of Medicine classification)
6. **Storage** for manual and computerized filing systems
7. **Recall/retrieval** of requested information
8. **Conversion into more usable forms** from microfilm or abstracts
9. **Synthesis**-evaluation, interpretation, and compilation
10. **Dissemination** in the form of newsletters, memos, and correspondence
11. **Interpretation** by the drug information pharmacist
12. **Utilization** by the practitioner

The drug information specialist should be able to evaluate, critically select, and utilize the drug literature from his or her knowledge of library facilities and the drug literature. Through written communications (newsletters, memorandums, correspondence, publication of papers, agendas and supportive information for the Pharmacy and Therapeutics Committee, and drug utilization studies) significant contributions can be made to all the health care professions through the promotion and monitoring of proper drug utilization. As a specialist in drug therapy, he or she should be an integral component in the provision of pharmaceutical care and of the education program of pharmacy practitioners. His or her services should be offered to other hospitals, community pharmacies, skilled care facilities, and the community in general.

In 1996, the American Society of Health System Pharmacists (ASHP) developed guidelines for the provision of medication information by pharmacists. ASHP listed the following medication information activities that should be provided depending on the particular practice setting and need. These activities should all be functions of the drug information service.

1. Providing medication information to patients and families, health care professionals, and other personnel
2. Establishing and maintaining a formulary based on scientific evidence of efficacy and safety, cost, and patient factors
3. Developing and participating in efforts to prevent medication misadventuring, including adverse drug event and medication error reporting and analysis programs
4. Developing methods of changing patient and provider behaviors to support optimal medication use
5. Publishing newsletters to educate patients, families, and health care professionals on medication use
6. Educating providers about medication-related policies and procedures
7. Coordinating programs to support population-based medication practices (e.g., development of medication-use evaluation criteria and pharmacotherapeutic guidelines)
8. Coordinating investigational drug services
9. Providing continuing education services to the health care professional staff
10. Educating pharmacy students and residents

ASHP guidelines continue to state that the pharmacist must not only accumulate and organize the literature, but also objectively evaluate and apply the information from the literature to a particular patient or situation. To do this properly, a systematic method for responding to the medication information needs must be followed. The systematic method is outlined as follows:

1. To probe for information and develop a response with the appropriate perspective, consider the education and professional or experiential background of the requester.
2. Identify needs by asking probing questions of the patient, family members, or health care professional or by examining the medical record to identify the true question. This helps in optimizing the search process and assessing the urgency for a response.
3. Classify requests as patient-specific or not and by type of question (e.g., product availability, adverse drug event, compatibility, compounding/formulation, dosage/administration, drug interaction, identification, pharmacokinetics, therapeutic use/efficacy, safety in pregnancy and nursing, toxicity and poisoning) to aid in assessing the situation and selecting resources. Refer to **Table 8–1** for a guide to locating reference sources.
4. Obtain more complete background information, including patient data, if applicable, to individualize the response to meet the patient's, family's, or health care professional's needs.
5. Perform a systematic search of the literature by making appropriate selections from the primary, secondary, and tertiary literature and other types of resources as necessary.
6. Evaluate, interpret, and combine information from the several sources. Other information needs should be anticipated as a result of the information provided.
7. Provide a response by written or oral consultation, or both, as needed by the requester and appropriate to the situation. The information, its urgency, and its purpose may influence the method of response.
8. Perform a follow-up assessment to determine the utility of the information provided and outcomes for the patient (patient-specific request) or changes in medication-use practices and behaviors.
9. Document the request, information sources, response, and follow-up as appropriate for the request and the practice setting.

TABLE 8-1
Guide to Locating the Reference Source of Choice

The following chart can be used as a guide to locating the best reference sources to answer a specific question. At the left are the "nature of request" categories. The numbers across the top refer to the texts listed at the bottom of the chart. The best references to answer each question are rated from 1 to 5; the answers to some questions, it will be noted, can be found in several books.

Reference	1	2	3	4	5	6	7	8	9	10	11	12	13	14	15	16	17	18	19	20
Adverse reactions		1			4		3				3			2	5	4		5		
Availability	1	4	1		1			2			5				2	3				5
Compatibility/stability		2			5				1	3					5		1	4		
Dosage		1			3		4	5	5		4		3		2	2		3		
Drug interactions		2			3	1	5	4							5	3		4		
Identification	1		5	5	1				3		3	4			4	2				
Pharmacology		1			3		2	4			4					4	5	5	5	
Side effects		1			4			5			3			2	5	4		5		
Therapeutic use		1			3		3	5	4		2		3		5	2		4	5	
Toxicology		2		1	4		3				3			5		4		4		

1 American Drug Index	**8** Handbook of Clinical Drug Data	**17** Remington's Pharmaceutical Series
2 ASHP Formulary Service	**9** Handbook of Nonprescription Drugs	**18** U.S.P., D.I., Vol. I: Drug Information for the Health Care Professional
3 Blue Book/Red Book	**10** Handbook on Injectable Drugs	
4 Clinical Toxicology of Commercial Products	**11** Martindale's Extra Pharmacopeia	**19** U.S.P., D.I., Vol. II: Advice for the Patient—Drug Information in Lay Language
5 Drug Facts and Comparisons	**12** Merck Index	
6 Evaluation of Drug Interactions	**13** Merck Manual	**20** U.S.P., D.I., Vol. III: Approved Drug Products and Legal Requirements
7 Goodman and Gillman's Pharmacologic Basis of Therapeutics	**14** Meylen's Side Effects of Drugs	
	15 Monthly Prescribing Reference	
	16 Physician's Desk Reference	

Role of the Pharmacy Technician in the Drug Information Service

The role of a technically trained person in the drug information service can be rewarding intellectually and personally for the individual and an asset to the drug information pharmacist. The technician can be of great assistance in the cataloging, filing, clerical retrieving, electric copying, collating, and organizing of the information selected by the pharmacist.

Specifically, the technician's major duties in the drug information service include the following tasks:

1. To become familiar with the textbooks, handbooks, abstracting services, computer databases, journals, catalogs, and filing systems and their locations in the drug information center
2. To catalog books, journals, and articles and to be able to retrieve pertinent drug information upon direction of the drug information pharmacist

3. To maintain accurate statistics on the types and numbers of questions received, references used, and so on
4. To maintain up-to-date filing systems for microfilm, abstracts, newsletters, correspondence, and so on
5. To assist in collation of drug usage data, drug utilization studies, adverse reaction reporting systems, and so on
6. To systematically record telephone requests for drug information
7. To assist the drug information pharmacist in any other technical or professional activities as necessary

An overview of the drug information technician's and the pharmacist's roles is provided in **Table 8–2.**

Keep in mind that drug information need not be confined to the hospital setting. However, most of the literature dealing with the subject places the service in this setting. Other areas where drug information center systems may be utilized include

1. pharmaceutical companies
2. governmental agencies
3. schools
4. community pharmacies
5. poison control centers

The properly trained technician should be able to function in any of these settings.

Other Technical Responsibilities

The technician assigned to a drug information service must be a responsible, mature, and motivated individual. As such, the technician must be able to participate in many of the service's functions. Some other areas of responsibility may include the following:

1. Pharmacy and Therapeutics Committee functions
   a. provide literature searches for drug evaluations
   b. maintain committee files and reference
2. Drug information newsletters
   a. maintain, file, and distribute newsletters
   b. maintain up-to-date mailing lists
3. Teaching functions
   a. maintain and coordinate schedules
   b. collect data
   c. maintain displays
4. Literature searches
   a. be familiar with various library indexes and bibliographies
   b. maintain filing systems
5. Facilities
   a. maintain and store references and equipment
6. Records
   a. maintain a filing system
   b. compile statistics from questions researched to serve as further reference

The responsibilities and assignments of the technician will be as diverse as the functions of the center itself. Without the aid of such a person the drug information service would not be able to function properly.

TABLE 8–2   **Comparison of Roles in the Drug Information Service**

Role Functions	Technician Assignment	Pharmacist Responsibility
Answering questions		X
1. Answer telephone	X	X
2. Document question	X	X
3. Categorize question	X	X
4. Refine question	X	X
5. Retrieve data	X	X
6. Evaluate and interpret question and data retrieval		X
7. Maintain statistics	X	
Provide drug information		X
1. Drug information newsletters		X
a. for physicians		X
b. for patients		X
c. for nurses		X
d. for pharmacists		X
e. others		X
2. Lectures		X
a. for professionals		X
b. for the community		X
3. Displays	X	X
Maintain and keep up-to-data		
1. Literature resources	X	X
2. Statistics	X	
3. Determine literature resources	X	
4. Maintain files	X	
a. abstract services		
b. adverse reaction reports	X	
c. current drug therapy and disease states	X	
d. microfilm	X	
e. question data	X	
f. AHFS files	X	
g. IND files	X	
h. committee reports	X	
i. reference catalogs	X	
j. poison files	X	
Pharmacy Therapeutics Committee	X	X
1. Collate data	X	X
2. Maintain statistics and files	X	
3. Prepare clinical data on products considered for formulary		X

(Continues)

TABLE 8–2   **Comparison of Roles in the Drug Information Service** (Continued)

Role Functions	Technician Assignment	Pharmacist Responsibility
Adverse drug reactions	X	X
1. Collect adverse drug reaction data	X	X
2. Document adverse drug reactions		X
3. Collate statistics	X	X
In-service education		
1. Establish resource data		X
2. Collect needed data	X	
3. Prepare and present material for		X
a. medical interns and residents		X
b. nurses		X
c. pharmacists		X
d. patients		X
e. other health professionals		X
Drug utilization studies	X	X
1. Determine study		X
2. prepare work sheet and initiate study		X
3. Evaluate results		X
4. Collate data and statistics	X	
Investigational drugs	X	X
1. Initiate control procedures		X
2. Maintain protocol files	X	X
3. Establish patient assignment "blind" studies		X
4. Participate in evaluation of drug results		X
Medical rounds		X
1. Attend and participate		X
2. Interview medical service representatives		X
3. Teaching functions		
a. maintain and coordinate schedules	X	X
b. collect data	X	X
4. Literature searches		
a. be familiar with various library indexes and bibliographies	X	X
b. maintain filing systems	X	
5. Facilities		
a. maintain and store references and equipment	X	
6. Records		
a. maintain a filing system	X	
b. complete statistics from questions researched to serve as further reference	X	X

Requests for Information

The major service provided by all drug information services is providing immediate drug information on request. This information may be patient-specific or drug-oriented information. Patient-specific information refers to inquiries ranging from dosage instructions to outlining specific therapeutic regimens. Drug-oriented information includes dosage forms and availability, product identification, and product compatibility.

The responsibility of answering drug information questions from the drug information center lies with the pharmacist. The dispensing of drug information, like the dispensing of drugs, is a professional responsibility that may not be delegated by the pharmacist to another individual. Therefore, technical personnel are responsible for assisting the pharmacist in the numerous auxiliary functions such as typing, filing, and cataloging that are essential services.

Documentation

When a question is received in the drug information center, it must be properly documented in writing. Most questions will be received via telephone, so a proper procedure for answering the telephone should be established.

Requests should be fully documented with the name and location of the inquirer. It is imperative that all drug information center personnel be polite, pleasant, courteous, and thorough in obtaining and documenting inquiries.

There are numerous variations of drug information center documentation forms. Each center will devise one to suit its needs. The request for information form is a mechanism for the collection of data to be used to keep statistics and evaluate and review the activities of the drug information center. The form must be utilized every time a request for information is received. In general, a single form should be used for a single question. Multipart questions should be broken down into their component parts and each question recorded separately. One example of a request for information form is shown in **Figure 8–1.**

After proper documentation of the form, it is then held for inclusion in the monthly statistics, filed and indexed, and put into a notebook, filing cabinet, or computer database.

Summary

Drug information is an essential aspect of the present-day practice of pharmacy. The pharmacist is held accountable for providing accurate knowledge as well as for providing the correct drug and dosage. The knowledgeable and trained technicians in the specialty of drug information can contribute significantly to the drug information service and assist the pharmacist in many ways.

We live in the information age supported by sophisticated computer capabilities. Effective drug therapy is based on timely and accurate drug knowledge and information.

Request for Information

Name _____   Date & Time _____

Address _____   Fax _____

Telephone _____   Beeper _____

e-mail _____

Requestor Category

_____ M.D.   _____ Patient

_____ R.N.   _____ Student

_____ R.Ph.   _____ Other

Classification of Request

_____ Adverse drug reaction   _____ Identification

_____ Availability   _____ Pharmacology

_____ Compatibility/stability   _____ Side effects

_____ Dosage   _____ Therapeutic use

_____ Drug interaction   _____ Toxicology

_____ Other _____

Request for Information

_____

_____

_____

Request received by _____

Response

_____

_____

_____

Response given by _____ (telephone, fax, etc.)   Date & time _____

Answered by _____

Outcome (if known)

_____

_____

QA

Response verified by _____ or _____

Comments _____

(Use reverse side of form for notes, patient data, and reference documentation.)

FIGURE 8–1 Drug information request form

ASSESSMENT

Multiple Choice Questions

1. The role of the pharmacist is to provide
   a. medications to ensure rational drug therapy
   b. accurate, up-to-date, and appropriate drug information
   c. filled prescriptions as quickly as possible
   d. a and b
   e. a, b, and c

2. Drug information is a service provided to
   a. physicians
   b. nurses
   c. patients
   d. a and b
   e. a, b, and c

3. Pharmacy technicians are responsible for all except
   a. cataloging drug information
   b. directly answering physicians' questions
   c. maintaining accurate statistics for the questions asked and the references used
   d. collating drug usage data
   e. all of the above

4. The best reference for adverse effects of drugs is
   a. American Society of Health System Pharmacists Formulary Service
   b. Facts and Comparisons
   c. Merck Manual
   d. Merck Index
   e. Drugs of Choice

5. The best reference to identify a drug is
   a. Pharm Index
   b. American Drug Index
   c. FDA clinical abstracts
   d. AMA drug evaluations

6. The collection of adverse drug reaction data is a function of the
   a. pharmacist
   b. technician
   c. both a and b

7. Areas where drug information center systems may be utilized include
   a. pharmaceutical firms
   b. government agencies
   c. medical and pharmacy schools
   d. poison control centers
   e. all of the above

8. Technicians may answer drug information questions if
   a. the pharmacist is not available
   b. the question is uncomplicated
   c. the technician is not sure of the answer
   d. none of the above
   e. all of the above

9. A technician assigned to a drug information service must be
   a. mature and responsible
   b. motivated to give service
   c. able to provide literature searches
   d. able to maintain filing system
   e. all of the above

10. A Drug Information Request form is
    a. documented and completed by the pharmacist
    b. submitted to and filled out by the physician who makes a request for drug information
    c. completed and verified by the pharmacy technician specialist

Bibliography

American drug index. (1999). St. Louis, MO: Facts and Comparisons.

American Society of Health System Pharmacists. (1996). ASHP guidelines on the provision of medication information by pharmacists. *Am J Health Sys Pharm, 53,* 1843–1845.

ASHP formulary service. (1998). Bethesda, MD: American Society of Health Systems Pharmacists.

Baker, D.E., Smith, G., & Abate, M.A. (1994). Selected topics in drug information access and practice: An update. *Ann Pharmacother, 28,* 1389–1394.

Blue book/red book. (1996). Montvale, NJ: Medical Economics.

Clinical toxicology of commercial products. (1984). Baltimore: William & Wilkins.

Drug facts and comparisons. (1998). St. Louis, MO: Facts and Comparisons.

Evaluation of drug interactions. (1991). St. Louis, MO: Professional Drug Systems Publishing Co.

Goodman and Gilman's pharmacologic basis of therapeutics. (1996). New York: McGraw-Hill.

Handbook of clinical drug data. (1993). Hamilton, IL: Drug Intelligence Publications, Inc.

Handbook of nonprescription drugs. (1990). Washington, DC: American Pharmaceutical Association.

Handbook of injectable drugs. (1996). Bethesda, MD: American Society of Health System Pharmacists, Inc.

Martindale's extra pharmacopeia. (1998). Englewood, CO: Royal Pharmaceutical Society of Great Britain.

Merck index. (1983). Rahway, NJ: Merck & Co., Inc.

Merck manual. (1992). Rathway, NJ: Merck & Co., Inc.

Meylen's side effects. (1975). Amsterdam: Excerpta Medica.

Monthly prescribing reference. (1998). New York: Prescribing Reference, Inc.

Physician's desk reference (PDR). (1998). Montvale, NJ: Medical Economics Co.

Remington's pharmaceutical series. (1980). Easton, PA: Mack Publishing Co.

Troutman, W.G. (1994). Consensus-derived objectives for drug information education. *Drug Inf J, 28,* 791–796.

U.S.P., D.I., Vol. I: Drug information for the health care professional. (1997). Rockville, MD: U.S. Pharmacopeial Convention, Inc.

U.S.P., D.I., Vol. II: Advice for the patient—Drug information in lay language. (1997). Rockville, MD: U.S. Pharmacopeial Convention, Inc.

U.S.P., D.I., Vol. III: Approved drug products and legal requirements. (1997). Rockville, MD: U.S. Pharmacopeial Convention, Inc.

Watanabe, A.S., & Conner, C.S. (1978). *Principles of drug information services.* Bethesda, MD: Drug Intelligence Publications.

CHAPTER 9

Organizations in Pharmacy

COMPETENCIES

Upon completion and review of this chapter, the student should be able to

1. Identify the major groups in pharmacy that have specialized associations.

2. Describe the two major issues that have brought about the formation of national pharmacy organizations.

3. Explain the historical aspects and identify the first college of pharmacy founded in the United States.

4. Discuss the early problems associated with the issue of drug quality in this country.

5. Match the acronyms to the full names of the various pharmacy associations.

Introduction

One of the characteristics of a profession is the organization of the membership into professional associations. Associations act through the collective voice of the members to set standards of practice and conduct for the profession. If the quantity rather than the quality of associations were an indicator of professionalism, pharmacy would certainly be near the top of the list. One of pharmacy's strengths—its diversity of practice environments and opportunities—is also one of its weaknesses. Each group of practitioners formed national associations (and numerous state and local associations) to further their professional objectives. Independent owner pharmacists, hospital pharmacists, long-term care pharmacists, academic pharmacists, and many other groups have formed into associations, each with its own distinctive name and set of initials or acronym (**Table 9–1**).

The goal of this chapter is to familiarize the reader with pharmacy associations and the important role they play in the profession in the United States. Finally, the professional journals that function as the voice of the various associations will be listed.

Historical Development

Two major issues caused the formation of the first local and national pharmacy associations in the United States: the development of educational standards for practice, and the quality of drugs available to the pharmacist for use in preparing prescriptions.

TABLE 9–1

Association Abbreviations

AACP	American Association of Colleges of Pharmacy
AAPS	American Association of Pharmaceutical Scientists
AAPT	American Association of Pharmacy Technicians
ACA	American College of Apothecaries
ACCP	American College of Clinical Pharmacy
ACPE	American Council on Pharmaceutical Education
APhA	American Pharmaceutical Association
ASCP	American Society of Consultant Pharmacists
ASHP	American Society of Health System Pharmacists
NABP	National Association of Boards of Pharmacy
NACDS	National Association of Chain Drug Stores
NAPM	National Association of Pharmaceutical Manufacturers
NCPA	National Community Pharmacists Association
NPA	National Pharmaceutical Association
NWDA	National Wholesale Druggists Association
PA	Proprietary Association
PRMA	Pharmaceutical Research Manufacturers Association
PTCB	Pharmacy Technician Certification Board

The first issue—education—has continued to be a primary concern of all pharmacy associations, since it affects both future and current practitioners. The formation of the Philadelphia College of Pharmacy in 1821, the first formal educational program in pharmacy, was one result of the organization of the first professional association of pharmacy. Additionally, the Philadelphia College of Pharmacy inspected drugs for quality and acted to arbitrate disputes between members of the college. Following the lead of Philadelphia pharmacists, other associations or colleges of pharmacy were formed in Boston, New York, Baltimore, Cincinnati, and St. Louis. Formal educational programs were not provided in the early years by these other "colleges," but eventually each evolved into a true college of pharmacy, providing a regular curriculum leading to education of pharmacy practitioners.

The issue of drug quality was an important concern to the early practitioners of pharmacy and medicine in the United States, because the drugs available to the physicians and pharmacists of the nineteenth and early twentieth centuries were mostly of natural origin. These animal and vegetable preparations were often imported into the United States. There was no U.S. pharmaceutical industry. The pharmacist would utilize these crude drugs to prepare the medications prescribed by the physician. Because these animal and vegetable products were so costly, it was not uncommon for drug merchants to adulterate (dilute) the desired material with worthless plant or animal by-products. The early pharmacy associations provided inspection committees to examine these imported materials. They also lobbied vigorously for governmental inspection at the major ports of entry. It was not until 1906, with the passage of the Food and Drug Act, that the federal government became involved with ensuring drug quality and purity.

Drug production and drug quality are still a major concern of pharmacy professional associations because of the many sources of drug products now available. The Drug Product Reporting Program, a mechanism by which the pharmacist can communicate drug-product quality problems to the Federal Food and Drug Administration, is cosponsored or endorsed by many of the major pharmacy associations and is promoted by many colleges of pharmacy through use in various courses in their curricula.

Organizations or associations are a way of life for Americans. There are approximately 23,000 national associations in the United States. Associations have become an industry and this industry spends about $48 billion per year. The American Society of Association Executives is the national association representing 9000 associations.

Although there are many organizations in pharmacy, some are of greater importance to the pharmacy technician. These include the ASHP, formed in 1942, which now has almost 30,000 members. Housed in its new quarters in suburban Washington, it has an annual budget of $28 million. ASHP is a major publishing house and a major provider of educational programming.

The American Pharmaceutical Association (APhA) is 146 years old and today has a membership of almost 50,000. APhA provides continuing education programs for pharmacists and technicians. APhA has been the birthplace for many pharmacy associations.

The training and recognition of pharmacy technicians in the United States has been a slowly evolving process which began in the mid-1960s. In this country, however, pharmacists over the years have engaged assistance to carry out ancillary tasks to expedite the preparation and dispensing of medication. European pharmacies, on the other hand, have a history of long-established and recognized pharmacy technician education programs. The first textbook specific to pharmacy technician education was published by Mosby Publishers in 1968 and authored by Durgin and Hanan. Formal technician training programs were established in that same era by Mercy Medical Centre in Long Island, New York, and in the Rhode Island Hospital in that state. Throughout the country, formal and informal programs were emerging to better train technicians who were already on the job. In 1979 the Association of Pharmacy Technicians was formed. In 1983 the ASHP accredited the first pharmacy technician training program at Thomas Jefferson Hospital in Philadelphia.

Today there is a Voluntary Technician Certification Program adopted by 24 states as of 1995. It is estimated that in the United States there are between 75,000 and 100,000 pharmacy technicians (Flanagan, 1995).

National Associations of Pharmacists

The first national association of U.S. pharmacists was the American Pharmaceutical Association (APhA). Formed in Philadelphia in 1852, APhA has grown into the largest of the national associations in pharmacy, with approximately fifty thousand members. The original objectives of the association, written over 100 years ago, addressed the major concerns of the profession then and surprisingly the major concerns now. They are improvement and regulation of drug supply and quality, inter- and intraprofessional relations, improvement of the scientific knowledge base of the profession and dissemination of that new knowledge through publication, educational standards for practice of the profession, restriction of drug-dispensing functions, and creation of ethical standards of practice. APhA supports voluntary certification of technicians by the pharmacy profession but opposes licensure, registration, or certification by state law or regulation.

In addition to being the first national professional pharmacy association, APhA is also considered to be the "parent" of many other pharmacy associations. The American Society of Health System Pharmacists (ASHP), the National Community Pharmacists Association (NCPA), the American College of Apothecaries (ACA), and the American Association of Colleges of Pharmacy (AACP) were all initiated by special interest groups originally a part of APhA. Most recently a large number of pharmaceutical scientists broke off from APhA's Academy of Pharmaceutical Sciences to form the American Association of Pharmaceutical Scientists (AAPS). These offspring of APhA have kept varied relations with the parent organization.

Recently APhA reorganized again into three academies: the Academy of Pharmacy Practice and Management, the Academy of Pharmaceutical Research and Science, and the Academy of the Students of Pharmacy. APhA has also added a political action committee or PAC to its structure.

The American Society of Health System Pharmacists (ASHP) represents pharmacists who practice in organized health care settings, primarily hospitals. More recently, ASHP membership has expanded to include pharmacists in various long-term care facilities, health maintenance organizations, and home health agencies. ASHP was founded at the 1942 meeting of APhA, and from its founding until 1972, membership in the parent organization (APhA) was required for membership in ASHP. ASHP has been a vigorous proponent of the role of the pharmacist as the drug-use control expert in organized health care settings. ASHP has taken strong positions regarding education of pharmacists and technicians and has accrediting standards for pharmacy residencies designed for pharmacy graduates, and for pharmacy technician training programs.

Education has been a hallmark for all organizations in pharmacy, but APhA and ASHP have been exceptionally strong. APhA now provides a framework for specialty certification of pharmacists. Their annual meeting is well organized and of benefit to pharmacists and technicians as well as to the industry.

ASHP holds two large meetings annually. The annual meeting, like the one at APhA, provides general education. The midyear clinical meeting provides a forum for pharmacists and technicians, but also has special educational programming for clinical specialists.

NCPA, formerly the National Association Representing Independent Retail Pharmacy, developed from the parent APhA's Section on Commercial Interests as an independent organization in 1898. NCPA has strongly represented the interests of the independent pharmacy owner since its inception and has championed the independent practice alternative to students of pharmacy. In 1991 NCPA created the National Home Infusion Association (NHIA). One recent focus of NCPA has been training and certification of pharmacists in the various areas of home health care. NCPA has a reputation for being a vigorous defender of the independent owner's rights on Capitol Hill. NCPA lobbied for over a decade for legislation to make armed robbery a federal offense. The NCPA PAC was also the first in pharmacy and has the slogan "Get into politics or get out of pharmacy." While many attempts to get APhA and NCPA to work together in the past floundered, the two organizations appear to be cooperating on a more regular basis.

The American Society of Consultant Pharmacists (ASCP) includes pharmacists who provide clinical consulting and/or distributive services to institutional and ambulatory health care settings, such as nursing homes and other long-term care facilities.

The American College of Clinical Pharmacy (ACCP) consists primarily of Pharm.D. clinical practitioners and faculty members. Its stated mission is to facilitate the creation, transmission, and application of new knowledge in the science of pharmacotherapy.

The American College of Apothecaries (ACA) is a small, selective association of community-based practitioners. Membership is granted only if the practitioner and his or her pharmacy complies with certain standards of professional service and appearance. Dual membership in APhA is required.

The National Pharmaceutical Association (NPA) is an association of black pharmacists. It was organized in the late 1940s to promote the economic position of black pharmacists.

The Pharmacy Technician Certification Board (PTCB) was established in January 1995 through the efforts of APhA, ASHP, the Illinois Council of Health System Pharmacists (ICHP), and the Michigan Pharmacists Association (MPA). It provides a voluntary mechanism for a national certification program.

PTCB offers the certification examination several times each year. To be eligible to take the examination, the candidate must have a high school diploma or GED. The cost for the application fee is currently $105. Recertification and continuing education are required by the board. As of January 1997, more than 18,000 technicians are certified. These individuals make up a valued group and are a powerful contribution to the mission of pharmacy.

Other Associations

Many other national associations in pharmacy represent special segments of the profession. These are presented here, with a brief description of their membership and mission.

The National Association of Chain Drug Stores (NACDS) is an organization of corporations, generally represented by their chief executive officers, many of whom are not pharmacists. The title is misleading because NACDS represents a variety of businesses, not only chain or multioutlet pharmacies. Grocery chains, department stores, and a variety of discount outlets that have pharmacies belong to NACDS. The strength of this organization lies in its size and large financial capabilities. Chains are the largest employer of practicing pharmacists. While nonpharmacy merchandising has been a large concern of NACDS, recent consumer trends have suggested that chains pay more attention to the pharmacy department and the employee pharmacist. Often at odds with APhA and NCPA in the past, NACDS has more recently found its interests are often best served by supporting pharmacy's interests and has joined with these other organizations in legislative efforts.

The American Association of Colleges of Pharmacy (AACP) is an organization of pharmacy colleges and schools. Representation of deans and faculty members is accomplished through membership on their respective councils, which have equal representation in the House of Delegates. The AACP is primarily concerned with educational issues, such as curricula and teaching methodology. One major issue debated over the past decade by the AACP is the proper length and title of the initial degree required to practice pharmacy. The 6-year doctor of pharmacy degree (Pharm.D.) or the 5-year baccalaureate degree (B.S.) was approved as the single entry-level degree for pharmacy at the July 1992 meeting. No final implementation date was set. The AACP recently adopted a policy of supportive personnel (pharmacy technicians), which states that the training of such personnel be based on sound educational principles. The AACP also recommended that its member schools offer their assistance for the development of those objectives.

The American Council on Pharmaceutical Education (ACPE) is the independent, government-recognized accrediting agency of degree and continuing education programs in pharmacy. Formed in 1932 through the efforts of APhA, AACP, and the National Association of Boards of Pharmacy (NABP), the ACPE has through its representative membership proposed and published the standards that schools must meet to obtain accreditation. Criteria such as budget, governance, faculty quality and quantity, admission standards, physical facilities, library, curricula, and student achievement are all considered during the accreditation process. Accreditation is voluntary, but inasmuch as all states require graduation from an accredited school of pharmacy as a prerequisite of licensure, an unaccredited program could not survive. Accreditation is also needed to qualify for a variety of state and federal financial aid programs.

The National Association of Boards of Pharmacy (NABP) is an organization of the members of the individual state boards of pharmacy, which are generally charged with the licensure of pharmacies and pharmacists and in many states with inspection and law enforcement activities. The NABP, since its inception in 1904, has worked to standardize the requirements for pharmacist licensure, while maintaining the posture of individual states' rights. Through its efforts, reciprocity—transfer of licensure among most states—has been facilitated and a national licensing exam for pharmacists, the NABPLEX, is used as a major part of all but several states' licensing examinations. The NABP works closely with the AACP and the ACPE in its activities but has maintained a degree of independence as it is responsible first and foremost to the public and the legislature of the states it serves.

The National Wholesale Druggists Association (NWDA) includes those companies that provide pharmacies with the drug and nondrug products required for practice. In the past, wholesalers were often locally based companies that mainly serviced the independently owned pharmacies. Recently, extensive consolidation has occurred in this sector, with fewer national companies controlling most of the wholesale drug business. Wholesalers are now providing more hospitals with their drug needs through primary wholesaler contracts.

The Pharmaceutical Research Manufacturers Association (PRMA) consists of the large drug manufacturers that provide the majority of prescription drugs sold in this country. The PRMA lobbies extensively with government agencies that regulate research, development, and production of new drugs and drug products. The PRMA also sponsors several academically based researchers and research projects through fellowship programs.

The Association of Pharmacy Technicians (APT) is an association of pharmacy technicians whose mission is the advancement and enhancement of pharmacy technicians and the profession of pharmacy. The APT conducts regional and national meetings and like other professional associations publishes a journal.

Association Publications

One of the first actions of a professional association is the publication of a journal for the dissemination of scientific and professional information for the membership and the profession. The founders of the Philadelphia College of Pharmacy were responsible for the publication of the first American pharmacy journal, the *Journal of the Philadelphia College of Pharmacy,* in 1825. In 1835 the title was changed to the *American Journal of Pharmacy* and as such has been published continually to this day. Since that initial effort the many national associations of pharmacy have continued and expanded on this effort, each with its own journal and newsletters (**Table 9–2**). In addition, several associations—most notably APhA and the ASHP—have produced publications providing pharmacists and other health professionals with needed drug information, such as the *Handbook of Nonprescription Drugs* and the *American Hospital Formulary Service.* The ASHP also publishes the *International Pharmaceutical Abstracts,* which is a semimonthly abstracting service of the world's pharmaceutical literature.

TABLE 9–2   **Organizational Publications**

AACP	American Journal of Pharmaceutical Education
AAPS	Pharmaceutical Research
ACA	Voice of the Pharmacist
APhA	American Pharmacy; Journal of Pharmaceutical Sciences
APT	Journal of Pharmacy Technology
ASHP	American Journal of Health System Pharmacy; Clinical Pharmacy
NCPA	NCPA Journal
NPA	Journal of the National Pharmaceutical Association
ASCP	Consultant Pharmacist

Summary

There are a number of professional organizations that meet the specialty needs of their membership.

Organizations represent members practicing in community, chain, hospital, consulting, and clinical pharmacy practice. Colleges of pharmacy, accrediting agencies, state boards of pharmacy, wholesalers, and more comprise additional specialty membership groups in pharmacy practice.

The various organizations in pharmacy link together pharmacists who are engaged in the numerous aspects of the profession. As a result all pharmacists have the opportunity to enter the mainstream of the constantly evolving growth and development of the profession of pharmacy.

ASSESSMENT

Multiple Choice Questions

1. An identifying characteristic of a profession is
   a. the organization of the membership into professional associations
   b. that all members agree on all professional policies regarding education and other important matters
   c. that all members have the same professional, academic degree
   d. that financial objectives are of primary importance

2. The two major issues that gave us the first national association of pharmacists were
   a. educational programs required
   b. means of expanding profitability
   c. quality and purity of drugs
   d. a and c
   e. a, b, and c

True/False Questions

3. ___T___ An organization represents the special interests of the membership.

4. ___T___ The American Society of Health System Pharmacists has taken a strong position regarding education of pharmacists and technicians.

5. ___T___ The National Community Pharmacists Association (NCPA) represents the interests of independent retail pharmacy owners.

Matching

6. ___c___ ASHP   a. open to all pharmacists

7. ___b___ NCPA   b. independent community retail pharmacists

8. ___d___ AACP   c. hospital pharmacists

9. ___e___ PRMA   d. pharmacy educators

10. ___a___ APhA   e. drug firm associates

Bibliography

Flanagan, M.E. (1995). Voluntary technician certification program reflects changes in practice. *American Pharmacy, NS35*(5), 18–23.

Murer, Melissa M. (1996, August). Technician certification leads to recognition, better patient care. *Journal of the American Pharmaceutical Association, NS36,* 514–520.

Smith, Joe E. (1995). The national voluntary certification of pharmacy technicians. *American Journal of Health System Pharmacy, 52,* 2026–2029.

10 Pharmacy Practice in the Third Millennium

COMPETENCIES

Upon completion and review of this chapter, the student should be able to

1. Identify the major influences shaping pharmacy practice.

2. Describe the impact of changes occurring in other health care disciplines and the broad socioeconomic and technological trends that are likely to influence pharmacy's future.

3. Describe how professional and social changes will likely influence the education and training expectations of pharmacists and pharmacy technicians.

Introduction

Where will you be at the end of the century and the start of the new millennium? What will you be doing and how will you be doing it? We would all like to know the answers to these questions and whether we will find ourselves fulfilled professionally. Economic and sociopolitical changes of the first half of the 1990s have had significant influence on the structure and mission of health care in the United States. Moreover, such changes will undoubtedly continue to alter the way in which both pharmacy and other health care disciplines achieve their social mandates in the new millennium.

Periodic introspection of any profession's progress and current status can be quite useful. Through history, we are often allowed to frame our perceptions of the causes and effects in our professional and personal lives. History, per se, offers no refuge for us—it is only helpful to the extent that it confirms our current position and provides the initiative and resolve for making rational choices as we proceed into the future. Ultimately, we have no alternatives other than to forge ahead, engage, and adapt to the forces influencing us in the pursuit of our goals as pharmacists and pharmacy technicians. Our only "hedge" for coping with the future may be our common understanding of changes, their significance, and the mutual support and interdependence of pharmacists and technicians.

The goals of this chapter are

■ to provide a brief historical perspective of pharmacy's evolution, particularly in the context of practice and education

■ to describe the major influences that have resulted in the most significant changes to the profession of pharmacy and health care in general and the attendant implications

■ to explore how current forces in pharmacy and health care's operating environment may shape opportunities and threats in the profession

■ to identify some of the future career path options available to pharmacists and technicians, particularly in the context of current trends

■ to describe levels of educational and training preparedness required to meet professional and societal needs in the third millennium.

Historical Overview of Pharmacy Practice and Education

From a historical viewpoint, pharmacy practice and education in the United States have been aptly described as evolving in three distinct "waves" or eras. These are the empirical era, the industrialization era, and the patient care era.

Empirical Era

The first such wave began in the mid-1800s and extended through 1940 (Hepler, 1987). This period has been described as the empirical era. The practice of pharmacy was largely cast in the image and role of the traditional apothecary—the drug store and/or pharmacy served as the apothecary's shop for processing and compounding natural products (drugs mostly derived from natural sources) into prescribed medicinals. Subjects such as pharmacognosy and galenical pharmacy were the mainstays of the pharmacy school's curriculum during the era. In fact, it was not until 1932 that a 4-year baccalaureate degree was mandated for pharmacists.

Industrialization Era

The period from 1940 to 1970 ushered in a new era of industrialization for the pharmaceutical industry and pharmacy practice, as well as a new dawn for pharmaceutical education. Advances in the physical and biological sciences became the basis of contemporary pharmacy practice and education. The pharmacy school's curriculum became a hybrid of theoretical basic science and applied "pharmaceutical sciences." The compounding and processing of pharmaceutical products shifted to a new and dominant sector: the American pharmaceutical industry. The practice role of the pharmacist during this period became largely that of a dispenser of prefabricated prescription products.

Patient Care Era

The third wave began in 1970 and continues to the present time. It is the "patient care" era in which the concepts of clinical pharmacy and pharmaceutical care reached maturation and became the mainstream function of pharmacists. Patients and their effective treatment with drugs are now central to the pharmacist's role. The role of providing a significant cognitive component or patient-specific knowledge and skills to patients receiving drug therapy reached maturity. The pharmacist's role as a "therapeutic advisor" subsequently began to emerge.

The era that began in 1970 has since positioned pharmacy and pharmacists in a strategically critical role in health care, especially in light of the importance of drug therapy.

Major Factors Influencing Health Care and Pharmacy's Future

A range of influences, both external and internal, are greatly affecting the future of the profession for both pharmacists and technicians. External influences such as structural change in the health care economy, the growth of managed care, changes in health care financing, telecommunications and automated technologies, and breakthroughs in drug research and biotechnology are only a few of the forces that will undoubtedly shape the environment of pharmacy practice.

Research into the molecular basis of disease and its treatment, multiple disease morbidity and chronicity in an aging population, and the critical nature of interdisciplinary health care relationships and collaboration will impose major challenges that will change our sense of purpose as professionals. Another influence on the profession may well be the heightened expectations of an increasingly informed and demanding public.

Many of these external influences may be beyond our control. On the other hand, certain factors may have even more influence over our destiny. These factors include internal forces such as competency expectations and assessments, continuous education, training and retraining, the differentiated nature of pharmacy practice and growth of specialization, and the achievement of the mission and vision of pharmaceutical care.

Economic Influences

A wide array of economic and market influences continue to shape the direction and nature of the health care delivery sector and pharmacy.

Market-driven reforms

Glacial yet profoundly fundamental changes have been occurring in health care since the mid-1980s. The Executive Summary of Third Report of the Pew Health Professions Commission poignantly describes the fact that, since 1990, the financial, organizational, and legal framework of American health care has been undergoing a transformation to systems of integrated care combining primary, specialty, and hospital services. "These systems attempt to manage the care delivered to enrolled populations in such a manner as to achieve some combination of cost reduction, enhanced patient and consumer satisfaction, and improvement of health care outcomes. Within another decade 80–90% of the insured population of the United States will receive its care through one of these systems" (Hepler, 1987). The failure of the federal government and political system to successfully enact comprehensive health care reform legislation has given way to de facto market-driven reforms energized by consumer and employer demands for more services and more intense technology. This problem is further compounded by a growing market trend of health care payers (public and private) refusing to pay the true and full economic costs of health care (ASHP Reports, 1993).

Cost containment

A continuing focus on cost containment in health care delivery has led to a fiercely competitive marketplace. In some instances, the vision of success through providing care at the lowest possible cost may well be outpacing the quest for quality outcomes in health care. The continued market penetration of managed care and consolidation and integration of health care provider systems may well result in a survival of the fittest scenario in which only those systems that can produce the expected stakeholder results will survive.

Public demand for health care services

Heightened public demand for a broader and improved spectrum of health care continues unabatedly as a result of availability of consumer-focused education and the virtually instantaneous world of information access through telecommunications and the personal computer. As more information about health-related issues, breakthroughs in science and technology, and disease treatment advance, public demand spirals upward. Although health care's future will ultimately be defined by public expectations, it will at the same time mandate that health care providers continually and systematically assess, ensure, and improve the quality and effectiveness of services provided.

Hospital reorganization

The 1990s have ushered in a frenetic pace of price-driven competition among hospitals for the business of third-party payers, managed care organizations, and large employers for the services of physicians, and other hospital services. Hospitals must now compete on the basis of providing levels of care and services at predetermined prices (ASHP Reports, 1996). Financial risk continues to be shifted to *providers* of health care as opposed to those that *pay* for such care. Much of this shift is a result of the growth of managed care and its impact on exposing excess hospital capacity.

As a result of such trends, some hospitals that have not planned effectively or failed to recognize impending change have been forced to close. Hospital closures and consolidations are expected to continue into the next century.

Many hospitals are pursuing various forms of horizontal or vertical integration. Horizontal integration is usually achieved when hospitals and other health care provider delivery systems combine their operations to share any number of administrative, business, and technological capacities and opportunities to become more effective and efficient in their markets. For example, it is not unusual for community hospitals to integrate with academic medical centers to share the use of high-cost consultative medical expertise and/or capital-intensive high technology and other resources. Such integration can also provide a steady and continuous source of referred high acuity patients for the tertiary care hospital or academic medical center. Consolidation and integration may well continue as business strategies for the survival of many smaller hospitals. Whether these strategies will be a future mainstay in the United States will depend largely on such hospitals meeting the health care needs of markets while controlling their cost structures.

Vertical integration attempts to provide potential powerhouses of health care services with a bundled "seamless" approach to providing care and service (ASHP, 1996). This approach is usually accomplished by providing a continuum of care from hospital to ambulatory, home, and long-term care settings. In either horizontal or vertical integration, the resulting benefits evolve from economies of scale and market share gains. Most experts agree that any accrued benefits to providers and payers of services, and patients, are as yet indeterminable.

Unquestionably, the successful evolution of integrated health care will be determined economically. Yet, the health care industry must not lose sight of its mission to satisfy the needs of patients in the process. The interests of cost and profit cannot be allowed to supersede optimal patient outcomes. In the final analysis, demand for health care services will be satisfied at the price its consumers are willing to pay. Pharmacists and technicians must market themselves to remain a part of such a demand structure and ultimately demonstrate their roles in optimizing patient care outcomes and value.

Effect of economic influences on pharmacy

How do such trends affect pharmacy? Many of the economic changes and trends discussed thus far characterize the health care industry as a whole and are not focused on the profession of pharmacy per se (Biles, 1991). Nonetheless, these changes have compelled pharmacists to further constrain their operating costs to the extent that is within their control. This has resulted in meticulous scrutiny of contractual arrangements with suppliers, increased justification for formulary additions, and adjusting or "flexing" manpower requirements as hospital census and patient day volume vary.

All too often, for large purchasers of prescription drug services (large employers or managed care organizations), the determining factor quite often is the lowest cost without consideration to the pharmaceutical service component provided by pharmacists and technicians. Current efforts to advance the concept of pharmaceutical care through improving patient outcomes has often been difficult to quantify in economic terms. Nonetheless, demonstrating the value of pharmaceutical care remains perhaps the singular challenge in influencing pharmacy's future in terms of role justification, marketing, and meeting the demands of an increasingly discerning public.

The new order in health care economics is being felt in hospitals and in hospital pharmacies; but independent community pharmacies also have long been under competitive pressures to survive in the face of heightened price competition with chain pharmacies. It has been estimated that within the last 50 years the volume of payment by third parties for outpatient medications and service has grown from 0 to 30 percent. Mandated co-payments for the insured population help to decrease third-party expenditures for medication. "Since drugs are both highly valued and increasingly expensive, third-party coverage will grow" (Cocolas, 1989). The imposition of maximum allowable costs for prescriptions by third-party payers continues. Independent community pharmacy survival, and that of many chain pharmacies, is increasingly threatened by competition for contractual agreements with third-party payers and managed care organizations. With the burgeoning technologies of the coming millennium, the traditional independent and chain pharmacy settings will be challenged by competing mail-order prescription services which will offer added convenience to consumers. The central question facing pharmacy is whether pharmacists can successfully shift the focus of their service from competing on the basis of product costs and delivery to a focus on its pharmaceutical care mission of reducing the growing problem of medication misuse and the resulting adverse consequences of drug therapy.

Public Expectation and an Aging Population

Just as scientific and technological breakthroughs are accelerating, so, too, are consumer expectations. It seems that everyone wants everything instantly—information, service, treatment, medication. Such demands are not limited to the United States. They are truly global in nature. The world population continues to expand at a rate that is estimated to double every 50 years. International political changes are leading to global economic changes that will undoubtedly impact world consumer demand for drug products and other health-related products and services.

The elimination of classic geopolitical boundaries resulting from a global economy and advances in telecommunications and technology transfer have redefined national cultures in most developed countries. Increased cultural diversity places greater complexity and expectations on health care providers to meet personal and cultural expectations of patients. The most poignant example of this is the expectation for instructions for medication use to be provided in multiple languages as a means of reducing the potential for medication misuse.

It is estimated that during the next decade, one in five United States citizens will be over 65 years of age. As a result, demand for health care services and products will grow dramatically. Chronic diseases and disabilities such as AIDS, mental health issues, and heart disease will undoubtedly lead to increased demands for elder care, subacute care, long-term care facilities, and assisted living retirement centers. An informed and highly educated aging population will demand technology that provides them with new drugs to treat chronic diseases and multiple organ problems. Unchecked increases in medication use and polypharmacy will further heighten existing problems of medication misuse. Pharmacists need to be prepared to service these pharmaceutical care needs by identifying, reducing, and preventing drug-related morbidity. Pharmacists will, by definition, need to manage a patient's "drug therapy across all environments of care, including home, acute, long-term and intermediate care facilities" (Biles, 1991).

In short, an increasingly aging and knowledgeable population will demand that new health care technologies be developed to further extend life expectancies. This demand, in turn, will necessitate further enhancements of educational standards for health care providers, including pharmacists and pharmacy technicians.

The Impact of Accelerating Technology

Take a moment and look at the things around you. How many tasks that used to be manually performed are now being performed by a machine or some other labor-saving device? Does everything seem to be moving at a greatly increased pace? How many new sources of information are available to you for use that were not routinely available even 10 years ago? Unquestionably, the world is moving at a greatly accelerated pace as a result of a "cyber-cultural" revolution. That is, computerization and telecommunications have redefined access to knowledge and its attendant power. We can gather and transmit vast amounts of information and data arrayed in an almost infinite variety of ways. We can receive information through wire, fiber optics, CD-ROM, satellite, the Internet, and smartcards. Major work elements can now be performed, in part, by computer. In some instances, computers are able to direct and maintain entire manufacturing operations. Some industries in the manufacturing sector have transformed their facilities into robot-controlled processes that employ only minimal numbers of individuals.

Is this the future direction that health care will take? To what extent will computerization and automation replace conventional face-to-face contact with patients?

This broad social trend has transcended the industrial sector and now includes health care. There are more sophisticated and less invasive diagnostic devices available than ever before.

Technology in the pharmacy

Pharmacy is by no means immune from the rapid assimilation of such technology. The adaptation of computer-driven medication and filling devices, automated parenteral compounding devices, robotics units, and automated point-of-use dispensing units are commonplace phenomena in the pharmacy of the 1990s. Much of this has been driven, in part, by cost-cutting pressures in hospitals and by consolidations of operations. Although the reasons for such technological acceleration have been largely economic, the profession of pharmacy, at the same time, adopted a vision and mission to embrace a new philosophy and concept—*pharmaceutical care*.

The principle focus of pharmaceutical care is on patients and the consequences of their drug therapy rather than the preparation and delivery of products in isolation. It is postulated that technological advances will facilitate most of the production elements of preparation and distribution of drug products while pharmacists will assume active responsibility in identifying, resolving, and preventing drug-related problems in patients. Are pharmacists and technicians ready to assume their new roles in a practice environment defined by pharmaceutical care? Can this concept be economically and rationally supported? Can dispensing information and the direction of drug usage also be automated? Pharmacists and technicians who fully embrace the concept of pharmaceutical care have a noble and laudable cause. Creating a mainstream demand for such services, however, may be pharmacy's ultimate challenge in the upcoming millennium.

Many functions currently performed by technicians and pharmacists will be substantively changed or eliminated by automation in the not too distant future. For example, in hospitals or long-term care facilities, unit-dose cart filling will no longer be performed manually, but by computer-driven technology or robots, or precluded entirely by point-of-use dispensing devices located in patient care areas. Highly skilled technicians will be required to troubleshoot and operate such complex automated equipment and to ensure that the adequate supplies of product are available from vendors or outsourced partners who are committed to the same goals as the institution. The maintenance and stocking of these devices might also be accomplished by technicians employed by such outsourced vendors.

In ambulatory prescription service settings, much of the prescription filling will be mediated through electronic transmission and processing of prescriptions in area dispensing centers. These centers will, in turn, deliver medication by mail or overnight courier, or be made available on-site yet be controlled by pharmacists from remote locations. In concept, the automated centralization and/or regionalization of prescription filling may well offer unique and highly effective means for pharmacists to impact the health status of patients by providing pharmaceutical care.

The capacity to almost instantly convey vast amounts of information electronically, even interactive information, may well become the principal means by which health care professionals track complete patient clinical histories, summaries of hospital stays, and other critical information needed for effective treatment.

Smartcards that encode and capture portions of this information already exist in various formats (Crawford, 1987). It is conceivable that we will all have personal compact discs that contain all of the necessary information pertinent to our health care needs, including histories, scans, and X rays of various sorts that can be interactively manipulated for different three-dimensional views. Perhaps such a disc may provide access to sources of medical information that answer questions about medical treatment alternatives and information about drug use on an interactive basis.

Will drug therapy as it is known today be eclipsed by other forms of treatment? Will we begin to see the accelerated use of "gene splicing" technologies and the curing of selected diseases through advances in gene therapy? Will discoveries be made that lead the way to organ and/or tissue regeneration? How far can biotechnology take us? Will the diseases of today be eliminated through such therapies? Will pharmacists and technicians be involved in the proper use of new drugs or substances that act like drugs in the *curing* of disease rather than the *treatment* of its symptoms?

Unprecedented advances in the treatment and/or elimination of diseases are predicted for the next millennium. The enormous speed with which the science and technology of such treatment are accelerating is virtually exponential as a result of the continued improvement of computer processors. The vast amount of information that can now be handled greatly facilitates the work of research and subsequently hastens its availability and applications. Such discoveries and advances that demonstrate patient benefit and cost savings will undoubtedly foster more research and development with attendant escalating costs. An informed and demanding U.S. population will demand the use of the most current technology and will be willing to pay the price. Third-party payers and government may bear the costs for their customers (Cocolas, 1989), but at the expense of much of the current labor component of health care services.

The future of drug therapy is trending toward a single and minimally invasive dose or minimal number of doses of an agent to achieve desired outcomes. Costs for such agents and the expertise required for their administration will also be costly. Misuse and waste of such novel therapeutic agents will not be tolerated in light of their costs. Highly skilled pharmacists assisted by technicians will be vital in ensuring the appropriate and efficient use of such therapies.

Pharmacists and technicians may also be involved in the procurement, preparation, storage, and distribution of genetically altered substances (Pew Health Professions Commission, 1995). Gene therapy is still quite controversial and will likely remain so for some time. This procedure will undoubtedly require further specialized education and training on the part of both pharmacists and technicians.

Influences of Internal Professional Differentiation

Currently, pharmacy practice is primarily differentiated by service and/or delivery setting (hospital, independent community and chain pharmacies, home care, managed care, nuclear, and industrial pharmacist). Pharmacy technicians practice in all of these settings. For a variety of reasons each of these groups has, for quite some time, found it difficult to embrace common professional goals. Pharmaceutical care, however, appears to have become the unifying influence that minimizes such differentiation.

All sectors of the health care industry will face a range of threats and opportunities. The 1995 *Pew Health Professions Commission Report* has made some stark projections for the future. According to the report, the potential closing of many hospitals and the reduction of as many as 60 percent of currently available hospital beds, the expansion of primary care in ambulatory settings, shrinking demand for specialties, automation and greater centralization of health care functions may result in a labor surplus in many health care disciplines. It is estimated that there will be a surplus of 100,000 to 150,000 physicians, a surplus of 200,000 to 300,000 nurses, and a surplus of 40,000 pharmacists. The Pew Report suggests that many other allied health professionals will need to be retrained as multiskilled professionals. Moreover, there will be a public mandate for restructured educational programs for research and patient care. According to the Report, pharmacy can expect to see reductions of 20 to 25 percent in several pharmacy schools within 10 years. Increased support of underserved areas and more emphasis on integration and working as a member of a health care team will be an expectation of all health care disciplines in the future.

Regardless of the Pew Commission's predictions and recommendations, a newly defined and demand-driven health care market will require pharmaceutical care as a mainstream professional function.

Delivering pharmaceutical care will in turn mandate a true team approach to care—a team that must include pharmacists and technicians, with physicians and other health care professionals. The extent and impact of pharmacy's role in providing pharmaceutical care will, in the final analysis, rest within pharmacy's membership ranks. More specifically, it will evolve through creative reengineering of mutual understanding among technicians and pharmacists.

Educational Direction and Influence

"Those who teach us and those who learn must contend with the constantly changing world of health care. The knowledge base will change, the technology will change, and the practice environment will change, perhaps profoundly" (Ebert, 1991). Such a scenario for health care appears virtually certain as we hasten our stride into the next millennium. How will health care education need to change to meet the future demands of consumers of health care? What will be needed to achieve the outcomes that we as pharmacists and technicians are designing for our future?

The bedrock of pharmacy education has typically been the ability to teach and demonstrate scientific principles (Green, 1992). With a redirected educational focus toward pharmaceutical care and caring, it will be critical to supplement science with the study of human behavior as it relates to health and the treatment of disease. More specifically, learning to deal with patients and family members on a more humanistic rather than on purely scientific terms will be an essential skill and tool to be used in case management. Effective written, verbal, and listening communication skills will be pivotal in the survival of the pharmacist, technician, and other health care team professionals. Both problem-solving and analytical skills will also be critical in a practice environment that is constantly changing.

The pharmacist in the third millennium will be required to be a clinical resource manager. That person will need to be skilled in the management of proper drug use and in the development of treatment protocols and their administration, and serve as the gatekeeper for high-cost biotech and genetic forms of therapy.

Treatment protocols will be so complex that effective management of coordination with other health disciplines will be the norm. Health professionals working independently will no longer be able to produce optimum patient outcomes or provide the level of professional satisfaction they once did. Coordinated efforts will produce cognitive economies of scale as well as provide, if managed appropriately, the desired economic efficiencies that will be essential. Efforts to educate health care teams in role differentiation, tolerance, diversity, professional interdependence, and teamwork will be paramount.

Pharmacy education will be mandated to provide educational opportunities that embrace the mission of pharmaceutical care. Pharmacist and technician educational opportunities need to encompass the entire spectrum of pharmacy practice and to involve all types of practice settings. This education will facilitate the movement of pharmacists and technicians on a common path toward our patient-focused mission. Ambulatory care pharmacists can serve as the first line of defense in the development and application of treatment protocols (Hepler & Strand, 1989). They can serve as sentinels of recognition for determining when to involve or refer patients to other specialized pharmacies. Ambulatory care pharmacists will become more involved in adjusting doses, therapy selection, prevention programs, and protocol management. They will be responsible for monitoring drug usage and its associated patient care outcomes. The volume of work necessary to manage this multibillion dollar problem of appropriate drug use will also require the use of highly trained technicians.

Technicians will need to have broader backgrounds in pathophysiology and information management skills. Their skills will be utilized to obtain patient medical and drug histories and to gather other medical data to be reviewed by case managers.

Managed care organizations will use pharmacists to screen patients on an outpatient basis as a means of referral for initiation of therapy and routing of medical complaints to other health care team members. They will, in many instances, order and interpret laboratory tests. How pharmacists, technicians, and health care teams will likely function in the future is contingent upon effective marketing, the advancement of educational efforts, and the ability of pharmacists to be recognized and reimbursed for their cognitive services by third-party payers.

How can the educational process better prepare its students for the realities that await them? How can the focus be changed from traditional science to human behavior, economics, communications, analysis, and management training that will be necessary? Significant progress has already been made. Incorporating health care faculty members in real-time practice settings can serve as a model for future educators. What better way to train students than to train them in real-time settings? Simulated settings in a laboratory or classroom are only marginally effective. Key elements of human behavior, communication, management, and other problem-solving skills can be experienced first hand. *Real* outcomes, favorable or unfavorable, can be observed. Training students in a broad continuum of various health care settings will undoubtedly provide the most effective role models.

Summary

As a profession, pharmacy's destiny in the new millennium is unquestionably linked to the broader social, economic, and technological trends that are shaping the entire health care sector. As key participants in health care delivery, pharmacists and pharmacy technicians have a new set of challenges that have been, in part, molded by these broader trends in health care and a new and exciting mandate to add value to health care services through the provision of pharmaceutical care. The extent to which pharmacists and technicians can add such value to health care services is a function of qualified and competent practitioners with both the will and skill to provide pharmaceutical care.

ASSESSMENT

Multiple Choice Questions

1. External factors influencing health care and pharmacy's future include
   a. structural changes in health care economics
   b. managed care
   c. drug research and biotechnology
   d. health care expectations of a well-informed public
   e. all of the above

2. Which of the following is NOT an internal factor impacting pharmacy's future direction?
   a. competency expectations
   b. continuous education, training, and retraining
   c. differentiated and specialized pharmacy practices
   d. development of automated technologies
   e. the mission of pharmaceutical care

3. The intent of managed care development is to
   a. achieve health care cost reductions
   b. enhance patient and consumer satisfaction
   c. improve health care outcomes
   d. all of the above

4. Which of the following are included in hospitals' attempts to integrate horizontally?
   a. sharing of administrative and business services
   b. shared technological capacity
   c. combining of community hospitals and academic medical centers to form a network
   d. all of the above

5. When health care providers attempt to integrate vertically, they
   a. benefit from economies of scale from sharing common services
   b. combine community hospitals and academic medical centers to form a network
   c. provide care over a continuum from hospital to ambulatory, home, and long-term settings
   d. a and c
   e. all of the above

6. Which of the following are challenging the future of the retail pharmacy sector?
   a. maximum allowable costs paid by third-party payers
   b. managed care contracts
   c. mail-order prescription operations
   d. all of the above
   e. none of the above

7. The 1995 Pew Health Professions Commission Report
   a. is optimistic about the future direction of the health care industry and of pharmacy
   b. states that the role of heath care providers in the future will need to remain highly differentiated and specialized
   c. states that pharmacy schools will continue to increase in numbers for another 10 years
   d. indicates that pharmacists in the future will need to become a part of an integrated health care team

8. Future pharmacy technicians will need to develop skills that include
   a. the ability to interact with various health care professionals as part of a multidisciplinary team
   b. their ability to use information technology and analyze data
   c. the development of good verbal, written, and listening communication
   d. a broader knowledge base in pathophysiology
   e. all of the above

9. Future pharmacist and technician education needs to change to a system that includes
   a. only the teaching and demonstration of scientific principles
   b. more cognitive-based skills
   c. education incorporating the mission of pharmaceutical care
   d. laboratory settings to simulate real-life health care problems
   e. b and c

10. The future of pharmacy for technicians and pharmacists will be concerned with
    a. the provision of care to prevent drug misuse and abuse
    b. the ability to provide health care services as part of an integrated health care team
    c. the educational changes to develop skills to use future technologies and to be communicators on a variety of levels
    d. serving a highly informed public about health care provision and expected outcomes
    e. all of the above

Bibliography

ASHP Reports. (1993, January). ASHP accreditation standard for pharmacy technician training programs. *American Journal of Hospital Pharmacy, 50,* 124–126.

ASHP Reports. (1996, January). Vision statement. American Society of Health-System Pharmacists. *American Journal of Health-System Pharmacy, 53,* 174.

Biles, J.A. (1991). Beyond our walls: Part II. Culture-science-profession. *American Journal of Pharmaceutical Education, 55,* 345–348.

Crawford, D.S. (1987, October). Planning for the future. *American Pharmacy, 10,* 654–655.

Critical challenges: Revitalizing the health professions for the twenty-first century. The Third Report of the Pew Health Professions Commission, November 1995.

Ebert, R.H. (1991). Health professions education for year 2000. *American Journal of Pharmaceutical Education, 55,* 356–360.

Green, L. (1992, January). Gene therapy: Medicine for the future. *American Journal of Hospital Pharmacy, 49,* 172–173.

Hepler, C.D. (1987, Winter). The third wave in pharmaceutical education: The clinical movement. *American Journal of Pharmaceutical Education, 51,* 369–385.

Hepler, C.D., & Strand, L.M. (1989). Opportunities and responsibilities in pharmaceutical care. *American Journal of Pharmaceutical Education, 53.* 7S–15S.

Hughes, E.F.X. (1989). Trends in health care systems delivery. *American Journal of Pharmaceutical Education, 53,* 49S–54S.

Kalman, M.K., Witkowski, D.E., & Ogawa, G.S. (1992, January). Increasing pharmacy productivity by expanding the role of pharmacy technicians. *American Journal of Hospital Pharmacy, 49,* 84–89.

Knapp, D.A. (1992, October). Pharmacy practice in 2040. *American Journal of Hospital Pharmacy, 49,* 2457–2461.

Koda-Kimbel, M.A., & Herfindal, E.T. (1991, April). Impact of specialization on pharmacy education. *American Journal of Hospital Pharmacy, 48,* 700–706.

Manasse, H.R. (1992, January). Facing the future: Issues in pharmacy manpower. *American Pharmacy, 32,* 72–74.

McCombs, J.S., Nichol, M.B. et al. (1995, June). Commentary: Is pharmacy's vision of the future too narrow? *American Journal of Health-System Pharmacy, 52,* 1208–1214.

Miller, W.A. (1990). Agenda for change: The central issues. *American Journal of Pharmaceutical Education, 54,* 341–344.

Miller, W.A., Campbell, W.H. et al. (1991). The choice is influence. The 1991 Argus Commission Report. *American Journal of Pharmaceutical Education, 55,* 8S–11S.

Murawski, M.M., & Miederhoff, P.A. (1994). Pharmaceutical caring. *American Journal of Pharmaceutical Education, 58,* 310–315.

Newton, G.D. (1991). Pharmaceutical education and the translation of pharmaceutical care into practice. *American Journal of Pharmaceutical Education, 55,* 339–344.

Penna, R.P. (1994, November). Commentaries: Creating your future. *American Journal of Hospital Pharmacy, 51,* 2714–2715.

Rough, S.S., Reid-Ganske, L.M. et al. (1996, August). Work redesign and role restructuring in a pharmacy department with pharmacist assistants. *American Journal of Health-System Pharmacists, 53,* 1928–1933.

Schwartz, M.A. (1990). Envisioning pharmacy's future: A further commentary on strategic planning. *American Journal of Pharmaceutical Education, 54,* 167–174.

Schwartz, M.A. (1994, October). Creating pharmacy's future. *American Pharmacy, NS34* (10) 44.

The third strategic planning conference for pharmacy practice: Executive summary. (1995, October). *American Journal of Health-System Pharmacy, 52,* 2217–2233.

Zellmer, W.A. (1995, October). At large: Planning for the future of pharmacy practice. *American Journal of Health-System Pharmacy, 52,* 2362.

Administrative Aspects of Pharmacy Technology

11 The Policy and Procedure Manual

COMPETENCIES

Upon completion and review of this chapter, the student should be able to

1. Define and differentiate a *policy* and a *procedure*.
2. Give five reasons to justify the need for a policy and procedure manual.
3. List the basic format requirements for such a manual.
4. Explain the steps involved in the manual approval process.
5. List five topics that could be included in each of the following pharmacy areas: administrative, distributional, and clinical.
6. Indicate three problems that may be encountered in the interpretation and implementation of departmental policies and procedures.

Introduction

In every organization there are rules or policies to accomplish the objectives of the organization. There are also specific ways in which these policies are to be carried out. These ways of carrying out policies are called *procedures*. The formal definitions are as follows:

■ A policy is a definite course or method of action selected from among alternatives; a high-level, overall plan embracing the general goals and acceptable procedures.

■ A procedure is a particular way of accomplishing something or acting; a series of steps followed in a regular definite order; a traditional or established way of doing things.

In summary, a policy is a decision by an organization or a department to do something; a procedure is a step-by-step method used to accomplish that policy.

Need for Policies and Procedures

When new employees begin work in a pharmacy, there are literally hundreds of things to learn. Not only must the newcomers learn the work, but they must also learn about lunch hours, benefits, hours of operation, the chain of command, what scope of services is provided by the department, and so on. By reading a manual in which policies and procedures are described, new employees should be able to learn a considerable amount about their respective jobs. So the first reason for having a policy and procedure manual is to use it in the training of new employees.

If written policies and procedures did not exist, employees would have to be trained and instructed verbally by other employees. Because not everyone is a good teacher or can explain things fully or clearly, it is helpful to have information in writing in a clear and consistent manner. Therefore, the second reason to have a written policy and procedure manual is to prevent errors from verbal communication.

People handle different situations in different ways. In a pharmacy, however, to ensure that the same accurate and consistent results occur and that people and situations are treated the same way every time, a set way for doings things is established and set forth in a policy and procedure manual. Therefore, another reason for having a policy and procedure manual is consistency—to ensure that the same policy is followed in the same situation all the time.

The pharmacy department uses a large number and variety of drugs and supplies. Although many drugs are expensive, labor and supplies used in compounding, packaging, and labeling in a pharmacy can also comprise a considerable amount of the costs of bringing drugs to patients. If procedures are performed in a consistent, efficient, and economical manner, waste can be minimized. This is accomplished by having thought-out policies and procedures. Thus, a policy and procedure manual can eliminate the waste of both materials and manpower.

A good manager is responsible for seeing that the work is done and that employees are aware of how well they are performing in their jobs. One way in which this is accomplished is through periodic evaluations of personnel job performance (i.e., how well an employee is following procedures). Evaluations can be accomplished only if there are written policies and procedures by which job performance can be measured. Policy and procedure manuals are therefore used to evaluate job performance.

Because of potential harm to patients, pharmacy departments take considerable care to ensure that medications are purchased, stocked, packaged, compounded, labeled, dispensed, administered, and charted accurately. However, in health care, lawsuits are not uncommon and it is sometimes necessary to determine what took place during a specific procedure. Policy and procedure manuals therefore often serve as legal documents in the event of a lawsuit to protect the individual and the institution.

Finally, it must be recognized that pharmacies and hospitals are highly regulated establishments. They are governed by laws, rules, regulations, standards, and guidelines that they must follow. Many of these federal, state, and local regulating agencies require written policies and procedures. During inspections these written policies and procedures must be shown, and therefore it is necessary to ensure that they are accurate and current.

In summary, policy and procedure manuals exist for the following reasons:

- to train new employees or retrain existing employees
- to prevent errors that occur due to verbal communication
- to ensure consistency of policy and job performance
- to eliminate the waste of human resources and materials
- to evaluate job performance
- to serve as legal documents in the event of a lawsuit
- to comply with regulatory and accreditation agencies

An example of an evaluation form for a technician is illustrated in **Figure 11–1.**

EVERBROOK UNIVERSITY HOSPITAL & MEDICAL CENTER

Performance Review

Review Form Name:	Technician
Employee Name:	Joe Technician
Address & Telephone No:	111 Main St._240-5991
Date of Hire:	8/1/98
Employee ID:	1234
Position Number:	99
Position Title:	Technician
Position Code:	1234
Division:	Pharmacy
Last Review Date:	8/1/98
Review Period Start:	8/2/98
Review Period End:	8/1/99
Next Review Date:	8/1/99
Next Review Due By:	Jane Chieftech
Reviewer Title:	Chief Technician

PERFORMANCE ELEMENTS

Personal Appearance   *Meets job requirements*

Joe dresses appropriately for the position and he presents a well-groomed appearance.

Initiative   *Meets job requirements*

Joe is quick to volunteer whenever others need help and he often seeks out additional responsibilities beyond the normal scope of his job. He takes independent actions and appropriate, calculated risks. Joe is resourceful at taking advantage of opportunities. He undertakes self-development activities on his own initiative and he usually indicates when he needs help.

Accountability   *Meets job requirements*

Joe responds promptly and reliably to requests for service and assistance. He follows instructions conscientiously and responds well to management directions. He is usually very punctual and he makes an effort to schedule time off in advance. In most situations, he assumes responsibility for his own actions and outcomes. He usually puts forth extra effort when asked and he generally keeps his commitments without delay or follow-up.

Interpersonal Skills   *Meets job requirements*

Joe regularly displays a positive outlook and pleasant manner. He usually establishes and maintains good working relationships. He exhibits tact and consideration in his relations with others. Joe assists and supports his co-workers. He works cooperatively in group situations and he takes responsibility to help resolve conflicts.

Technical Knowledge   *Meets job requirements*

Joe demonstrates competency in the skills and knowledge required. He learns and applies new skills within the expected time period. He is knowledgeable about current developments in his field and he works within the normal scope of supervision. Joe displays a good understanding of how his job relates to other jobs. He effectively uses the resources and tools available to him.

Accuracy   *Meets job requirements*

The work Joe produces is usually highly accurate and thorough. He displays a strong dedication and commitment to excellence. He looks for ways to improve quality. Joe applies the feedback he receives to improve his performance and he monitors his work to meet quality standards.

Productivity   *Exceeds job requirements*

Joe usually produces more work than expected and he often completes his work ahead of schedule. He demonstrates a strong commitment to increasing productivity and he works at a faster pace than normally expected for the position. Joe strives hard in the achievement of established goals.

Ability to Learn New Skills   *Meets job requirements*

Joe usually adapts well to changes in his job or his work environment. He normally is able to manage competing demands on his time and he generally accepts criticism and feedback well. Joe can adjust his approach or method to fit different situations.

Presentation Skills   *Meets job requirements*

Joe presents information and ideas clearly and persuasively. To better understand others, he listens well, displaying interest and asking questions. He responds well to questions and he has good presentation skills. Joe actively participates in meetings.

MANDATED IN-SERVICE ATTENDANCE & RETENTION

Has completed all mandated in-service education programs.

CONTINUING EDUCATION PARTICIPATION

Has participated in departmental educational programs designed for technicians.

FIGURE 11–1 Technician evaluation form *(continues)*

POSITION-SPECIFIC RESPONSIBILITIES
Complies with position-specific responsibilities as outlined in policies and procedures.
SUMMARY
Meets all required criteria and job requirements.
PLANS FOR IMPROVEMENT
No recommendations at this time.
EMPLOYEE COMMENTS

Employee Acknowledgment
I have reviewed this document and discussed the contents with my manager. My signature means that I have been advised of my performance status and does not necessarily imply that I agree with the evaluation.

_____
Employee Signature/Date

REVIEWER COMMENTS

_____
Reviewer Signature/Date

FIGURE 11–1 Technician evaluation form *(continued)*

Composing a Policy and Procedure Manual

Let us now examine how the policy and procedure manuals are written and what information can be found in a pharmacy department's manual.

Format

To avoid confusion and for the sake of consistency, it is best if all policies and procedures follow a similar **format.** Some institutions use special preprinted blank forms on which to write their policies and procedures. Most institutions, however, follow some kind of standard format that contains the information required. Let us examine some of the items that should be part of every policy and procedure manual.

Title

First, every policy and procedure should have a title. This tells the reader what subject is covered in the policy and procedure. This title is also used in a **table of contents** or an **index.** Examples of policy and procedure titles include "Hours of Operation," "Drug Recalls," "Labeling of Outpatient Prescriptions," and "Organizational Chart—Pharmacy Services."

Date

Every policy and procedure should be dated. Initially, a date of implementation indicates when the policy and procedure went into effect. Often, however, it is necessary to change, update, expand, or modify an existing policy and/or procedure. Therefore, additional dates indicate when the policy and/or procedure was revised. These dates often also appear on the specific policy and/or procedure. Many institutions use just the original and latest revision dates. For example:

Approved and Implemented: 1-19-99
Revised: 10-25-99

Occasionally some departments use a code for a date composed of the year (two digits), the month (two digits), the day (two digits), and a letter (*A* for the first policy prepared that day, *B* for the second, etc.). For example, the second policy and procedure prepared on October 25, 1999, would be coded with the alphanumeric: 991025B.

Some hospitals use a classification number or letters on each policy so that the particular department, type of policy, and other facts can be determined from this information. Unless the system is easy to understand, however, it can often confuse staff members.

Signatures

Polices and procedures should also contain at least two signatures. The first should be the originator of the policy and procedure, most often the administrative pharmacist who is responsible for a specific area of the pharmacy where the policy and procedure is most frequently carried out. The second should be the director or associate director who is responsible for the area in which the policy and procedure will be followed and enforced. These signatures are valuable because they indicate who is the person responsible for generating the policy and procedure and document the agreement of the administrative personnel on the highest level.

Many policies and procedures affect other departments as well. These policies and procedures should also bear the approving signature of an administrative person in that department to ensure agreement and cooperation. For example, pharmacy department policies and procedures on the requisitioning, distribution, control, and documentation of controlled substances should bear the signature of the director of nursing services. Similar policies regarding controlled substances to anesthesia personnel should bear the signature of the director of anesthesia. Policies and procedures that involve the monitoring of food-drug interactions should bear the endorsing signature of the director of the department of food and nutrition services.

Formal statement of policy

The body of the policy and procedure must contain the formal statement of policy, and is usually followed by the step-by-step, logical, and detailed procedure for carrying out that policy. Sometimes background material is included to explain why the policy exists. The body of a policy and procedure should designate the person who is responsible for carrying out the policy and procedure and the administrative staff titles of those responsible to ensure proper compliance. This section clearly delineates the chain of command and the responsibility for ensuring compliance. For example, policies and procedures carried out by staff personnel are supervised by a pharmacy supervisor or assistant director.

If possible, all policies and procedures should be prepared using the same typewriter or computer printer to ensure a uniform and consistent appearance. It has been suggested that a useful policy and procedure manual must answer the following questions regarding a specific activity.

- What must be done?
- Who should do it?
- How should it be done?
- When should it be done?

Figure 11–2 is an example of a format used in a large teaching hospital. This format has a place for all the elements described previously.

THE EVERBROOK UNIVERSITY HOSPITAL
AND MEDICAL CENTER
DEPARTMENT OF PHARMACY SERVICES
POLICY AND PROCEDURE MANUAL

CODE NAME: JDPHMTEK.ADM	SUBJECT: PHARMACY TECHNICIAN - JOB DESCRIPTION	
PREPARED BY: L. ZUCKER	REVISED BY: S. KATZ	APPROVED BY:
ORIGINAL DATE OF ISSUE: MAY 9, 1986	REVISION DATE: AUGUST 6, 1999	TOTAL PAGES: 4

A. **POSITION SUMMARY**

Pharmacy technicians (also referred to as pharmacy specialists) are paraprofessional members of our pharmacy department. After training and verification of competencies in sterile technique, unit dose distribution, packaging, unit inspections, brand and generic names, and pharmacy calculations, persons in this position perform routine, manipulative and supportive tasks as allowed by New York State Law under the close supervision of a licensed pharmacist. This frees the pharmacist to provide more clinical services.

B. **POSITION REPORTS TO**

The Assistant Director of Pharmacy for Training and Research is the immediate supervisor of the technicians; however, they may also be supervised by any member of the administrative group while working in various pharmacy areas.

C. **AREAS OF SPECIALIZATION**

Prepackaging, inventory control, centralized and decentralized pharmacy distribution, sterile product preparation, and miscellaneous supportive functions.

D. **MAJOR DUTIES AND RESPONSIBILITIES**

1. Prepackaging Area Responsibilities
   The pharmacy technician will
   1.1 Initiate prepackaging protocols.
   1.2 Prepackage medication using unit-dose and bulk packaging equipment under the supervision of a pharmacist.
   1.3 Make labels for packaged medication using labeling equipment under the supervision of a pharmacist.
   1.4. Complete all required packaging records.
   1.5. Ensure that all policies and procedures are followed and counterchecked by a pharmacist to avoid errors.
   1.6. Service and maintain equipment.
   1.7. Keep equipment clean and properly stored.
   1.8. Service label printing machine.
   1.9. Ensure that work is checked by a registered pharmacist and released by an Assistant Director.
   1.10. Perform routine quality control as per policy and procedures.
   1.11. Prepare dilutions of soaps and antiseptics as per established protocol.

2. Inventory Control Responsibilities
   The pharmacy technician will
   2.1 Review storage area and prepare the prepackaging inventory sheets.
   2.2 Order stock and supplies from the storeroom in the main Pharmacy for pharmacy areas in which they are working on a regularly scheduled basis.
   2.3 Deliver completed stock orders from the main pharmacy to the satellites and other pharmacy areas.
   2.4 Place the stock orders on the shelves and drawers in the satellite pharmacy areas.

FIGURE 11–2 Job description for pharmacy technician (continues)

2.5 Check the inventory in the pharmacy areas regularly for outdated medications, return outdated items to the main pharmacy, and make sure that all items are stored according to light and temperature requirements.

2.6 Inform the Assistant Director of the appropriate area if bulk items are not available for prepackaging and make out reorder cards for out-of-stock items.

3. Centralized and Decentralized Satellite Pharmacy Responsibilities
   According to the "Pharmacy Handbook" September, 1994, Section 29.7 (22)(i), unlicensed persons may assist a pharmacist in the dispensing of drugs by
   3.1 Receiving written prescriptions.
   3.2 Typing prescription labels.
   3.3 Keying prescription data for entry into a computer-generated file or retrieving prescription data from the file in accordance with the above stated provisions.
   3.4 Getting drugs from stock and returning them to stock.
   3.5 Getting prescription files and other manual records from storage, and locating prescriptions.
   3.6 Counting dosage units of drugs.
   3.7 Placing dosage units of drugs in appropriate containers.
   3.8 Affixing the prescription label to the containers.
   3.9 Preparing manual records of dispensing for the signature or initials of the pharmacists.
   3.10 Handling or delivering completed prescriptions to the patient or the patient's agent.
   3.11 Filling patient cassette drawers from a written order.

4. Sterile Products Preparation
   4.1 The technician shall prepare sterile products (e.g., total parenteral nutrition solutions, antineoplastics and intravenous admixtures) under aseptic conditions following established protocols. Technicians shall also display the following skills and perform the following related tasks:
       4.1.1 Proof of knowledge and ability. This will be ensured by preliminary training and testing by the area Assistant Directors.
       4.1.2 All nonjudgmental aspects of maintaining the sterile product areas in the pharmacy shall be undertaken by the technician, e.g.,
           4.1.2.1 Clean and maintain sterility of laminar-flow hoods.
           4.1.2.2 Assist in sterility testing.
           4.1.2.3 Replenish supplies as needed.
   4.2. Prepare labeling for admixtures.
       4.2.1 Primary labeling and calculations of flow rate for routine volumes according to protocol. The technicians must ensure that all labels and calculations are countersigned by a registered pharmacist.
       4.2.2 Providing auxiliary labeling according to protocol.

5. Miscellaneous
   The pharmacy technician will also have responsibilities that include, but are not limited to
   5.1 Rounding to the patient care units to pick up stat and regularly scheduled physician medication orders.
   5.2 Delivering patient unit floor stock medications to the areas covered by satellite service.
   5.3 Delivering stat and regularly scheduled medications to the patient care units serviced by satellite pharmacies.
   5.4 Preparation and profiling of premature nursery oral syringes as per protocol and assurance that the above are checked by a pharmacist.
   5.5 Maintaining par level medications for patient units including, but not limited to, the neonatal nursery.
   5.6 Making emergency trips to the main pharmacy to pick up medications required by the satellite pharmacists.
   5.7 Delivering controlled drug floor stock in sealed bags to the nursing stations serviced by the satellite pharmacies on designated controlled drug requisition days.

FIGURE 11–2 Job description for pharmacy technician *(continued)*

5.8 Performing nursing unit inspections as delegated to do so.

5.9 The pharmacy technician will perform other delegated duties assigned to him/her that are in accordance with New York State Pharmacy Laws and Regulations.

6. Education Inservice

The technician will

6.1. Undergo periodic evaluations and training on new equipment, machinery, or techniques used in the pharmacy.

6.2 Attend all in-service education seminars held for pharmacy technicians and nonpharmacist personnel to develop and maintain his/her competency in assisting the pharmacist (e.g., I.V. additives, reconstitution of oral and parenteral medications, prepackaging of medications, and reviewing physician orders) if present.

6.3 Give at least one (1) in-service per year or more than one per year if so scheduled.

6.4 Participate in all pharmacy technician journal clubs.

E. SCOPE AND EFFECT ON WORK

The performance of the above tasks directly affects the internal daily operation of the department and alleviates the pharmacist of much of the routine manipulative and non-judgmental tasks involved in many pharmacy department activities, allowing the pharmacist more time for clinical work.

F. SUPERVISION RECEIVED

1. The technician works under the direct supervision of a licensed pharmacist who has the final responsibility for all the technician's activities.

2. The technician is supervised by the pharmacy department's administrative staff.

G. EXPERIENCE REQUIRED

Experience in a hospital pharmacy is highly desired and experience in community pharmacy is helpful; however, neither are required.

H. PROFESSIONAL AND EDUCATIONAL REQUIREMENTS

1. The technician must be a high school graduate.

2. The technician must have completed an acceptable technician training program, or must have completed or be enrolled in some higher education program. Requirements of the above programs are as follows:

2.1 Technician Training Program

2.1.1 The training program must be formal and structured. It must be a minimum of five (5) months and 600 hours duration of course work and/or workshops.

2.1.2 The training program must have included the following:

2.1.2.1 Sterile Product Formulation (preparation)

2.1.2.2 Unit-Dose Medication Distribution Systems

2.1.2.3 Pharmaceutical Calculations

2.1.2.4 Pharmacology

2.1.2.5 Printing, Packaging, and Labeling

2.2 Higher Education Program - must be accepted by the administrative staff.

3. An associate degree is desirable, but not required.

FIGURE 11–2 Job description for pharmacy technician *(continued)*

In summary, policies and procedures should follow a uniform appearance and format, have meaningful titles; possess dates of approval, implementation, and revision; be signed by the appropriate personnel; and be clear and logical.

The Approval Process

In most hospitals, the Pharmacy and Therapeutics Committee serves as the liaison between the medical staff and the department of pharmacy services. The Joint Commission on Accreditation of Healthcare Organization (JCAHO) requires that the Pharmacy and Therapeutics Committee annually review and approve the policies and procedures of the pharmacy department. Although some pharmacy departments indicate the approval of the Pharmacy and Therapeutics Committee on each policy and procedure itself, most pharmacy departments use a cover page at the beginning of the manual which indicates all approvals. Additional approvals may also come from such individuals as the administrator responsible for the pharmacy department and/or the hospital's chief executive officer, as well as the chairman of the hospital's medical board.

Many hospitals or other health care institutions have a subcommittee of the Pharmacy and Therapeutics Committee that deals with medication procedures and also serves as a pharmacy-nursing liaison committee. Many policies and procedures dealing with medication distribution, control, administration, and documentation are developed by the nursing and pharmacy department members of this committee jointly. The minutes of these meetings are then approved by the parent Pharmacy and Therapeutics Committee. Therefore, approval of many policies and procedures are accomplished before formal implementation.

Policies and procedures developed jointly with other departments should also have a unique and consistent format. Often different professional services utilize drastically different formats for structuring and filing their policies and procedures. Because the recent trend by the JCAHO is to have patient-focused standards, they have shifted the emphasis from individual department standards to one that concentrates on the needs of the patient. They therefore are more concerned with the services provided to patients rather than which specific professional provides the care. This focus, therefore, encourages a multidisciplinary approach to patient care and the development of policies and procedures that involve several disciplines.

Figure 11–3 is an example of a multidisciplinary policy and procedure format with space for three professional departments. Each department has a space for its code numbers in its specific system of filing. Every hospital department must be diligent in ensuring that all policies and procedures comply with governmental regulations and laws and that they are consistent with the requirements of all accrediting agencies.

Contents of a Policy and Procedure Manual

The format and contents of a policy and procedure manual will vary from hospital to hospital. In some institutions there may be two manuals: a policy and procedure manual (containing hospital-wide policies and procedures) and an **operational manual** (containing only those policies and procedures that affect the internal workings of the pharmacy department). Under such a system it is often confusing where a particular policy and procedure is to be found. Such a system has fallen into disfavor in recent years.

**THE EVERBROOK UNIVERSITY HOSPITAL
AND MEDICAL CENTER**
MULTIDISCIPLINARY POLICY & PROCEDURE

SUBJECT:	PAGE OF

ORIGINAL:	REVISED:	REVISED:	REVISED:
DEPARTMENT:			
CODE NAME:			
SECTION:			

POLICY:

PROCEDURE:

FIRST PAGE

THE EVERBROOK UNIVERSITY HOSPITAL AND MEDICAL CENTER

MULTIDISCIPLINARY POLICY AND PROCEDURE

SUBJECT:	CODE:
	PAGE: OF

DISTRIBUTION:

REFERENCE:

INDEX:

LAST PAGE

FIGURE 11–3 Multidisciplinary policy and procedure format

The most common methods for organizing policy and procedure manuals fall into two main groups. The first has policies and procedures placed in a book in alphabetical order by title, for example, Abbreviations; Absenteeism; Administrative Services; Alcohol, Dispensing, and Control; Ambulatory Care; and Assay and Quality Control.

A second, more common method of organizing a manual is to group policies and procedures into categories and then divide the manual into separate sections for each category. Two examples of this format are outlined here.

The first example involves a format that is composed of five major categories.

■ *Section I: Organization.* This section contains information on the hospital itself; organizational charts for both the hospital and the department; services offered; pharmacy department participation on hospital committees (e.g.,

Pharmacy and Therapeutics Committee, the infection control committee.); interdepartmental relationships, and so forth.

■ *Section II: Personnel Policies.* This section contains job descriptions; staffing information; policies on benefits, holidays, sick leave, disciplinary procedures, payroll periods, vacations, medical and maternity leaves, educational benefits, and so forth.

■ *Section III: Administrative Policies.* This section contains policies and procedures on the department's hours of operation; purchasing policies and procedures; inventory control; drug charging to patients, employees, and third parties; interdepartmental requisitions; alcohol and controlled drug record keeping; administrative reports; annual reports; statistics gathered; and so forth.

■ *Section IV: Professional Policies.* These policies and procedures involve the compounding, labeling, packaging, dispensing, and control of medications; patient profiles; drug therapy monitoring; pharmacokinetics consultation services; drug information services; investigational drugs; drug ordering; automatic stop orders; in-service education services; antineoplastic, parenteral nutrition, and intravenous admixture services; and so forth.

■ *Section V: Facilities and Equipment.* These policies and procedures pertain to the use and maintenance of the department's physical facilities and equipment, their maintenance and repair, service contracts, requisitioning, and security.

This system requires a comprehensive table of contents and/or index so that any policy and procedure can be easily and readily located.

A second system that has been recently developed uses only three main sections for all policies and procedures: Administrative, Distributional, and Clinical.

The **administrative section** contains those policies and procedures that pertain to the operation of the department, its personnel, and its place within the total organizational structure of the hospital. Policies and procedures that fall into this category include the following:

■ job descriptions
■ confidentiality of records
■ hospital table of organization
■ department table of organization
■ formulary operation
■ infection control
■ incident reporting
■ personnel policies
■ continuing education
■ personnel evaluations
■ quality assurance
■ orientation of personnel
■ telephone operation
■ others, depending on the institution and/or department

The **distributional section** contains those policies and procedures that deal with the acquisition, storage, ordering, dispensing, documentation, and disposition of drugs and supplies. Examples include the following:

■ drug ordering
■ unit-dose drug distribution
■ pharmacy services to specialty areas
■ dispensing to ambulatory patients
■ sterile product preparation and dispensing

- compounding and manufacturing
- emergency boxes and crash carts
- investigational drugs
- interdepartmental requisitions

The **clinical section** contains those activities involved in patient-related monitoring and other activities of a clinical nature. Examples include the following:

- clinical monitoring of profiles
- discharge counseling
- interaction screening
- drug information services
- thrombolytic monitoring and control
- pharmacokinetic consultations

This system lends itself well to the use of electronic data processing. Traditional computer operating systems permit files to be saved using the 8-3 system, that is, eight letters (or select symbols), a period, and then three additional letters. Each policy and procedure is given a file name that ends in an appropriate three-letter designation that computer operating systems allow for file names. In the 8-3 system, the three last letters permit policies and procedures to use the following: "ADM" for administrative policies and procedures, "DIS" for distributional policies and procedures, and "CLN" for clinical policies and procedures. The use of such file names permits easy backup and the sorting of files by major categories.

Distribution

A policy and procedure manual is a dynamic entity, as it is constantly changing. Policies and procedures are being revised, added, or deleted on a continuing basis. Therefore, the more copies of a manual that are available, the more difficult it is to keep each issue current. A copy of the policy and procedure manual, however, should be readily available to every employee, so that it may be used as a reference in handling both new and repeat situations. A copy should be available in every pharmacy area to ensure easy access. In addition, a number of copies should be available for the orientation of new employees.

In hospitals where pharmacy departments have a modern computerized information system, it is now possible to place the policy and procedure manual on the system's computer network. This permits access to the policy and procedure manual from any terminal and makes updating the policy and procedure manual quick and easy since the network file can be easily modified. Individuals can also generate a hard copy of any policy and procedure when necessary.

Updates to the policy and procedure manual should indicate if the new policy and procedure being distributed is a revision of an existing policy and procedure or a completely new policy and procedure. If it is a revision, it should indicate which policy and procedure it is replacing. Many hospitals put a cover sheet at the front of the manual on which revisions and updates are indicated. A space is provided for the signature of the person who placed the update in the manual.

In addition to this procedure some hospital pharmacies post each new policy and procedure on a bulletin board, with a signature sheet. Each employee is expected to review the posted policy and procedure and sign the posted sheet. The sheets are then filed. A permanent record is maintained showing that the employee has acknowledged the policy and procedure. If the institution has a good e-mail system, staff can be alerted to a new or revised policy and procedure in that manner.

Problems

In addition to the problem regarding distribution, policy and procedure manuals have other problems relating to their successful use. First, if policies and procedures have no method to ensure enforcement, they have no value. It is therefore necessary for all employees to understand the reason behind each policy and procedure. Supervisory personnel must ensure that policies and procedures are followed. If particular policies and procedures are not being followed, the supervisor must determine if they should be changed for some reason or if disciplinary action is warranted. At times, policies and procedures are very difficult to accomplish under certain circumstances. In this case, each employee has an obligation to bring this matter to the attention of supervisory personnel so that the procedure can be modified. Many times there are valid reasons for not following a particular procedure. Unforseen circumstances may require recourse to an alternative action.

Another major problem with policy and procedure manuals involves their update and distribution. In the past, modification on any one part of a long policy and procedure often meant that the entire policy and procedure had to be retyped, then photocopied and distributed. The advent of the relatively low-cost **personal computer (PC)** has changed this procedure significantly. Many pharmacy departments today maintain their policy and procedure manuals on computer disks or on the hard disks that are an integral part of the computer. Computer disks, also referred to as "floppy disks," can easily be duplicated so that copies can be transported and utilized in any other computer in which the common software program resides.

When policies and procedures are stored on a computer disk, they can be readily retrieved and modified in any way, and a revised copy can be printed out. Word-processing software programs permit easy changes, deletions, insertions, and other modifications of any policy and procedure. The newly revised policy and procedure are then stored on the computer disk in place of the old. Additional copies of the revised policy and procedure can be generated, if necessary, or can be photocopied and distributed. Making the policy and procedures available on a computer network simplifies any changes.

The newer computers use small 3½″ disks that can hold approximately 75 to 100 typewritten pages, more than enough for most policy and procedure manuals. Recently disks and disk drives with two to ten times that capacity have become available. Internal hard disks are now standard and can accommodate many thousands of typewritten pages.

As the utilization of computers has increased, costs have decreased. Therefore, computers have become almost universal. Presently it is estimated there are over 100 million personal computers in use and millions more larger computers and terminals being utilized. This growth has led to a trend of placing the policy and procedure manual into the computer's memory where it can readily be accessed by any user, at any time. As a result, except for a master copy, there may be no written policy and procedure manual at all. In these cases, security must be considered. The ability to modify any policy and procedure on a personal computer or computer network must be limited to authorized personnel.

One additional problem that many pharmacy departments must address concerns "memos" versus "policies and procedures." When some new activity or service begins or if there is a modification of some long-standing activity or procedure, there is often a tendency to send out a memorandum instead of finding, updating, and distributing the appropriate policy and procedure. Memorandums are easy to generate, often take only a few minutes, and do not require the thought and effort needed to revise a policy and procedure. However, they are just as easily discarded, do not become part of the official departmental manual, and tend to make the appropriate policy and procedure obsolete and useless. Therefore, what may appear to be the easier way of handling a change should be avoided in favor of the more efficient and established way of revising the policy and procedure in question.

Summary

Policy and procedure manuals that are comprehensive and current are necessary and useful tools in the proper management of any well-managed organization. They should be current and dynamic because the roles and responsibilities of the department change. They should be viewed as helpful guides in providing efficient and consistent service to the patients and staff whom the pharmacy department serves.

ASSESSMENT

Multiple Choice Questions

1. A policy is
   a. a series of steps to follow in a definite order
   b. a traditional way of doing things
   c. a high-level overall plan
   d. an educated way of accomplishing a task
   e. all of the above

2. A procedure is
   a. a step-by-step method used to carry out a direction
   b. a decision to do something
   c. a plan of general goals
   d. a and b
   e. a, b, and c

3. New employees must become familiar with
   a. the work (job description)
   b. the hours of work
   c. the benefits
   d. the chain of command
   e. all of the above

4. Policy and procedure manuals are used to
   a. train and inform new employees
   b. prevent errors from verbal communications
   c. ensure that the same policy is followed in the same situation
   d. serve as legal documents in the event of a lawsuit
   e. all of the above

5. Which of the following is not true regarding policy and procedural manuals?
   a. Many regulating agencies require written policies and procedures.
   b. Any change requires approval of the chief operating officer of the institution.
   c. They prevent waste of manpower, time, and materials by providing direction in repetitive tasks.

   d. They provide a new employee with valuable information about his/her new job.

   e. They ensure accuracy and consistency in routine operational activities.

True/False Questions

6. _____ Policy and procedural manuals are used to evaluate job performance.

7. _____ Every policy and procedure should have a title.

8. _____ Policies and procedures should be signed by all persons affected by the policy.

9. _____ Every 5 years the members of the Pharmacy and Therapeutics Committee review and update the manual.

10. _____ Technicians should be familiar with policies and procedures that pertain to the administrative and technical aspects of the manual.

Matching

11. _____ operational manual

12. _____ policy

13. _____ memo

14. _____ policy and procedure manual

15. _____ procedure

   a. guidelines that contain goals and methods of carrying out the goals

   b. a particular way of acting

   c. a directive in message form

   d. overall plan of general goals

   e. internal workings of the pharmacy department

Bibliography

Brown, T. R. (Ed.). (1992). *Handbook of institutional pharmacy practice* (3rd ed.). Bethesda, MD: American Society of Health-System Pharmacists.

Hospital pharmacy management: Forms, checklists & guidelines. (1992). Aspen Reference Group, Kenneth E. Lawrence, Director. Frederick, MD: Aspen Publishers.

Hospital pharmacy policy and procedure manual. (1985). Tarzana, CA: AMI Pharmacy Management Services.

Policy and procedure manual of the Department of Pharmacy Services of the Brookdale University Hospital and Medical Center. (1998). Seymour Katz, M.S., R.Ph., FASHP, Director. Brooklyn, NY.

Trudeau, T. (Ed.). (annual). *Topics in hospital pharmacy management.* Frederick, MD: Aspen Publishers.

12 Materials Management of Pharmaceuticals

COMPETENCIES

Upon completion and review of this chapter, the student should be able to

1. List the functions involved in the drug procurement process in the institutional pharmacy.

2. Explain the major methods used to distribute drugs in the hospital.

3. Describe the function of the Pharmacy and Therapeutics Committee in drug selection.

4. Distinguish between generic drugs and brand-name drugs.

5. Enumerate the seven basic principles that are essential for group purchasing.

6. List the records/reports required to be maintained in the materials management section.

7. State the information that must be included in a pharmacy purchase order.

8. Describe checkpoints to be observed when a drug order is received in the hospital.

9. List the environmental considerations required in the storage of drugs.

10. Define the following temperature requirements for drug storage: cold, cool, room temperature, warm, and excessive heat.

11. Name the drugs and pharmaceutical products that require special safety precautions.

12. Calculate an inventory turnover rate, and state the desirable turnover level range.

Introduction

This chapter will address the methods used to select, acquire, and organize a drug inventory for institutional use; describe the various systems of drug distribution and control; recognize the impact of cost-containment strategies used by pharmacy personnel; and describe the scope of activities that can be assumed by qualified pharmacy technicians.

Health care costs, at both the federal and state levels, have increased more rapidly than any other category of products or services used in our society. Private insurance companies and government agencies have been overwhelmed with requests for payment of expensive charges for state-of-the-art diagnostic procedures and sophisticated treatments and therapies. The costs associated with pharmaceuticals continue to increase at astronomical rates, due to a constant flow of costly new **bioengineered therapies** resulting from advances in research and to sophisticated marketing programs. As a result of increased costs for health care services and a decrease in resources to pay for them, it has become essential for pharmacy department managers to assess cost containment in all aspects of pharmacy service.

The objective of this chapter is to identify and describe the methods used by pharmacy personnel to deliver the appropriate drug to the right patient, at the right time, and at the most reasonable cost. Another way of stating this objective is, "to identify pharmacy services that are both effective and affordable."

Controlling the costs associated with a complete pharmacy service includes not only the acquisition cost of drugs but also the total cost of the "managing" materials. An institutional pharmacy **materials management** program includes the following:

- *Procurement*—drug selection, source selection, cost analysis, group purchasing, **prime vendor** relationships, purchasing procedures, record keeping, and receiving control.
- *Drug storage and inventory control*—storage conditions, security requirements, proper rotation of inventory, computerized inventory control
- *Repackaging and labeling considerations*—unit-dose and extemporaneous packaging, labeling requirements
- *Distribution systems*—unit-dose, floor stock, compounded prescriptions, intravenous admixtures, emergency drugs
- *Recapture and disposal*—unused medication, returns and reuse, environmental considerations

In a hospital the overall responsibility for the materials management of pharmaceuticals lies with the director of the pharmacy department. The Pharmacy and Therapeutics Committee selects drugs and therapeutic agents that are to be available in the institution. This committee is chaired by physicians who are appointed by the medical board, and the secretary is the director of the pharmacy services. The committee consists of representatives from the medical board, the pharmacy, nursing, and dietary departments, quality assurance, and the hospital administration. It is essential to have the clinical and technical knowledge of pharmacists, physicians, and nurses available when making decisions regarding which drug products should be included in the formulary to ensure adequate and appropriate therapy.

The director of pharmacy delegates certain aspects of the pharmacy materials management program to trained pharmacy personnel to deliver effective and efficient pharmacy services. The official list of drugs available is known as the hospital formulary, which is reviewed and modified on an ongoing basis as required.

Procurement

Drug Selection

The drug selection process may begin with a physician's request for a new drug. The pharmacist processes the request and prepares an objective review of the medication requested. If the drug required is similar to other drugs on the formulary, it is important to determine if the benefits justify admission to the formulary. Guidelines for the evaluation of drugs are provided by the ASHP Technical Assistance Bulletin on the Evaluation of Drugs for Formularies (Appendix C).

The pharmacy department's objective review includes cost analysis information—an important factor in this age of cost containment. The Pharmacy and Therapeutics Committee considers how much a drug costs per dose, per day, or even per treatment cycle. The decision regarding whether to add a new drug to the formulary is not based solely on whether it is a better therapeutic agent but whether the perceived benefit is worth the additional cost (cost-benefit analysis). The pharmacy department's research and presentation can have a profound effect on whether a new drug is added to the hospital formulary.

The most cost-effective materials management programs are the result of combining the required expertise and specialty knowledge of a pharmacist with the materials management and systems expertise of a trained pharmacy technician. The pharmacist selects the brands or generic equivalents that are acceptable. The trained pharmacy technician may negotiate price, monitor inventory levels, input purchase order and receiving information into a computer system or manual record-keeping system, and organize inventory. Under supervision of the pharmacist, the technician will fill and deliver floor stock orders, repackage medication for unit-dose distribution, and may inspect medication storage areas for proper environmental conditions. The degree of supervision by a pharmacist will vary, depending on the ability of the technician and the policy of the pharmacy department. The pharmacist responsible for materials management supervises the entire process.

Source Selection

Another aspect of procurement deals with source selection. One aspect of source selection deals with the concept of **generic drugs** versus **brand-name drugs.** The pharmacist determines if the generic product is a **therapeutic equivalent** of the brand-name product and then makes the source selection.

The Food and Drug Administration regulates the manufacturing of generic drug products to make every effort to ensure therapeutic efficacy. To minimize therapeutic inadequacies, the pharmacist carefully considers the reputation of the generic drug manufacturer and reviews drug analysis data and information. Although cost savings associated with the use of generic drugs have proven to be of great value, selection is made on quality assurance of the product. Therapeutic equivalence is sometimes difficult to ascertain. However, the reputation of the generic manufacturer and an ongoing surveillance of the professional literature assist the pharmacist in determining if the amount of savings realized by purchasing a generic drug is cost-justified. Guidelines are provided by the ASHP Guidelines for Selecting Pharmaceutical Manufacturers and Suppliers (Appendix C).

Cost Analysis

Source selection also includes cost considerations. Drug product cost analysis is an essential step in assessing cost-containment strategies. Information regarding acquisition cost of the product is readily available and a price comparison of therapeutically equivalent drugs can be studied. Nonacquisition costs may include costs related to storage, time required to prepare products for patient use, and even packaging considerations. Nonacquisition costs include those related to getting the medication to the patient, not simply getting the drug to the pharmacy.

Group Purchasing and Prime-Vendor Relationships

Group purchasing and prime-vendor relationships are two important strategies utilized in an attempt to control the purchase price of drugs. In general, as a result of group purchasing, the unit cost of a drug is lowered as the projected quantity of the drug to be purchased is increased. Simply stated, group purchasing allows each participating hospital the benefit of quantity discounts as a result of pooling the projected quantities of each hospital and negotiating one contract that applies to all participating members. The seven basic principles that are essential for group purchasing to be effective are as follows:

1. Most hospitals should have generic formularies allowing across-the-board evaluation opportunities to all vendors.
2. All group members should be committed to buy from the awarded agreement.
3. The group should normally award each item to only one supplier.
4. A pharmacy committee should be established to ensure thorough product quality and vendor review. The pharmacy committee, when it addresses issues for the entire group, can direct the group to many years of successful agreements.
5. The management of individual hospitals should support group programs, especially pharmacy purchasing.
6. The group director should maintain open communication with vendors through newsletters, cooperation in dealing with compliance issues, and approval of regular visits.
7. The group should be willing and able to consider the addition of new products to the bid.

A prime-vendor relationship allows the pharmacy to reduce the size of inventory. This reduction frees dollars to pay other outstanding debts or to pay bills on time, which will minimize the amount of costly premiums associated with late payments. This is accomplished when the pharmacy department purchases as many products as possible from one single supply source, usually a drug wholesaler. A drug wholesaler can make same-day deliveries, and acts as a local warehouse and distributor for various manufacturers. Some manufacturers maintain their own direct shipment service as well as a wholesaler distribution program, whereas others distribute exclusively through wholesalers thereby eliminating the need for their own distribution facilities.

Purchasing Procedures

Most wholesalers sell products at established contract prices plus an additional handling fee that can vary from –2 percent to 4 percent depending on the payment terms established with the hospital. The shorter the payment period, the lower the wholesaler markup. Prepayment schedules are usually necessary to realize discounts. If the hospital minimizes the markup charge by maintaining an efficient accounts payable schedule, the cost benefits realized from reducing the pharmacy inventory will far outweigh the additional cost associated with the wholesaler's fee. The following questions will assist the pharmacy technician to understand the intricacies of purchasing pharmaceuticals:

1. Is a single-brand purchasing policy in effect for the pharmacy department?
2. Has the Pharmacy and Therapeutics Committee approved a written generic substitution policy?
3. Has the Pharmacy and Therapeutics Committee approved a written therapeutic substitution policy?
4. Is competitive bidding used for high-cost items? For high-volume items?

5. Is either of these methods used to set prices: guarantee of bid prices or price ceiling set for the term of the contract?
6. Are the following considered when evaluating bids: prompt payment discount, terms of payment, nonperformance penalties, delivery time limitations, returned and damaged goods policy and services?
7. Are contracts negotiated when appropriate?
8. Are contracts renegotiated on a regular basis (e.g., annually)?
9. Is group purchasing used when advantageous?
10. If group purchasing is used:
    a. Are prices guaranteed?
    b. Is there a mechanism for determining that group prices are competitive?
11. Are primary wholesalers or wholesale contracts used for specific drugs when appropriate?
12. Are the wholesaler costs equal to or less than the costs of purchasing the same drugs directly? (Consider all factors such as increased investment revenues, decreased number of purchase orders, reduced inventory value, and receiving costs.)
13. Have inventories been adequately reduced?
14. Have ordering and receiving costs been adequately reduced?
15. Do outages that require payment of premium prices occur frequently?
16. Are there frequent outages?
17. Are volume discounts evaluated for net savings before purchase (i.e., gross savings minus increased carrying cost)?

Record Keeping

The pharmacy department must also establish and maintain adequate records to meet government regulations, standards of practice requirements, accreditation standards, hospital policies, and management information requirements. These records include budget reports, productivity and workload documents, purchase orders, inventory, receiving and dispensing reports, and controlled substances and alcohol records. The pharmacy's materials manager should be intimately involved with the development and maintenance of many of these documents.

The purchase order

The purchase order document should be prepared at the time the order is placed by telephone, mail, computer, or fax. The information included on the purchase order includes the following:

- the name and address of the hospital
- the shipping address
- the date the order was placed
- the vendor's name and address
- the purchase order number
- the ordering department's name and location
- the expected date of delivery
- shipping terms (e.g., FOB, Net 30)
- the account number or billing designation
- a description of items ordered
- the quantity of items ordered
- the unit price
- the extended price
- the total price of the order
- the buyer's name and phone number

Receiving Control

Accepting the responsibility for receiving drugs for the pharmacy department is another important role that can be filled by the pharmacy technician. When receiving deliveries, the pharmacy technician should follow these basic rules.

- Check the shipping address to be sure the package received was intended for delivery to the pharmacy department.
- Check the outside of the package for visible signs of damage to the carton or the contents. Note any damage on the receiving document before you sign for the delivery.
- Look for any shipping documents attached to the outside of the package and determine if special handling is required (e.g., store in freezer; controlled substance).
- Carefully open the package and check each item for breakage.
- Check each item for expiration date and make note of any short-dated material for immediate use or return.
- Verify the order received against a copy of the purchase order. Make a notation of any variation. Refer to the shipping document or packing slip to determine if items are back ordered or out of stock.
- Refer any order discrepancies to the supervising pharmacist.

Complete accountability of drugs from receiving to patient administration requires a tightly controlled, coordinated effort on the part of all pharmacy and nursing personnel.

All drugs should be delivered directly to the pharmacy department or a secured pharmacy receiving area to prevent diversion of drug orders. Controlled substance and tax-free alcohol require special handling and must be closely supervised by a licensed pharmacist to minimize loss or adulteration. The pharmacist prepares purchase orders, receives and secures shipments, and monitors the inventory of controlled substances and tax-free alcohol. These practices are required by law in most states.

Drug Storage and Inventory Control

Storage

After drugs have been selected, ordered, and received, they must be properly stored. Appropriate storage requires environmental considerations, security issues, and safety requirements.

The inventory may be divided into an active drug inventory and a backup storeroom inventory for large, bulky items that require much space. The inventory may also be divided by how the drugs will be used. For example, parenteral medication for intravenous (I.V.) administration may be stored in the I.V. admixture room only.

Environmental consideration

Environmental considerations include proper temperature, ventilation, humidity, light, and sanitation. Standards have been developed and are referenced in various statutes as a basis for determining appropriate storage requirements since they affect strength, quality, purity, packaging, and labeling of drugs and related articles. These important standards are contained in a combined publication that is recognized as the official compendium, the *United States Pharmacopeia* (U.S.P.) and the *National Formulary* (N.F.).

For example, the U.S.P. defines *controlled room temperature* as the acceptable temperature when a variation is not specified. In addition, specific requirements are stated in some drug monographs where it is considered that storage at a lower or higher temperature may produce undesirable results. Specific storage conditions are required to be printed in product literature and on drug packaging and **drug labels** to ensure proper storage and product integrity. The conditions are defined by the following terms:

1. *Cold*—any temperature not exceeding 8°C (45°F). A refrigerator is a cold place in which the temperature is maintained thermostatically between 2° and 8°C (36° and 46°F). A freezer is a cold place in which the temperature is maintained thermostatically between –20° and –10°C (–4° and 14°F).
    a. Protection from freezing—When freezing subjects an article to loss of strength or potency or to destructive alteration of its characteristics, the container label bears an appropriate instruction to prevent the article from freezing.
2. *Cool*—any temperature between 8° and 15°C (46° and 59°F). An article for which storage in a cool place is directed may alternatively be stored in a refrigerator, unless otherwise specified in the individual monograph.
3. *Room temperature*—the temperature prevailing in a working area. Controlled room temperature is a temperature maintained thermostatically between 15° and 30°C (59° and 86°F).
4. *Warm*—any temperature between 30° and 40°C (86° and 104°F).
5. *Excessive heat*—any temperature above 40°C (104°F).

When no specific storage directions or limitations are provided in the individual monograph, it is understood that the storage conditions include protection from moisture, freezing, and excessive heat.

Additional standards regarding the preservation, packaging, storage, and labeling of drugs are described in the "General Notices and Requirements" section of the U.S.P./N.F. Persons involved in any aspect of materials management of pharmaceuticals must be familiar with the official standards and definitions as they relate to the proper storage and handling of drugs. The pharmacy technician shares this obligation with all other members of the health care team involved in medication-related activities.

Security Requirements

Security requirements that restrict access to drugs to "authorized personnel only" are often the result of legal requirements, hospital policy, and established standards of practice. All medications must be maintained in restricted locations so that they are only accessible to professional staff who are authorized to receive, store, prepare, dispense, distribute, or administer such products.

Legend drugs (those that require a prescription) must be dispensed by a licensed pharmacist. However, a pharmacy technician under the direct supervision of a pharmacist can receive and fill floor stock orders and deliver the medication to a drug storage location. Medication storage areas located on nursing units must also be secured and restricted to authorized personnel only.

Controlled substances and tax-free alcohol require additional restrictions. Only a licensed pharmacist can order, receive, prepare, and dispense these drugs. However, a qualified pharmacy technician under the direct supervision of a pharmacist can assist in storing and delivering these products. Special security procedures, such as daily physical counts of pharmacy and nursing units inventories, are essential to ensure that there is no diversion or misuse of controlled substances. Tax-free alcohol, which is most often used only by the pathology department, is controlled by performing periodic record audits and physical inventories.

Safety precautions must also be carefully considered when handling materials that have a high potential for danger. For example, when storing volatile or flammable substances, it is important to have a cool location that is properly ventilated and has been specially designed to reduce fire and/or explosion potential. Another consideration would be to store caustic substances, such as acids, in a location that would reduce any potential for the container being dropped and broken (e.g., in a locked cabinet instead of an open shelf). Oncology drugs used to treat cancer are often cytotoxic themselves and therefore must be handled with extreme care. They should be received in a sealed protective outer bag that restricts the dissemination of the drug if the container leaks or is broken. These drugs should also be stored in a secure area that has limited access and a restricted traffic flow. When the potential exists for exposure to chemotherapy, all personnel involved must wear protective clothing and equipment while following a hazardous materials cleanup procedure. All exposed materials must be properly disposed of in chemohazardous waste containers.

Proper rotation of inventory

Segregating inventory by drug category also helps to prevent errors that could increase the potential for harm. For example, the standards of the Joint Commission on Accreditation of Healthcare Organizations (JCAHO) require that internal and external medications must be stored separately to reduce the potential for someone dispensing or administering an external product for internal use. Rotating inventory and checking expiration dates on products when drugs are received helps to reduce the potential for dispensing and/or administering expired drugs and also maximizes the utilization of inventory before drugs become outdated.

Computerized inventory control

Many of these functions can be better controlled with the use of computer programs dedicated to monitor the purchasing, receiving, and dispensing functions on an ongoing basis. Perpetual inventory systems are now being utilized to indicate when predetermined reorder points are reached. Most dedicated pharmacy systems can generate management reports that allow the materials manager to review drug use. For example, the monthly usage rate of each drug can be monitored, and utilization can be tracked to determine which clinical department or patient population is using specific drugs. Computers also enable the materials manager to closely monitor budget trends and year-to-date purchases by drug category. It is important for the pharmacy technician to remember that computer systems are only as effective as the users are accurate when inputting information. Therefore, the materials management technician must have a basic understanding of how the pharmacy computer works and must be properly trained to maximize the potential benefits of inventory control programs. More detail on pharmacy computerization is discussed in Chapter 14.

Turnover rate

Determining the pharmacy's inventory turnover rate is a good method of measuring the overall effectiveness of the purchasing and inventory control programs. The inventory turnover rate is calculated by dividing the total dollars spent to purchase drugs for 1 year by the actual value of the pharmacy inventory at any point in time. The number produced by this calculation offers an indication of how many times a year the inventory may have been used or replaced. The larger the number of inventory turnovers, the stronger the indication that the inventory control program is efficient.

In the 1980s a turnover rate of 6 to 7 percent was considered to be acceptable. In the 1990s, turnover rates of 10 to 12 percent were easily achievable because of more efficient methods of purchasing, such as prime-vendor programs and computerized order-entry systems. Even higher turnover rates will be achieved in the twenty-first century due to new materials management techniques and business strategies such as consignment of inventory programs.

The following questions may further assist the pharmacy materials manager in his or her attempt to maintain adequate controls on a very large and complex inventory.

1. Has an inventory turnover rate been calculated for your hospital?
2. Is this rate optimal for the facility?
3. Is the storeroom checked at regular intervals to verify that appropriate purchasing and inventory methods are being followed?
   a. Are reorder points adjusted as needed?
   b. Is this rate optimal for the facility?
4. Are inventories controlled in dispensing areas?
   a. Are minimum and maximum inventories maintained?
   b. Is the space allotted for each product restricted?
   c. Is there a routine check for outdated drugs and excesses?
   d. Are exchange systems used when appropriate (e.g., carts, self-units, and boxes)?
5. Are nursing-unit drug inventories controlled?
   a. Is an approved floor-stock list used for drug items?
   b. Are there maximum allowable quantities for each item?
   c. Are inventory dollar limits set for each nursing unit?
   d. Are units checked monthly for excesses and outdated drugs?
6. Are inventories controlled in the emergency, operating, and recovery rooms?

Repackaging and Labeling Considerations

In-house packaging and labeling are sometimes necessary when required dosage forms are not available commercially. The pharmacy technician is often directly involved in preparing unit-dose packaging that utilizes automated packaging equipment. The pharmacy technician must be adequately trained to ensure the stability of the product and appropriate labeling. Accordingly, the pharmacy technician must receive detailed training in this regard.

Depending on the product, the desired route of administration, and the method of dispensing, there are different container types from which to choose. For example, unit-dose packaging for solid oral forms (e.g., tray-fill blister packaging, cadet foil packaging) and oral liquids (e.g., Baxa® cups, oral syringes). In addition, some of the new automated dispensing technologies require packaging unique to their dispensing design (e.g., APS Robot®-ready cards, Envoy® and SureMed® dispensing cartridges).

Regardless of which type of packaging container is used, it should be clean and special precautions and cleaning procedures may be necessary to ensure that extraneous matter is not introduced into or onto the drugs being packaged. It is also essential to be sure that the container does not interact physically or chemically with the drug being placed in it so as to alter the strength, quality, or purity of the article beyond the official requirements.

Some drugs may have special packaging requirements as described in the manufacturer's literature and in official monographs published in the U.S.P. and N.F. The following requirements for use of specified containers may apply when in-house packaging is required:

- *Light-resistant container*—protects the contents from the effects of light by virtue of the specific properties of the material of which it is composed, including any coating applied to it. Alternatively, a clear and colorless or a translucent container may be made light resistant by means of an opaque covering, in which case the label of the container bears a statement that the opaque covering is needed until the contents are to be used or administered. When it is directed to "protect from light" in an individual monograph, preservation in a light-resistant container is required.
- *Tamper-resistant packaging*—required for a sterile article intended for ophthalmic or otic use, except when extemporaneously compounded for immediate dispensing on prescription. The contents are sealed so that they cannot be opened without obvious destruction of the seal.
- *Tight container*—protects the contents from contamination by extraneous liquids, solids, or vapors, from loss of the article, and from efflorescence, deliquescence, or evaporation under the ordinary or customary conditions of handling, shipment, storage, and distribution, and is capable of tight reclosure.
- *Hermetic container*—is impervious to air or any other gas under the ordinary or customary conditions of handling, shipment, storage, and distribution.
- *Single-unit container*—is one that is designed to hold a quantity of drug product intended for administration as a single dose, or a single finished device intended for use promptly after the container is opened. Each single-unit container shall be labeled to indicate the identity, quantity and/or strength, name of manufacturer, lot number, and expiration date of the drug or article.
- *Single-dose container*—is a single-unit container for articles intended for parenteral administration only. Examples of single-dose containers include prefilled syringes, cartridges, fusion-sealed containers, and closure-sealed containers when so labeled.
- *Unit-dose container*—is a single-unit container for articles intended for administration by other than the parenteral route as a single dose, direct from the container.

Each label must at least include the following information:

- generic name of the product (brand name optional)
- strength in units (e.g., mg, ml, oz)
- drug form (e.g., tablet, capsule, suppository)
- lot number and manufacturer's name
- expiration date for repackaged drug

The expiration date used on repackaged drugs should be based on the prevailing community standard of practice or based on an evaluation of scientific information. In all cases a maximum expiration date should be adhered to as identified in law and regulation. The seventeenth addition of the U.S.P. states, "In the absence of stability data to the contrary, such date should not exceed (1) 25% of the remaining time between the date of repackaging and the expiration date on the original manufacturer's bulk container, or (2) a 6-month period of time from the date the drug is repackaged, whichever is earlier."

All repackaged drugs must be carefully checked by a licensed pharmacist and approvals must be documented in writing before repackaged drugs are put into active inventory. Documentation of the repackaging process should include the following information:

- date of repackaging
- name and strength of drug
- quantity of drug repackaged
- manufacturer's name
- manufacturer's lot number
- manufacturer's expiration date
- in-house code number
- in-house expiration date
- initials of packaging technician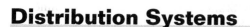
- initials of pharmacist

Distribution Systems

Drug distribution systems have changed considerably in the last 10 years. In the past it was acceptable to dispense large containers of drugs (bulk packaging) to be stored at the nursing unit for use whenever a nurse needed to administer a drug to a patient. This method, known as a floor stock system, does not allow the pharmacist to review drug therapy before it is administered to a patient. It is therefore potentially dangerous. Also, floor stock medication cannot be reused once it is removed from the original container because there is no way to guarantee product integrity. As a result this method increases the potential for waste. Today the JCAHO and most state agencies require unit-dose dispensing and pharmacy-based intravenous additive programs. (The importance of these programs is discussed in Chapter 24).

Certain emergency drugs are still maintained as floor stock because they may be urgently needed. Emergency drugs may be stored in mobile units for quick transfer to a patient's bedside when resuscitation techniques are required. Emergency drugs are stored in a medication cabinet at the nursing unit for use when rapid blood levels are necessary in patients who cannot wait for drug orders to be processed and delivered by the pharmacy department. Determining when it is appropriate to circumvent a pharmacist review of drug therapy to have medication available for immediate administration is a difficult undertaking. It constantly challenges pharmacy and nursing relationships. The best way to minimize controversy regarding this consideration is to have comprehensive pharmacy services that meet the requirements of patient needs in a timely manner. Traditionally, emergency drugs are immediately available as circumstances require.

Recapture and Disposal

Returned Medications

Properly processing medication that is returned to the pharmacy department is an important role that can be fulfilled by a pharmacy technician. When unit-dose packaging is used, the pharmacy technician can check return medication for package integrity and proper dating before putting the drug back into stock. In case of a manufacturer's recall, each dose of medication can be located by lot number to ensure its removal. Records of all recall information should be maintained to ensure that a proper review of all potentially dangerous drugs has been completed.

Expiration Dates

All drug packages have expiration date notations that identify the date when the medication is no longer suitable for use. The expiration date will be designated in one of two ways: month and year (e.g., June 1999), which means that the packaged material, if properly stored, is good until the last day of the month; or more specifically as month, day, and year (e.g., June 15, 1999). Every hospital pharmacy must have a system whereby drugs are checked for expiration dates on a regular basis to guarantee that only properly dated drugs are available for use. Expired drugs must be segregated from active inventory to prevent a potentially dangerous dispensing error. Many pharmaceutical companies will give full credit for expired medication. It is essential for the pharmacy materials manager to determine the return policy for each company.

Environmental Considerations

When disposing of partially used drugs or expired drugs that cannot be returned for credit, it is important to consider the negative impact that certain drugs may have on the environment. For example, many oncology drugs used for the treatment of cancer are carcinogenic (i.e., they have the potential to cause cancer themselves). It is essential that strict precautions be taken and procedures followed to properly dispose of these items. Another concern is related to partially used injectable medication that may have come in contact with a patient who has a communicable disease. Once again the drug, needle, and syringe must be disposed of in a special puncture-resistant container that can be handled safely and then properly destroyed.

Materials management personnel must not only be concerned about the products they are obtaining, but they must also consider the type of packaging materials used by the manufacturers to ship their products. Many plastics and Styrofoam materials are not biodegradable and will have a detrimental effect on our environment for years to come.

Summary

It is important for the pharmacy technician to realize that the responsibilities of materials management are comprehensive and must be carried out in an organized and consistent manner to ensure patient safety and guarantee cost-effective pharmaceutical care.

ASSESSMENT

Multiple Choice Questions

1. An institutional pharmacy materials management program includes
   a. procurement
   b. drug storage
   c. inventory control
   d. drug distribution
   e. all of the above

2. In a hospital, overall responsibility for the materials management of pharmaceuticals lies with the
   a. chairman of the Pharmacy and Therapeutics Committee
   b. director of pharmacy services
   c. materials manager
   d. hospital administration
   e. chief pharmacy technician

3. Brand-name drugs are those drugs
   a. developed and marketed by the drug firm that did the original research and production
   b. that fall under a particular category of drugs
   c. developed by a drug firm after the original patent has expired
   d. b and c
   e. a, b, and c

4. A drug distribution system includes
   a. unit dose
   b. floor stock
   c. compounded prescriptions
   d. emergency drugs
   e. all of the above

5. Therapeutic equivalency indicates that the drugs
   a. are the same size, shape, and color
   b. have the same amount of active ingredient
   c. are equally effective in the same dose
   d. b and c
   e. a, b, and c

6. Environmental considerations in the storage of pharmaceuticals include
   a. proper temperature and ventilation
   b. proper humidity
   c. appropriate light
   d. proper sanitation
   e. all of the above

7. The pharmacy department is responsible for
   a. preparing purchase orders
   b. receiving and securing shipments of pharmaceuticals
   c. monitoring the inventory of controlled substances and tax-free alcohol
   d. coordinating the distribution of medical surgical supplies
   e. a, b, and c

8. Inventory control may include
   a. minimum and maximum reorder points maintained
   b. return of outdated stock
   c. restricted usage of pharmaceuticals
   d. drug usage report
   e. all of the above

True/False Questions

9. _____ A legend drug is one that requires a prescription and must be dispensed by a licensed pharmacist.

10. _____ The calculation of the pharmacy turnover rate is a good indication of the effectiveness of a purchasing and inventory control program.

Matching I

11.	_c_ cold temperature	a.	–20° to –10°C (–4° to 14°F)
12.	_a_ freezer	b.	15° to 30°C (59° to 86°F)
13.	_b_ room temperature	c.	not exceeding 8°C (46°F)
14.	_e_ refrigerator	d.	30° to 40°C (86° to 104°F)
15.	_f_ excessive heat	e.	2° to 8°C (36° to 46°F)
16.	_d_ warm	f.	above 40°C (104°F)

Matching II

17.	_a_ select the drug source	a.	pharmacist's responsibility
18.	_a_ prepare the drug order		
19.	_b_ check the incoming drug products	b.	technician's responsibility
20.	_b_ maintain a proper drug storage environment		
21.	_a_ prepare formulary revision		

Bibliography

Abramowitz, P.W. (1984). Controlling financial variables—changing prescribing patterns. *American Journal of Health Systems Pharmacists, 41,* 503–515.

Comprehensive accreditation manual for hospitals. (1996–1997). Joint Commission on Accreditation of Health Care Organizations, pharmacy services (various sections).

General notices and requirements: Preservation, packaging, storage, and labeling. (1995). *The United States Pharmacopeia XXIII/The National Formulary XVIII,* 10–13.

Powers, J.R. (1987). Hospital pharmacy buying groups: The perspective of a contract sales manager. *Topics in Hospital Pharmacy Management, 7,* 12–13.

Rich, Darryl S. (1996, September). Expiration dating of pharmacy packaging. *Hospital Pharmacy, 31,* 1159–1160.

The Pharmacy Formulary System

COMPETENCIES

After completion and review of this chapter, the student should be able to

1. Outline the five core attributes of the formulary system.
2. List at least three strategies to gain the consensus of the medical community.
3. Explain why a formulary should be selective.
4. List three surveillance activities fostered by the formulary system.
5. Give an example of how the formulary system can define policy.
6. Illustrate why it is important to revise the formulary regularly.

Introduction

Throughout much of the history of pharmacy, the term *formulary* has referred basically to a listing of drugs. The spectrum of sophistication of a formulary can range from a simple list for use in a small institution to an elaborate compendium of detailed standards, which may in fact carry some official weight as a legally recognized standard. Formularies can be used for many purposes. Perhaps the most historically significant of the ancient formularies is the "Ebers Papyrus," a listing of complex prescriptions and cures from ancient Egypt. Formularies have documented the state-of-the-art therapeutic knowledge of the cultures that compiled them. Not all formularies are from the Old World. Some very complete ones, usually described as codices, are attributed to Central American native civilizations. In fact, some of the drugs, such as digitalis and cocaine, appeared in these formularies many years before they were "discovered" by Western or Oriental medicine. The most revered formulary in the United States is the *National Formulary*. Many pharmacists are familiar with the initials *"N.F."* following drug names. Formularies, then, are a continuation of a worldwide, centuries-old pharmacy tradition.

In their modern form, formularies are usually associated with hospitals or other organized medical care settings. The utility and effectiveness of formularies, despite their ancient heritage and pervasiveness, are not without controversy. Some agencies and organizations seem to depend on them increasingly more. For example, the Veterans Affairs system has adopted a "national" formulary (not to be confused with the official compendium, *National Formulary*) and uses it to optimize therapy and as a tool to negotiate price savings due to its effect on standardization. Conversely, recent comments in various publications refer to the whole idea of formularies as archaic and ineffective. Formularies are tools, and like any tool, how one uses it determines the overall judgment of its value. As part of this tradition, certain attributes come to mind when using the term *formulary*. It is interesting that some ancient concepts embodied in formularies are now being used to expand the role of the pharmacy profession for its technician practitioners as well as for pharmacists.

The Formulary System

The formulary system is another concept associated with formularies. Essentially the formulary system describes how formularies are derived and how the drug-use process can be guided, controlled, and accounted for when a particular formulary is in effect.

The core attributes of a formulary and formulary system include the following:

- The formulary system represents the consensus of the Pharmacy and Therapeutics Committee (P&T Committee) (Appendix C), which created it regarding the most effective therapeutic agents to be used in the practice.
- Formularies represent a selective list of the drugs available from the pharmacy (Appendix D).
- Formularies should also contain additional information about the drugs and their use.
- The formulary system defines the policies and procedures established by the medical staff concerning drug use and defines the scope of the formulary.
- Formularies must be continuously revised (Appendix D).

Consensus is important for the formulary to be effective. Thus, the members of the P&T Committee should be selected with this in mind. It would be frustrating if the committee failed to accurately reflect the feelings and expertise of the medical staff whom it represents. In that case, the drugs listed in the formulary or the policies established by the committee would not accomplish what was intended, or their effectiveness might be significantly reduced over what might have been, if the committee had been truly representative. The pharmacy department can play an important role in establishing consensus. Several strategies to gain consensus are provided next.

1. Additions to the formulary should be requested in a formal fashion through the use of a request form. This form can channel the thoughts of the requester by including some questions such as "Are there similar drugs on the formulary?" or "What are the advantages of this drug?"
2. Requests can be forwarded to the clinical chief of the department of the requester. Support of the chief eliminates a potential source of controversy.
3. The P&T Committee should prepare a "white paper" report on the advantages, disadvantages, therapeutic impact, and financial impact of the request. This task often falls to the drug information service. Subcommittees of the P&T Committee consisting of physicians and other professionals are often established, especially in large and complex institutions.
4. When the report of the committee indicates an unfavorable response to the request, it is advisable to share with the requester in writing the reasons why the drug will not be recommended for acceptance. Often the requester is asked to provide additional information in support of the request, or is invited to attend the meeting at which the request will be presented.
5. The actions of the committee and the reasons for them should be published as soon as possible after the meeting. If actions were not to include a drug, it is particularly important to specify why.

It is important for formularies to be inclusive (i.e., they should be more than a list of drugs in a particular institution). Rather, the formulary should be selective and represent the best drugs available for the institution. There are many therapeutic reasons supporting a selective formulary—the elimination of unnecessary and potentially confusing duplications is one. A second reason deals with economics. It is now much more important for hospitals to watch carefully how the money is spent. The advent of such high-tech drugs such as colony stimulating factors and monoclonal antibodies can literally precipitate an economic crisis for the hospital if the potential economic impacts of these agents are treated in a cavalier fashion. The pharmacy budget as a percent of the total hospital budget has increased dramatically in the past few years. All indications are that this trend will continue indefinitely because of the many hundreds of new, high-tech and innovative agents in the "pipeline." It is not unusual for the drug budget of a typical pharmacy to be 70 percent of the total pharmacy budget. You may read in other chapters about the challenges of the fiscal environment in hospitals today. The implications for the formulary are similar: There is less money to do more work at a higher cost. Selectivity, therefore, is becoming more important.

One method of viewing the economic impact of drug therapy is represented in the flow diagram shown in **Figure 13–1**. This figure represents a more global perception of pharmacoeconomic impact than merely considering the price of a drug or its impact on the "pharmacy budget." Impact and possible decision alternatives are divided into three case scenarios.

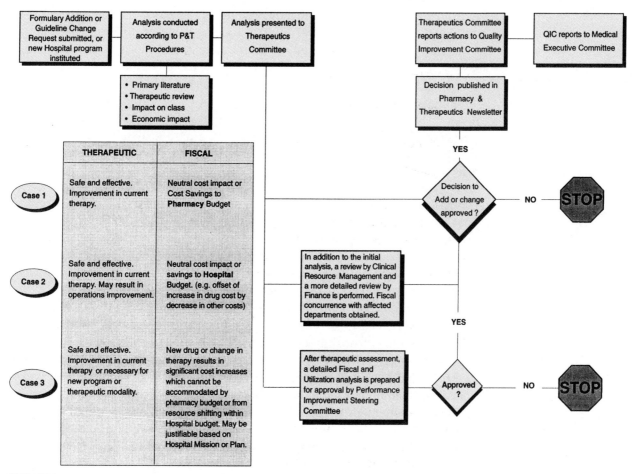

FIGURE 13–1   Flow diagram showing economic impact on drug therapy

Case 1 represents an uncomplicated situation when the proposed formulary change, in addition to being safe and effective, is cost neutral or represents a savings.

Case 2 becomes somewhat more complicated because the cost neutrality or potential savings of the choice involves another or several other departments. In this case it is important to get a clear consensus from all parties to ensure that a cost burden in one area is actually offset by a savings in another. The economic analyses in these types of cases can be complex and usually involve financial experts and the clinical expertise of the P&T members.

Case 3 represents a truly global situation within the institution and requires sign-off at the highest administrative and clinical levels. These issues usually involve significant cost increases (often in the six- and seven-figure range), which clearly cannot be accommodated in either the pharmacy or the hospital budget. They require an approval at the strategic level of the organization. Although such cases were rare or nonexistent only a few years ago, they are rather common today.

Complications can arise when trying to be selective and trying to reach a consensus at the same time. Little doubt remains that as pressure increases to become more selective, consensus will also become important and possibly more difficult to achieve.

The information a formulary contains, aside from the listing of the available drugs, can often be a decisive factor in determining its effectiveness and quality over another formulary. Pharmacy can be very effective when in consensus about how and which drugs are used. Reviewing formularies from similar institutions (e.g., university hospitals) would indicate a remarkable similarity in the drugs they contain. Although the additional information they convey is different, even in this aspect, uniformity seems to be more common. Additional information, for example, may list certain policies about drug use in a single place. Sample protocols for drug use can be listed. (Think of a protocol as a recipe for how to use a specific drug.) Often charts comparing the features or costs of an important drug class are included. Many large and small institutions have their formularies produced by outside vendors who prepare them from elaborate electronic databases. It is not surprising that many of these companies started in business producing cookbooks for various groups and organizations.

The formulary system defines the policies of drug use and can be effective in several aspects. For example, the system not only has the responsibility to select drugs and to foster rational drug therapy, but it can also function in an educational role as means of quality assurance. The educational role of the P&T Committee is carried out through the formulary system. Traditionally in the form of written communications, today's education involves more direct in-service programs sponsored and/or conducted by the P&T Committee.

Some surveillance activities fostered by the system have an educational and a quality assurance aspect. For example, monitoring nonformulary drug use can provide to the medical staff certain trends that would otherwise go unnoticed. Many monitoring activities, or drug utilization evaluations (DUEs), are discussed elsewhere that fall into this category. An exciting outgrowth of the formulary system linked to computer technology is the ability to track **adverse drug reactions (ADRs).** Sophisticated database management programs often allow a more rapid identification of trends that might not otherwise be obvious and thus result in interventions to avoid such reactions. Recent literature has provided data that quantify the cost of ADRs—and the number is remarkable! For example, an overall average of the additional cost involved in ADRs is $2000 per incident, but the range may vary from $6700 per case for "bleeding" to $9000 for "induced fever" (Classen et al., 1997). These observations support the view that there is more to the relationship of formulary management, drug therapy, and cost than may be at first apparent.

The traditional application of the formulary system could be described as occurring in two dimensions: mostly in writing and often "after the fact." However, the growing trend is to apply sophisticated computer techniques to how information is used. As a result, many of the formulary system's procedures and protocols can move away from the "scripture-like" status of written documents to a prospective and often interactive status. For example, in some computer applications, the program can alert the pharmacist to a drug's formulary status and to any restrictions that apply, and document special criteria for use—all while the order is being entered. In a growing number of cases, physicians enter their own drug orders into the hospital information system. In these cases certain checkpoints can be established that have to be answered before the order can proceed. You will no doubt hear more about the implications of such technology before too long, as more systems with these capabilities are installed.

We have included some examples of how the formulary system can define policy. Another aspect of the formulary system that should be discussed briefly is the relation of these concepts to the operation of the department of pharmacy. This relation involves some controversy, and certainly much variation from hospital to hospital. In general, the P&T Committee must avoid trying to deal with operational pharmacy issues and stick to issues of broad therapeutic concern. In many institutions the committee selects the drug entity to be included in the formulary, and the pharmacy determines the actual drug products to be procured.

Revision of the formulary is an important function, because its effectiveness depends on how current it is. Keeping formularies current is a difficult task, because they are created by the P&T Committee in hospitals, which meets several times a year or, in most cases, monthly. New drugs are also being introduced at a faster rate than in previous years. These factors combine to make formulary revision a constant activity.

Formularies are usually published once a year, even though they may be revised after each P&T Committee action. These changes that occur between official revisions can be communicated in several ways. Often the pharmacy department publishes them in a newsletter, or the P&T Committee releases a special publication when changes are made.

Summary

Formularies and the formulary system are ancient concepts that have been adapted to the dynamic environment of modern medical care. When sound therapeutic management principles are applied in a practical, scientific manner, they can also become very effective tools for clinical safety and quality of care.

ASSESSMENT

Answer True or False

1. The core attributes of the formulary system include:
   a. ___T___ It represents the consensus of the P&T Committee.
   b. ___F___ It guarantees the best drugs at the lowest cost.
   c. ___T___ Formularies represent a selective list of drugs available in the pharmacy.
   d. ___T___ The formulary system defines the policies and procedures established by the medical staff concerning drug use and defines the scope of the formulary.
   e. ___F___ A properly established formulary needs little or no revision.

2. Three effective strategies to gain a consensus of the medical community include:
   a. ___T___ The committee should hold a regular series of educational programs with free lunch.
   b. ___T___ The formulary process should be formal and encourage direct medical staff input.
   c. ___T___ When the evaluation process indicates an unfavorable response to a request, appropriate communications and additional participation should be solicited.
   d. ___T___ The actions of the committee and the reasons for them should be published as soon as possible.
   e. ___F___ Keep the important doctors happy at all times.

3. Appropriate surveillance activities of a formulary system might include which of the following:
   a. ___T___ a monitor of nonformulary drug use
   b. ___F___ a list of known "problem" salespeople who often interfere with the formulary
   c. ___T___ a system of drug utilization review (DUE) that is driven by criteria accepted by the medical staff
   d. ___F___ a report to administration of all physicians who prescribe expensive drugs
   e. ___T___ a system to tabulate and analyze adverse drug reactions (ADRs) and recommend steps to minimize them
   f. ___T___ incentive bonuses for physicians who use cheaper drugs

Bibliography

American Society of Health System Pharmacists. ASHP statement of the pharmacy and therapeutics committee. Practice Standards of ASHP 1996–1997, p. 4.

American Society of Health System Pharmacists. ASHP guidelines on formulary management. Practice Standards of ASHP 1996–1997, p. 60.

American Society of Health System Pharmacists. ASHP technical assistance bulletin on hospital drug distribution and control. Practice Standards of ASHP 1996–1997, p. 97.

American Society of Health System Pharmacists. ASHP technical assistance bulletin on drug formularies. Practice Standards of ASHP 1996–1997, p. 120.

American Society of Health System Pharmacists. ASHP technical assistance bulletin on the evaluation of drugs for formularies. Practice Standards of ASHP 1996–1997, p. 128.

American Society of Health System Pharmacists. ASHP technical assistance bulletin on assessing cost-containment strategies for pharmacies in organized health-care settings. Practice Standards of ASHP 1996–1997, p. 147.

Classen, D.C., Pestotnik, S.L., Evans, R.S., et al. (1997, January). Adverse drug events in hospitalized patients: Excess length of stay, extra costs, and attributable mortality. *Journal of American Medical Association, 277*(4).

Joint Commission on the Accreditation of Health Care Organizations, Accreditation Manual for Hospitals. Chicago, Illinois.

Computer Applications in Drug-Use Control

COMPETENCIES

Upon completion and review of this chapter, the student should be able to

1. List the pharmacy applications that automation has been designed to facilitate.

2. Describe how computer systems interact within the pharmacy, and with other systems in the health care delivery process.

3. Explain the concept of project management relating to the implementation of a computer system.

4. Describe the role of the pharmacist and pharmacy technician in the management of a pharmacy information system.

Introduction

The management of medication administration plays a crucial role in the patient care process. The information contained in pharmacy information systems is important to the management of the pharmacy. Keep in mind that this information is important beyond the walls of the pharmacy. Health care professionals who play a role in caring for patients rely on this information in the decisions they make concerning patients under their charge.

Pharmacy information systems have been successfully used in the management of its operations for many years. Hospitals and pharmacies have been using automation and information systems to improve productivity and ensure the quality of pharmaceutical care for some time. Finding a pharmacy operation that does not employ some level of automation is rare.

As the health care marketplace has evolved, information systems have grown in importance to assist pharmacy professionals in meeting the demands placed upon them. The continuing evolution of this marketplace is creating new opportunities for pharmacists and technicians in the health care delivery process. These opportunities can be augmented by the strategic use of information system technology.

The increasing penetration of health maintenance organizations (HMOs) into the marketplace has created new financial and competitive pressures for health care providers. As managed care penetration started to grow, hospitals were placed in the position of trying to deliver the best possible service for the lowest possible price, and remain viable as a business. As a result, we have witnessed a reduction in lengths of stay, lower patient census, and downsized hospitals.

As the competitive nature of the marketplace continued, we watched hospitals come together to form health care delivery networks to ensure their survival. These pressures have forced all constituencies within hospitals to become creative in redesigning the mechanisms for delivering care to patients more efficiently. The roles of pharmacies and pharmacy professionals have been critical components to this development.

The evolution of the marketplace has created a need for pharmacy operations to link more closely with other constituencies within the hospital (e.g., laboratory, dietary) as well as other hospitals, labs, and physicians who are participating in the health care delivery network. The effectiveness and efficiency of the health care delivery process are clearly impacted by having complete and correct information in the hands of the decision maker, regardless of where that individual is located. That person must also be given the ability to communicate the results of the decision to those health care professionals who are expected to react to it.

Partnerships have been formed between pharmacies and information systems professionals to meet the challenge of strategically deploying automation in a way that will better support pharmacy operations in a changing marketplace.

In this chapter we will review the evolution of information systems within the hospital pharmacy, and the role that pharmacists and technicians have played in their use. We will also review how that evolution is continuing to redefine how information technology and automation interact within the pharmacy, and the professionals working within the pharmacy.

Components of Computer Applications

Application Software

A good way to look at pharmacy computer systems, and computer systems in general, is that they are a collection of electronic features and functions designed to be used by nontechnical users. Each type of job or function for which a series of computer programs are written is referred to as an application. Computer applications are designed to perform a specific set of features and functions that, if implemented correctly, should improve the user's effectiveness in performing the job. These features and functions should be considered no differently than one would consider a good set of tools. Examples of computer applications in the pharmacy include purchasing applications, receiving and inventory management applications, and patient medication administration applications.

In delivering the desired features and functions, system developers employ computer hardware, software, and software development tools. They design these systems for use on varying types and brands of computer hardware. Different database technologies and different computer languages are utilized in the building of computer systems.

The user's knowledge of the system structure, hardware capabilities, features, and functions of the system in use will allow the user to take full advantage of the system's capabilities. This knowledge will allow more informed decision making in the system selection process, during the implementation of the system, and in managing day-to-day operations.

Files

From the standpoint of system structure, it is helpful to understand the files that a system contains, and the information contained in each file. A file is a collection of like elements of information, and this information is stored together under a common name (file name) on some storage medium (e.g., tape, disk). An example of a file could be the hospital's formulary file (or drug item master files). This file would contain such elements of information as drug name (generic), drug brand name, drug code number(s), units of purchase quantity, and units of issue quantity. Other files may include an inventory file (to account for inventory on hand) and files to account for purchases, receipts, and patient medication profiles.

Knowledge of the file structure, and the relationship of the data elements between the files, will provide a system's users with a good understanding of why and how a system works. Such information also will facilitate the maintenance of a system (e.g., adding/deleting items to/from the files) and the diagnosis of system problems.

Software license

When a buyer acquires application software (the computer programs) that provides the desired features and functions, the buyer is really obtaining a license to use the software products. This license is, in essence, a right to use the software only for an intended purpose, for example, to support the operation of a pharmacy. The licensee (person acquiring the rights to use the software) typically cannot sell the software to anyone else, cannot make copies for anyone else, and in many cases is restricted to using the licensor's programmers to make any modifications to the software.

Issues concerning software licenses are complex. The licensing of a system software product can be a complex transaction, which should be reviewed by competent legal counsel in conjunction with a senior information system's professional (usually the organization's chief information officer or information systems director).

Computer Hardware

The basic components of computer hardware necessary to operate a computer application are the central processing unit (CPU or processor), memory, disk storage, the operating system, and other peripheral devices (printers, tape drives, terminals, networking components, etc.).

CPU

The central processing unit (CPU) is the component of the computer that executes the software commands. The CPU is the brain of the computer. When a user requests a system function to be performed, it is the processor that receives and acts on the user's command by the instructions received from the application software and the operating system software.

Disk storage

The application software and related information (data) are stored in disk storage. As system users enter data (provide input), make queries (look for output), or execute any other command, the processor must seek out the necessary information and software instructions which reside on disk storage.

An interesting fact to keep in mind is that disk storage is one of the few mechanical, or moving parts, in a computer. When a user makes a request, disk arms move across the disk (magnetic platters) to locate the appropriate information or instructions, and make it available to the processor. Today's processors are able to absorb information at a far faster rate than the current disk drive technology can read it off of the magnetic storage media in the disk mechanism. Likewise, processors can process information for storage faster than disk drive mechanisms (read/write heads) can write it to disk. Accordingly, the computer's memory serves as the buffer to allow the computer to operate more efficiently. Upon the commencement of any process or query, the processor's instructions will cause the disk to fill the memory with as much (if not all) of the required information and instructions to allow as quick a response time as the hardware is capable of providing.

Server

Due to improved technology and miniaturization, computer processors, memory, and disk storage are delivered in a single self-contained unit referred to as a server. A server is a computer that collects and stores information for use by other computers. This information can consist of data or information files. It can also consist of application software files. Servers have particular applicability to situations when information needs to be shared among a number of users.

Servers can be anything from a high-end microcomputer, to a mid-range minicomputer, to a mainframe computer.

- A microcomputer is a single-user system, which means it can only be used by one user at a time.
- A mid-range computer has the capacity to handle a larger number of simultaneous users, who are accessing multiple computer applications located in the same system.
- A mainframe computer has even more capacity than a mid-range computer. It can serve more simultaneous users and run even more computer applications, all at the same time.

Depending on the system design, servers can exist as a self-contained physical unit or as component pieces that are connected. Servers perform such functions as home for a discrete database (pharmacy formulary, patient drug profiles, etc.), interface engine (to manage communications with other systems), and traffic control over a network.

Printer

Another mechanical device is an output device—the printer. Report production in a computing environment can be a long, slow, and tedious process. Printers capable of printing at speeds of 1200 lines per minute cannot operate as fast as a computer processor can output the information. Memory serves to store (or buffer) the required output so that the printer can work efficiently, within the boundaries of its capabilities.

Operating system

The operations of the processor, disk storage, memory, and peripheral devices attached to the processor are controlled by the operating system. The operating system is a set of software instructions and utilities that manage the interaction between the physical components of the computer. It regulates input and output between disk, memory, and the processor and provides the utilities that make the mechanical devices (disk, tape drives, printers) react to the appropriate instructions. It reports back to the operator (or system administrator) the percent of capacity at which the system is operating. The operating system allows technical computer staff to diagnose and begin corrective action should a problem occur with the computer's operation. Examples of operating systems in microcomputers include Microsoft Windows™ and Windows98™.

Hardware capabilities have a direct impact on such issues as processing speed, response time, and system capacity. When users turn on a computer, they have an expectation that it will work up to a minimum level of performance. A key exercise that must be undertaken with the procurement of a new system is sizing of the computer.

Critical information must be estimated in a reasonably reliable fashion to ensure that the computer equipment can meet the user's processing expectations. In a pharmacy application such information includes number of drugs in the formulary, number of prescriptions to fill (daily, monthly, annually), number of patients to track in the system, number of weeks/months/years of data to be maintained in the system, and number of desktop devices (terminals and microcomputers) that will be accessing the system in total and simultaneously.

Network

Until recently, computer systems were wired directly to each device (terminal, printer, or other computer) that relied on it. As a result, a pharmacy system computer terminal could only be used to access the pharmacy system. Modern computer technology has been engineered to allow intelligent workstations (or microcomputers) to access any one of a number of computer applications that a user is authorized to access. The technology that supports the connection of multiple computers (to include application processors, printers, and microcomputers) is networking.

A network consists of the wiring, electronics, software, and protocols that allow computers and computer devices to communicate with one another. A typical network has a high-capacity cable (copper or fiber) which serves as the main vehicle to transport information between locations. This vehicle is typically referred to as the network backbone. Computer devices tap into the backbone at key termination points known as hubs. For example, if the pharmacy application server (computer that houses the computer programs and data for the pharmacy system) is located in a different building from the pharmacy, a network cable will connect this server to a nearby hub. The microcomputers and printers in the pharmacy will be connected via cable to a hub near the pharmacy. A backbone network cable connects the hubs.

Multiple servers, computers, microcomputers, printers, and a host of other types of devices can be attached to a network. The ability to access given computer applications is governed by the level of security access granted to the user by the security system in each computer.

Client Server Technology

Client server, or distributed processing, is the use of a network to connect a number of computers that interact or manage the same information. Information (or data) may be pulled into one computer from another, a process is applied to that information, and the results of the process may be retained in one computer or returned to the original one. An example would be the calculation of a drug dose at a local workstation. The system user's workstation may pull in the patient's weight, height, sex, and related drug information. The calculation of the appropriate dose would then occur at the workstation level. The resulting dose would be communicated back to the database server and incorporated into the patient's medication administration record.

System Project Organization and Management Methodology

Systems that have successfully achieved the goals for which they were acquired share some important ingredients. They operate under the auspices of a senior executive of the organization—a system sponsor. A dedicated project manager manages the implementation of the system. A project team participates in the tasks necessary to implement the system project in accordance with a well-defined work plan. A systems administrator handles the ongoing management of the system once it is put into production. The implementation of the system follows a well-defined project management methodology. What is most important—the intent for the procurement and ongoing management of the system's operation—is well defined.

The system sponsor is the individual for whom the project is being undertaken. The sponsor is responsible for justifying and obtaining funding for the procurement and ongoing operation of the system. This individual also defends departmental initiatives with the system. Generally the project (or system) sponsor is the person to whom the pharmacy director is accountable. The sponsor also serves as the person whom the project manager is accountable to during the course of the system project.

The project manager is the field boss during the implementation or upgrade of a computer system. In the pharmacy, a pharmacist or pharmacy technician best fills this job. That person should have an intimate knowledge of the operation to be automated, and the goals and objectives of the project. In addition, this individual should possess sufficient skills to manage pharmacy staff, participating staff from other departments, vendors, and assigned technical personnel. The project manager develops the work plan and uses it to manage the project team through to its completion.

One job of the project manager is to manage the expectations of all who are involved in the project. The project manager must manage the expectations of the sponsor, the members of the project team, and the other members of the hospital community who will be relying on the system when it goes into production. The work plan developed by the project manager must be realistic. Project milestones and other deliverables should take into consideration all steps necessary to complete the assigned tasks in a professional manner.

The project manager becomes the principal architect in designing how the system will be used in the pharmacy, and how it will interact with other systems and departments throughout the hospital. The project manager also will coordinate the definition of terminology, how the work flow of the area(s) being automated will interact with the system, and the development of all related forms, policies, and procedures.

A computer system can serve as a change agent to facilitate improvements of the processes being automated. If a system project automates a manual process without materially improving that process, the benefits of the system investment may be subject to question. Through the work flow design process, and the development of policies, procedures, and forms, the project team has a real opportunity to effect positive change.

A well-managed system project is supported by a team working under the direction of the project manager. The project team should consist of people containing the right mix of skills, experience, and knowledge to build the desired system. The team usually consists of representatives of the areas being automated. They should be intimately familiar with the work flow in their areas of responsibility, and all relevant policies and procedures. Subject to the components of the system being implemented, the project team should include information systems staff with hardware, network, or programming expertise. Additional participants should be considered from areas with which the pharmacy interfaces on a regular basis (e.g., nursing, admitting, medical staff). These additional team members can assist in designing into the system those features and functions that will promote increased customer satisfaction through the use of the system.

To begin the discussion about pharmacy computer applications, we must first understand how they fit within the framework of the hospital's mission critical applications.

Hospital Information System Application Relationships

Patient Flow Cycle

The basic hospital information system (HIS) manages a process of patient admission, charge capture, and billing. Although this is an oversimplification, it is in essence the set of features and functions performed within the HIS.

The admission process is of course a more complex process which is often referred to as the admission/discharge and transfer system (ADT). The ADT is the system that first acknowledges a patient's existence in the hospital to every other system. The pharmacy system depends on the ADT system to know that a patient is a current patient of the hospital, whether on an inpatient or ambulatory basis. The ADT provides the pharmacy system with basic demographics on each patient (name, medical record number, bill/account number, date of birth, sex, etc.).

The ADT keeps the pharmacy system informed as to each patient's location in the hospital. The pharmacy then knows the room and bed location of each patient. The ADT lets the pharmacy know where to send medication orders, where to send reports concerning patients, and if the patient has been discharged and is no longer entitled to filled orders.

In addition, the ADT provides other systems with critical information necessary to manage other processes within the hospital. Insurance information is collected here to facilitate the billing process. Next of kin information is collected here to allow health care providers to contact the patient's family should there be a need to do so.

The ADT can be used to help the hospital collect other valuable information about its patients. Does the patient have a living will or durable power of attorney? Who referred the patient to the hospital? Who is the patient's physician?

The next component of the patient flow cycle is the charge capture system. A modern HIS system is referred to as the order entry system. Every time an order is entered on a patient, a charge is being captured for billing purposes, and a statistic is being captured for management monitoring purposes. Depending on the nature of an order, some charges are not computed until a test is resulted or the order is completed. In the case of physical therapy, an order for such a service typically is not finalized until after the physical therapist can assess the patient's condition and determine the amount of therapy required.

Medical records owns a piece of the patient flow cycle. At discharge, the medical records department codes the chart with procedure and diagnostic information. This information is required for regulatory and billing purposes. A linkage between this coded information, charge information, and admitting information forms the basis of the billing and accounting functions performed relative to the services rendered to each patient.

The patient accounting component forms the last piece of the patient flow cycle, which is the final piece into which all previously collected information flows, and allows the hospital to bill and collect for its services. Components of this system include charge capture, accounts receivable, collection system, and cash receipts system. This system, and its relationship to the other components of the patient flow cycle, forms the basis for compliance with regulatory reporting standards of state, federal, and other accrediting organizations.

Ancillary Systems

The pharmacy system is one of many ancillary departmental systems. Other departments have specialized systems that support their operations such as radiology, clinical pathology, surgical pathology, food and nutritional services, the operating room, and other procedure areas, and specialty labs. These systems relate to the patient flow cycle systems in the same manner as the pharmacy system.

Patient information is received via the ADT system. When a patient is registered in the ADT system, this information is made available to each ancillary system. Each time an inpatient transfers to another room or bed, each ancillary system receives a notification from the ADT system. Upon each patient's discharge, the ancillary systems also receive notification of this transaction.

The relationships of systems in many hospitals allow ancillary systems to communicate with one another to support patient care needs. For example, if a lab result indicates the need for an adjustment of a patient's medication, then such a result can be triggered to automatically place a notification in the pharmacy system for a pharmacist to review. As a dietician may have a similar need to manage patients' nutritional intake, certain lab values also can be automatically sent to the food and nutritional services system.

Services provided by the ancillary department are captured within the ancillary system. Each order entered is processed to interact with the inventory that the department manages. Issues result in a reduction of the inventory on hand. The item that has been ordered and issued to the patient, with the patient's identifying information, is communicated back to the hospital's billing system. To the extent that test results would accompany this communication from the ancillary system (in the case of radiology or laboratory systems), the result would be placed in a portion of the hospital's information system where it can be retrieved by caregivers who have a need to access such information.

Many HIS environments support order entry via the HIS. These orders can be transmitted directly to each ancillary system via an automated interface as a vehicle to speed the service delivery. Order entry interfaces and their implications in the pharmacy will be addressed later in this chapter.

Business Systems

Several other systems support the day-to-day activities of a hospital. For the purposes of this chapter, they are classified as business systems.

The finance department requires a number of systems to support its operations: payroll systems, accounts payable systems, general ledger and budgeting systems, and cost accounting systems. For the most part, the functions performed by these systems are self-evident by their names. It is also important to understand that the pharmacy interacts with each of these systems on paper, or in an automated sense as it relates to the business processes of the pharmacy.

The hospital's payroll system is the vehicle that will pay the employees of the pharmacy. Hours have to be collected for input at the end of each pay period. Adjustments, vacation time, sick time, and staffing shift differential pay (for evening and night shift staff) need to be collected and submitted by the pharmacy's management in a timely manner to get staff paid.

The accounts payable system processes the pharmacy's bills for payment, as it does for every other department of the hospital. This system requires that the pharmacy verify the purchases of supplies, products, or services on invoices prior to processing payment. Accounts payable systems are often linked to materials management systems to facilitate the linkage between purchasing and receiving, and the accounting for the payment for purchases.

The general ledger and budget systems allow the pharmacy to submit its budget for the coming year and track its actual expenditures against the approved budget.

Although only one system may reside in the pharmacy, it must interact with the vast majority of systems in the hospital to conduct its day-to-day business.

The Hospital Pharmacy Application

Pharmacy information systems are designed to support the specific needs of pharmacy operations. These systems support activities that fall into several broad categories: inventory management, purchasing, distribution/production, and clinical support.

Inventory Management

A good place to start is the maintenance of the pharmacy's inventory. The level or quantity of each item in inventory triggers the need to order more product. Items in inventory are ordered in quantities that may equal the same quantities of issue. Some items in inventory must be processed, and new items or products are created for inventory. The inventory system must be maintained in a manner that defines the relationship of the quantities of items purchased as compared with the quantities of issue for each item.

Inventory systems must also notify the purchasing component of the system when it reaches a reorder point with regard to each item of inventory. This reorder point is the result of a calculation that is typically performed by the pharmacy system. System users can elect to use the results of this calculation, or use their own reorder quantity. The inventory system requires a defined par level value, or the total quantity or level to which a reorder should bring each item in inventory.

When shipments are received, they must be checked against the purchasing documentation and then logged in to inventory. Many pharmacy systems employ bar code scanners which speed up the process of item identification and input into the system. These scanners allow the user to enter quantities to facilitate the process of receiving and issuing items from inventory. When an order received is incomplete, the pharmacy system will track open order, or back order, situations. When the inventory level dips to a critical low, it will notify the purchasing component of the system and the key system user that follow-up is necessary.

As patient medication orders are filled, stock levels are automatically reduced in the inventory system. As stock items are taken to create new products (e.g., I.V. admixtures), the inventory system reduces the inventory by the items removed and increases the quantities of the items manufactured. In each type of transaction it is critical for the pharmacist or technician to ensure that the transaction is recorded in the system.

The term *perpetual inventory* is best understood as the quantity count of items in stock, based on the computer's calculations of purchases, less medications dispensed plus the inventory item count at the last physical inventory. Its accuracy is dependent on several variables, including compatibility of the unit of issue with the unit of purchase, the accurate reporting of inventory shrinkage (e.g., items removed from stock due to expiration), and the accuracy of reporting of every item added to and removed from stock. It is up to the pharmacist or pharmacy technician to maintain the definitions in the inventory system in a manner that the system can correctly perform the necessary calculations. Periodic physical counts of the inventory in stock must be performed, and the results compared with the system inventory. This procedure will ensure the integrity of the information in the system and will alert the pharmacy as to any shrinkage of inventory that requires follow-up.

Purchasing/Receiving

When drugs, supplies, or other items in inventory require restocking, or new items must be purchased, the purchasing system is the vehicle that serves to facilitate the process. The purchasing system enables the management of orders placed, tracks open orders and back orders, and possesses the capability to electronically communicate new purchases to suppliers.

Whether the order for restocking is computed electronically (calculated by the system) or an item is entered for purchasing, the system will create a purchase requisition. Subject to the nature of the item(s) to be purchased, the system provides analysis tools to assist in analyzing supplier pricing. Once the supplier for each item is identified, requisitions are converted into purchase orders. Each purchase order contains those items to be acquired from one supplier. It contains all agreed terms and conditions of the purchase.

When a purchase order is generated by the system, and signed by an authorized signatory, it becomes a legally binding agreement when accepted by the supplier. Most suppliers will ship an order based only on receiving a purchase order number. Pharmacy computer systems are usually capable of generating purchase orders and transmitting them to suppliers electronically. In these instances, both the pharmacy (hospital) and the supplier usually agree to be bound by certain terms and conditions, as if a purchase order was duly signed by the purchaser and accepted by the supplier.

An electronically transmitted purchase order employs a technology referred to as electronic data interchange (EDI). EDI technology is commonly used for ordering merchandise, transferring funds (e.g., electronic payroll deposits), and billing.

Upon receipt of merchandise ordered, pharmacy personnel must count the items received and compare them with the items, quantities, and pricing ordered. Although the process can occur directly on-line on a computer terminal, it typically is more expeditious to check the order against the vendor's packing list, and then check the packing list against the order and the invoice. If there is any discrepancy in the shipment against the order, the system will facilitate correcting the error. It is important to understand that the system will not correct the error, but merely provide the pharmacist or technician sufficient information so that the discrepancy may be followed up. When ordered merchandise is acknowledged to the system as received, the inventory on hand is updated.

Clinical Support

The production side of pharmacy operations relates to the receipt of medication orders for patient care, the processing of the orders, and the tracking of patients' medication history. The features and functions of pharmacy information systems, and the relationship they bear to a hospital's order entry system, vary widely.

Most physicians generate medication orders in their own handwriting. The issues surrounding physicians entering orders directly into a system are complex, and will be discussed briefly later in this chapter. In most hospitals today, physician orders are keyed into systems in the pharmacy. Fax machines, pneumatic tubes, and couriers are all being used to transmit orders from nursing units to the pharmacy. In some instances, physicians are entering orders directly into the HIS, which is interfaced to the pharmacy system or order entry.

Upon entry of the medication order, some systems will immediately identify existing medication orders, laboratory test results, or allergies that may be incompatible with the order just placed. Other systems have functionality which will suggest to the user that certain laboratory tests should be ordered with the medication order, and other open orders should be discontinued based on the current literature. Still other features include suggesting more cost-effective medications than the one ordered. In such instances, the system is not designed to terminate the order, but merely suggest to the pharmacist or technician that the physician who wrote the order should be contacted to verify that the order is as intended.

The pharmacy system will generally receive relevant information on every patient from the HIS to facilitate the processing of appropriate doses. Date of birth, sex, height, weight, medical record number, and admitting (or billing) number are critical pieces of information. These data, coupled with the history of medications already ordered/dispensed to the patient, laboratory results, vital signs, diet orders/restrictions, and knowledge of procedures which have been ordered/scheduled provide the system and the pharmacist with critical information to assist in managing the patient toward a speedy recovery.

When orders are entered, the system queues up the orders for a regular production cycle. Pharmacists and technicians prepare medication doses in accordance with schedules prepared by the system. The system also generates the appropriate labels for the medication to be administered. When robotics is being utilized, pharmacy information systems can electronically pass the order to the robot.

As the orders are packaged for shipping to the patient units, the inventory system is automatically adjusted to reflect a reduction in stock. In addition, each patient's medication administration record is updated to reflect the order and the medications dispensed. Medication lot numbers are also tracked so as to facilitate patient identification in the event of a manufacturer's recall.

Orders issued are communicated to such other systems as the hospital patient accounting (or billing) system, cost accounting system, utilization review system, or other systems which have authorized access.

For a pharmacist to fill a medication order for a patient, the pharmacist must determine that the order was written by a physician, and that the medication, dosage, and frequency of its administration is in accordance with the physician's order. The two accepted mechanisms to accomplish this process are (1) the pharmacist visually inspects the physician's written order and then enters it into the system, or (2) the physician enters the order directly into the system and uses a secret password that only he or she would know. Medication orders that are transcribed by a unit secretary or other personnel may result in errors, and should not be considered reliable. Most of the HIS implementations to date have not been successful in inducing the medical staff to enter medication or other orders directly into the computer without transcription.

Over the years a number of information system vendors have designed order entry systems which have attempted to induce physicians to enter orders directly into the system. Some of the newer systems have simplified the number of steps necessary to input an order. Some vendors have linked the order entry process with other patient information and current literature concerning the medication order. As of this writing very few hospitals have successfully implemented systems into which medication orders are entered directly by the medical staff.

Drug information is published in the *Physician's Desk Reference®* (*PDR®*) and in other publications which are of enormous value to physicians and pharmacists on a daily basis. The ability to access this information on a timely basis is a perfect application for computerization to facilitate. Several leading pharmacy information system vendors incorporate some level of capability to perform searches for educational material about medications.

There is a vendor whose core business is the maintenance of current information concerning medications, general pharmacology, and other related health care information in the form of numerous computerized database products. Micromedex, Inc., a Denver-based company, sells a series of database services designed to provide access to medical information.

According to Micromedex's own literature, the features of their various product offerings include the ability to access "dosing, pharmacokinetics, cautions, interactions, clinical applications, comparative efficacy and place in therapy for investigational, prescription, FDA-approved, and over-the-counter medications" (Micromedix, 1998). Additional databases are maintained which provide valuable information in researching potential poisonous agents and general safety information.

The Future of Pharmacy Information Systems

The future of pharmacy information systems appears to be heading in two distinct directions. The first is the integration of the data and information-driven systems with robotics for drug dispensing. The second is the improvement of voice recognition technology to attract more physicians to enter their own orders directly into a system.

In a truly integrated environment the management of patient medications is closely tied with laboratory results and diet. Abnormal laboratory test results can trigger alerts to clinical decision makers, which can result in a change to the patient's medications or diet. As physician order entry occurs, integrated systems can provide educational reminders, or a series of cost-effective options, for physicians and other clinical decision makers to consider. When orders are about to be entered that are inconsistent with the patient's treatment plan, the system can also alert the system user to the potential problem.

An order system that is linked to a robotics system can then complete the automation loop by processing and filling the orders without human involvement from the moment the order is entered. These robotic systems must be managed by pharmacy personnel. Inventory levels within the robot must be periodically checked. The restocking of the robot's inventory levels also must be manually supervised.

True integration allows the hospital to operate as a whole. Information concerning all services provided to a patient can interact against a common data repository, which will form the true source for all patient information. These repositories will not only hold patient data, but also diagnostic images (X rays, lab slides, etc.).

Clinical data repositories will form the basis of becoming an on-line, computerized patient record. This record will contain information concerning the most recent patient encounter, and all information concerning a patient's medical history throughout a patient's life.

Voice recognition is the vehicle that holds a lot of promise for bringing more physicians into the world of automated order entry. Consider the fact that the effort required to write an order is much easier than the effort involved in signing onto a system, flipping through order entry screens, identifying medications from the formulary, and validating the entry. Many physicians are reluctant to undertake this responsibility. Once perfected, voice recognition will provide a vehicle that will require little training, and actually ease the effort for physicians.

Although the technologies described in this section do exist today, they are not widely used or are in early stages of development and/or release. By looking at what they are being designed to accomplish, they create a clear vision of what the near future will look like.

Summary

Early forms of automation dealt with speeding the processing of information so that productivity gains could be reached. As computers and technology have gotten more sophisticated, speeding the ability to access information has allowed decision makers to make more intelligent decisions. This is true for the pharmacy, as well.

This chapter was written with the goal of letting the reader understand that the role of the pharmacist and pharmacy technician is a critical one in the implementation and management of systems in a hospital pharmacy operation. A systems consultant can certainly play a role in managing a system, but ultimately leaves the project when it is completed. The pharmacists and pharmacy technicians are the individuals who will be responsible for the care and feeding of the system after the consultants leave. The pharmacists and pharmacy technicians are the people who are responsible for linking the features and functions of a system with the operational needs of the workplace.

Society has grown to be more dependent on automation over the years. Successful pharmacy professionals will be those who understand what automation can contribute, are able to harness its power, and are able to align its power with the tactical and strategic requirements of the business of pharmacy and hospital management.

ASSESSMENT

Multiple Choice Questions

1. The software that provides the desirable features and functions is the
   a. operating system software
   b. files
   c. application software
   d. data

2. Under a software license, a user typically can
   a. modify the software
   b. use the software
   c. copy the software for sale
   d. copy the software for others to use

3. A benefit of using a server for file storage is NOT
   a. to facilitate sharing common files
   b. to store computer programs
   c. to facilitate communications between different computer systems
   d. to provide improved access security

4. Which of the following is NOT typically provided by the admission/discharge/transfer system?
   a. validates a patient to the pharmacy system as a hospital patient
   b. identifies the patient's room and bed location to the pharmacy system
   c. identifies patients' allergies
   d. identifies patients' insurance coverage

True/False Questions

5. _F_ Any computer connected to a computer network automatically gains access to all other connected computers.

6. _T_ Automating a manual process will definitely result in process improvement. _They say_

7. _T_ A computer system can serve as a change agent to facilitate improvement.

8. _T_ Most technology can be interfaced to communicate between different computers and robots automatically.

If physicians would enter their medication orders themselves into the hospital's HIS, the benefits would include

9. _T_ gaining access to allergy information

10. _T_ gaining access to drug interaction information

11. _T_ gaining access to a patient's medication administration record

12. _T_ the ability to link changes in lab values with medications administered

13. _T_ gaining access to suggested alternative medication therapies to the medications being ordered

14. _T_ being alerted to lab tests which should be ordered to monitor a drug's impact

15. _T_ having orders entered more accurately than if transcribed by another

Bibliography

Ball, M. J., Simborg, D. W., Albright, J., & Douglas, J. (1995). *Healthcare information management systems: A practical guide* (Computers in Health Care Series). New York: Springer Verlag.

Boland, P. (Ed.). (1996). *Redesigning healthcare delivery: A practical guide to reengineering, restructuring, and renewal.* Berkeley, CA: Boland Healthcare, Inc.

Drazen, Metzger, Ritter, & Schneider. (1994). *Patient care information systems: Successful design and implementation* (Computers in Health Care Series). New York: Springer Verlag.

Micromedex, Inc. (1998). Healthcare product catalog.

Tan, J. K. H. (1995). *Health management information systems: Theories, methods, and applications.* Gaithersburg, MD: Aspen Publications.

15 Medication Errors

COMPETENCIES

Upon completion and review of this chapter, the student should be able to

1. Discuss the role of the pharmacy technician in preventing medication errors.
2. Determine the cause of system breakdowns that result in medication errors.
3. Define the types of medication errors that occur during the ordering and dispensing process.
4. State the eleven steps necessary for proper dispensing of medications.
5. List some commonly used drugs that result in medication error deaths.
6. Define *confirmation bias*.
7. List the steps that should be taken to minimize errors when taking verbal orders.

Introduction

Concern about medication errors has intensified in both the lay public and health care sectors, especially with an increasing number of media reports about accidents. Health professionals acknowledge that medication errors are a growing concern because of the increased numbers of critically ill patients, the evolution of drugs toward more potent—and potentially more dangerous—agents and methods of administration, and more emphasis on fiscal constraints which impact on hospital staffing. Protecting patients from inappropriate administration of medication and intravenous fluids has become an important area of focus for hospitals, with many of the hospitals developing multidisciplinary teams to deal with this problem.

In a modern hospital pharmacy, technicians play a major role. On the basis of a summary of several studies, Allan and Barker (1990) estimated that medication errors occur at a rate of about one per patient per day. Although most of these errors probably have minimal clinical significance and do not adversely affect patients, it stands to reason that the less controlled drug distribution systems are, the more likely patients are at risk of serious error. This chapter focuses on system enhancements and the checks and balances needed to provide the maximum degree of safety as we prepare, dispense, and control medications in health care institutions.

Background

When an error occurs, it is the result of a deficit in one of two areas: knowledge or performance. Because no one knows everything there is to know and everyone has occasional lapses in performance, we all will occasionally make errors. Therefore, a system must be in place to filter out errors and prevent them from reaching patients. The reader may find it useful to refer to the ASHP Guidelines on Preventing Medication Errors in Hospitals.

Health care professionals must apply the "five rights" of medication prescribing, dispensing, and administering for medications to be both safe and effective. The *right* medication in the *right* dose has to be administered by the *right* route at the *right* time to the *right* patient. We will discuss eliminating medication errors by examining the ordering and dispensing processes.

Ordering Medications

In nearly all hospitals, physicians initiate the drug-dispensing and administration process, although increasingly pharmacists, nurses, and physician assistants are legally permitted to prescribe. Errors due to lack of knowledge or poor performance can occur. Although computerized order entry systems are being developed and implemented in hospitals, most of us continue to rely on handwritten medical orders. Although computerization may help reduce certain types of errors, such as illegible handwriting errors, a new type of error, computer entry errors, can occur because the computer is only as good as the human who uses it. More commonly, handwritten orders that are illegible, ambiguous, or incomplete cause or contribute to many errors made by nurses, pharmacists, pharmacy technicians, and other health care professionals who carry out orders.

Illegible Handwriting

To minimize the chance of misinterpretation, physicians with poor handwriting should print their orders in block letters or review them with the nursing staff before leaving the patient care area. In addition, including the purpose of the medication as part of the order can help readers distinguish drug name pairs when the writing is less than ideal. Very few name pairs that are spelled similarly are used for similar purposes. Notebook computers, dictation, and direct order entry into the computer by physicians are solutions for poor handwriting and improper orders. The hospital quality assurance program is used to identify problem cases and seek appropriate remedy.

Because even skilled individuals can misread good handwriting, a system of transcribing orders should be in place in which several individuals interpret and transcribe an order before it can be implemented. In many hospitals, each order is read by a unit secretary and reviewed by a nurse. At the same time, an exact copy of the order is sent to the pharmacy either directly or by fax. There are a number of times the drug should be checked against the original order regarding drug identity, drug label, and proper drug container. A technician often screens the order first, then enters it into a computer. A label is printed and then a pharmacist interprets the order and verifies the technician's computer entry by comparing it with the label. Later the order and label will again be read by technicians and pharmacists as doses are prepared and dispensed. In outpatient settings, this system should include a final check when providing counseling to the patient. In no case should pharmacy technicians interpret orders on their own, because this process does not offer enough checks in the event an error is made. In addition, it is important that orders are filled not only from the label generated from the computer, but the original order must also accompany the label to serve as another check.

Look-Alike Drug Names

Medications with names that are spelled similarly can easily be mistaken for another drug. Technicians must be alert to this problem and should never guess when in doubt. Hospitals should establish policies that, except in emergencies, nurses' oral requests for medications will not be accepted until the pharmacy has reviewed a copy of the order, because it is more likely that pharmacists are aware of newly marketed drugs with names similar to those of familiar drugs. Fax machines on each nursing unit and in the pharmacy make the process of having a pharmacist review the order easier.

Sound-Alike Drug Names

Drug orders communicated orally are often misheard, misunderstood, misinterpreted, or transcribed incorrectly. Seldane and Feldene sound alike as do amrinone and amiodarone, Procardia SL (sublingual) and Procardia XL (extended release), Lanoxin and Levoxin (changed by the manufacturers to Levoxyl to avoid errors), Kemadrin and Coumadin, and probably thousands of other pairs. All of these have been confused at least once and resulted in a patient receiving the wrong medication. In many cases, serious injuries have occurred because of misinterpreted oral orders. Sound-alike drug names present many of the same problems as look-alike names. Obviously, when uncertainties exist, the pharmacist must contact the prescriber for clarification of the order.

To decrease the opportunity for misunderstanding, hospitals should seriously discourage oral orders. Greater use of fax machines between hospital areas and between medical offices, pharmacies, and nursing units will help. When oral communication is unavoidable, strict adherence to the following procedures for oral orders minimizes errors.

- Oral orders should only be taken by authorized personnel.
- If possible, a second person should listen in while the order is given.
- The order should be transcribed and read back, repeating exactly what has been understood, sometimes spelling the drug name for verification.
- The order must make sense for the patient's clinical situation.

To prevent sound-alike and look-alike errors, physicians must be encouraged to include in their orders complete directions, strengths, and the indication (purpose) for use. All of these elements can serve as identifiers. It cannot be stressed enough that even if such information is lacking on orders, by knowing a drug's purpose and the patient's problems, skilled health care professionals can judge whether the drug ordered makes sense for the patient in light of the context in which the order is written. Diagnostic procedures given with orders could also provide valued information, which explains why it is so important for pharmacists to verify all orders processed by technicians. Never guess on an order. Always check with the pharmacist, who can call the physician for clarification.

Ambiguous Orders

Errors can result when ambiguous orders are interpreted in a manner other than what the prescriber intended. Proper expression of doses is vital in a drug order.

You should be able to recognize improper expressions of doses—and the potential for error—when you see them, and bring them to the pharmacist's attention. When the prescriber's clarification is needed, the pharmacist must contact the prescriber. Technicians should avoid using improper expressions of doses as they process orders, type labels, and communicate with others. Several improperly expressed orders are analyzed and corrected in the following examples.

1. *Decreased doses.* A diabetic patient who had been on 80 mg of prednisone daily for several months was seen by her physician. The physician decided to decrease the daily dose by 5 mg, from 80 mg to 75 mg, and wrote the order, "Decrease prednisone—75 mg." The order was misinterpreted as meaning 80 mg *minus* 75 mg and was transcribed as, "Prednisone 5 mg p.o. daily." As a result, a 5 mg dose was given, and the unintentional sudden, large decrease in dosage caused the patient to collapse. "Decrease prednisone by 5 mg daily" would have been clearer, but the safest way would have been "Decrease prednisone by 5 mg daily. New dose is 75 mg daily."

2. *Tablet strengths.* Orders specifying both strength and number of tablets are confusing when more than one tablet strength exists. For example, "Propranolol 1/2 tablet 40 mg qid" appears clear enough; however, when you realize that this product is available in both 40 mg and 80 mg tablets, this order becomes ambiguous. What is the intended dose, 40 mg or 20 mg? Orders are clearer if the dose is specified regardless of the strengths available: "Propranolol 40 mg qid." For doses that require several tablets or capsules, the pharmacy label should note the exact number of dosage units needed. For example, the label on a 500 mg dose of Diabinese, which is available in 250 mg tablets, should read "2 × 250 mg tablets = 500 mg." For a 2.5 mg dose of prednisone, which is available in 5 mg tablets, the label should read "1/2 × 5 mg tablet = 2.5 mg." If the pharmacy prepares a computer-generated medication administration record (computer MAR) for the nurses, this same type of notation should be used.

3. *Liquid dosage forms.* Expressing the dose only in milliliters (or teaspoonsful) for liquid dosage forms is confusing. For example, phenobarbital elixir is available in two strengths: 15 mg per 5 mL and 20 mg per 5 mL. If the prescriber wrote "5 mL," the intended number of milligrams would be unclear, but "20 mg" is clear. The amount of drug by metric weight as well as the volume should always be included on the pharmacy label: "Phenobarbital elixir 20 mg/5 mL." Further, the patient dose should also be included; for a 30 mg dose the label should read, "30 mg = 7.5 mL." The same holds true for unit-dose labels and bulk labels.

4. *Injectables.* For injectables, the same rule applies. List the metric weight or the metric weight and volume—never the volume alone—because solution concentrations are so variable. An error occurred from this problem at a hospital where hepatitis B vaccines were being administered. A preprinted doctor's order form was used to prescribe the vaccine, listing only the volume to be given. When the clinic switched to another brand of vaccine, containing a different concentration, the same preprinted forms continued to be used, thus underdosing hundreds of children until the error was discovered. This situation could have been avoided if the amount of vaccine had been prescribed (using micrograms), not just the volume.

5. *Variable amounts.* A drug dose should never be ordered solely by number of tablets, capsules, ampules, or vials, because the amounts contained in these dosage forms are variable. Drug doses should be ordered with proper unit expression, for example, 20 mEq of magnesium sulfate. A patient whose doctor

orders "an amp" of magnesium sulfate might get 8 mEq, 40 mEq, or 60 mEq. Under certain circumstances the higher dose could be lethal.

6. *Zeros and decimal points.* When listing drug doses on labels or in other communications, never follow a whole number with a zero. For example, "Colchicine 1.0 mg" is a very dangerous way to express this dose. If a decimal point is not seen, the dose could be misinterpreted as "10 mg" and a tenfold overdose could result. The same could happen if "Dilaudid 1.0 mg" is written. The proper way to express these two orders would be "Colchicine 1 mg" and "Dilaudid 1 mg," respectively. On the other hand, always place a zero *before* a decimal point when the dose is smaller than one. For example, "Synthroid .1 mg" may be seen as "Synthroid 1 mg," especially when a poor impression of the decimal is written, such as on order copies of faxes. Avoid using decimal expressions when recognizable alternatives exist, because whole numbers are easier to work with. In the previous example, "Synthroid 0.1 mg" would be good, but "Synthroid 100 mcg" would be better. Use "Digoxin 125 mcg" rather than "Digoxin 0.125 mg." Use "500 mg" instead of "0.5 grams."

7. *Spacing.* When typing labels, always place a space after the drug name, the dose, and the unit of measurement. It is difficult to read labels when everything runs together. Do not type "Inderal40mg" which can be misinterpreted as "Inderal 140 mg." Instead, type "Inderal 40 mg."

8. *Grams and milliliters.* On labels, "grams" should be abbreviated "g" and milliliter should be abbreviated "mL," not "ml." The abbreviation "cc" instead of "mL" is discouraged.

9. *Apothecary system.* Use the metric system exclusively. Although you have learned about the apothecary systems and its grains, drams, minims, ounces, and so on, the system is very inaccurate and is not used in modern expression of drug doses. The apothecary system is no longer official in the U.S.P.

Abbreviations to Avoid

Certain abbreviations are easily misinterpreted. Controlling dangerous abbreviations will reduce communication errors. Although many hospitals have lists of abbreviations that are approved for use by the professional staff, it would be far safer if each hospital also developed a list of abbreviations that should never be used. In fact, a negative list is easier to maintain and enforce.

A number of abbreviations are easily misinterpreted. These abbreviations should never be used on pharmacy labels, in newsletters or other communications that originate in the pharmacy, or in pharmacy computer systems, because they may find their way to medication orders, labels, and reports. Several examples of misinterpreted abbreviations are described.

The abbreviation "U" for unit is an example of what can go wrong; it should be on every hospital's list of unacceptable abbreviations. It can easily be confused with the numerals 0, 4, 6, and 7, and even "cc," resulting in disastrous drug overdoses with insulin, heparin, penicillin, and other drugs measured in units.

Another example of an abbreviation that should not be used is "d/c." It has been written to mean either discontinue or discharge, sometimes resulting in premature stoppage of a patient's medications. The "d/c" order can be incorrectly interpreted as discontinuation of a medication that the patient had never even received. In reality, the "d/c" means that the drug was approved for use by the physician.

Do not abbreviate drug names. For example "MTX" means "methotrexate" to some health professionals; others understand it as "mitoxantrone." "AZT" has been misunderstood as "azathioprine" (Imuran) when "zidovudine" (Retrovir) was the intended meaning. This misinterpretation led to an AIDS patient receiving azathioprine, an immunosuppressant, instead of the AIDS drug. The patient's immune system worsened, and he developed an overwhelming infection. In another example, the abbreviation "AZT" was used to prescribe aztreonam (Azactam), but zidovudine was incorrectly dispensed.

Do not use apothecary abbreviations and symbols. The symbol ℔ (for "minim") has been read as "mL" (there are 16.23 minims in 1 mL). When written as "3ĭ," the dram symbol 3 has been mistaken for a numeral 3, and the symbol ĭ, meaning "1," as the letter *T,* or 3T, and thus three tablespoonsful (45 mL) of drug were administered instead of 5 mL (1 dram = 5 mL). The abbreviation for grain (gr) and gram (g) can also be confused.

Dispensing

An important safety enhancement for preventing dispensing errors is the development of a system of multiple checks from the time an order is first written on the nursing unit, to receipt in the pharmacy, through dispensing and administration. Such a system is suggested in this section. Obviously, the more "looks" at the order, while efficient work flow is still maintained, the better. There are several checkpoints where various health professionals can review orders and maximize the chances of discovering errors. Hospitals with computerized drug distribution systems have an advantage, because labels and reports can be printed so that at various steps the order interpretation and entry can be checked. Even hospitals without computer systems should review the following suggested work flow, because many of the options are available in a manual system.

1. The physician sees the patient; performs an assessment; determines appropriate medication, dose, and frequency; and writes the order. Unusual orders or orders for new drugs not yet on the hospital formulary are also communicated orally to nursing personnel.
2. A unit secretary reads and transcribes the order onto the medication administration record (MAR). This step is unnecessary in hospitals where computers generate the MAR or where physicians can enter orders by computer, but the nurse and the pharmacist must still verify the order.
3. A nurse checks the unit secretary's transcription for accuracy.
4. Simultaneously with steps 2 and 3, a direct copy of the order is carried or faxed to the pharmacy, or the physician's computer entry reaches the pharmacy. The pharmacy technician reads the order and enters it in the pharmacy computer system. In some hospitals, orders are entered in the pharmacy computer system by pharmacists or technicians working on terminals located on nursing units. If the technician finds a duplicate order, incorrect dose, an allergy, or the like, it is documented and called to the attention of the pharmacist during the clinical screening (step 5).
5. A pharmacist reviews the technician's computer entry and does a clinical screening.
6. A label or a medication profile is printed. A copy of the medication order accompanies the label or medication profile while the order is filled. No orders are filled solely on the basis of what appears on the label or medication profile, as the patient profile entry may have been in error.
7. To choose an item for dispensing, a technician reviews both the label and the medication order for possible discrepancies.

8. A pharmacist checks the technician's work, reviewing the label against the medication order copy and the dose that has been prepared. The drug is dispensed.
9. The nurse receives the drug and compares the medication and pharmacy label against the copy of the physician's order and the handwritten transcription made earlier in the MAR.
10. The nurse administers the dose, explaining the drug's purpose, side effects, and so on, and answers questions and concerns raised by the patient.
11. Carts are returned to the pharmacy. The pharmacist or technician determines what doses, if any, have been returned, to make sure no omission errors have occurred.

Following are some ways that computerized drug order entry systems enhance routine drug-dispensing activities.

■ For routine bin filling, the pharmacy technician prints out the medication profile and fills labeled patient medication bins for the medication administration carts with doses to be used the following day. The pharmacist uses the medication printout to check the accuracy of bin filling by the technician and approves bins for transfer to the floors.
■ For drug administration, the nurse receives a computer-generated MAR each day listing all current items. The new MAR is compared with the previous day's MAR for accuracy.
■ For physician review, physicians receive an MAR printout each day for their review. They check the MAR to be certain that medical orders have been interpreted properly by pharmacists and nurses, that no orders have been accidentally discontinued, that no duplications exist, and so on.

Selecting the Medication

The importance of reading the label cannot be overemphasized. When the wrong drug or wrong strength is dispensed, the error may stem from failure to read the label. During drug preparation and dispensing, the label should be read three times: when the product is selected, when the medication is prepared, and when either the partially used medication is disposed of (or returned to stock) or product preparation is complete.

Selecting the correct item from the shelf, drawer, or bin can be complicated by many factors. Similar labeling and packaging is a common trap that leads to medication errors. Restocking errors are quite common and can lead to repeated medication errors before being detected.

Automated dispensing machines have become more common on the nursing units of many hospitals. The nurse must punch in a security code and a password into the dispensing device, with the name of the patient and the name of the medication before the machine will allow access to it to remove the medication. This system allows more control of items kept on the nursing unit and serves as a check for the nurse who retrieves the medication, more so than for regularly stocked floor stock items. In some cases, on-line communication with the hospital computer information system or pharmacy system allows a pharmacist to review medication orders prior to nursing access.

There are several places where a medication error can occur in this process. The automated machines are restocked daily and the incorrect restocking of items can occur. Also, when some of the devices are accessed, the drawer that opens may contain several medications in a matrix, creating the potential for the nurse to retrieve the wrong item. These are errors that also occur during the process of selecting floor stock items that are not in a machine. Errors can also occur in those systems where a pharmacist does not have access to the order before the nurse administers it, so that no double check is performed.

Such mix-ups occur primarily due to lack of correctly reading the label. The problem is compounded by what is referred to as "confirmation bias": When choosing an item, you see what you are looking for, and once you find what you are looking for, you stop looking. Often the health professional chooses a medication container based on a mental picture of the item. You may be looking for some characteristic of the drug label, the shape and size or color of the container, or the location of the item on a shelf, in a drawer, or in a storage bin instead of reading the name of the drug itself. Consequently, you may fail to realize that you have the wrong item in hand. Physically separating drugs with look-alike labels and packaging will also reduce the potential for error. Some technicians also separate drugs with similar names and overlapping strengths, especially those labeled and packaged by the same manufacturer, because they also look alike. For example, thiamine 100 mg tablets and thioridazine 100 mg tablets, both from the same unit-dose packager, might pose a problem, as well as quinidine 200 mg and quinine 200 mg. Pharmaceutical companies are aware of labeling and packaging problems, and many have responded to suggestions made by technicians and pharmacists. You can alert manufacturers about errors related to commercial packaging and labeling problems by using the USP-ISMP (Institute for Safe Medication Practices) Medication Errors Reporting Program (MERP). All reports are forwarded to the company and the U.S. Food and Drug Administration (FDA), and ISMP provides follow-up when appropriate. Call 1-800-23-ERROR, or complete a USP-ISMP MERP report (**Figure 15–1**). All reports are confidential.

All health care professionals should have input in deciding how and where drugs are available, how doses are prepared, who is responsible for preparing them, what the storage containers look like, and how they are labeled. Procedures to ensure their safe use must be written, and there must be an understanding of the importance of adhering to the guidelines that are developed.

Auxiliary Labels

To help prevent errors, the pharmacy should apply auxiliary labels in certain circumstances. For example, amoxicillin oral suspension is available in dropper bottles for pediatric use. When the suspension is used for an ear infection, some parents have been known to place the suspension in the child's ear rather than give it properly, that is, orally. An auxiliary label "For oral use only" would help prevent this error. Other such labels are "For the ear," "For the eye," and "For external use only."

Effective Medication Error Prevention and Monitoring Systems

The chance of dosage calculation or measurement error is minimized by systems designed with procedures that require a double check. The double check might be required for all calculations or measurements or only for those falling in special categories. Special categories may include dosage calculations for any child under 12 years, for certain situations such as critical care drug infusions requiring a dose in micrograms per kilogram per minute, insulin infusions, chemotherapy, and patient-controlled analgesia compounding. Calculators and computer programs may im-

USP MEDICATION ERRORS REPORTING PROGRAM

Presented in cooperation with the Institute for Safe Medication Practices

The USP Practitioners' Reporting Network℠ is an FDA MedWatch partner

MEDI-CATION ERRORS

REPORTING PROGRAM

❑ ACTUAL ERROR ❑ POTENTIAL ERROR

Please describe the error. Include description of sequence of events, personnel involved, and work environment (e.g., code situation, change of shift, short staffing, no 24-hr. pharmacy, floor stock). If more space is needed, please attach separate page.

Was the medication administered to or used by the patient? ❑ Yes ❑ No

Please describe outcome (e.g., death, type of injury, adverse reaction)._____

When and how was error discovered? _____

If practitioner intervened, what type of staff discovered the error? _____

Where did the error occur (e.g., hospital, outpatient or retail pharmacy, nursing home, patient's home)?_____

At what time of day? _____

What type of staff or health care practitioner made the initial error? _____

Was the error perpetuated by another practitioner? _____

Was patient counseling provided? ❑ Yes ❑ No If yes, before or after error was discovered? _____

Please complete the following if a product was involved.

	Product #1	Product #2
Brand Name of Product Involved		
Generic Name		
Manufacturer		
Labeler (if different from mfr.)		
Dosage Form		
Strength/Concentration		
Type and Size of Container		

If available, please provide patient information that may be relevant, including age, gender, diagnosis, etc. (pt. identification not required).

Reports are most useful when relevant materials such as product label, copy of prescription/order, etc., can be reviewed. Can these materials be provided? ❑ Yes ❑ No Please specify _____

Please retain these materials/samples for 60 days, if possible.

Do you have any recommendations to prevent recurrence of this error, or have you instituted policies or procedures to prevent future similar errors?

A copy of this report is routinely sent to the Institute for Safe Medication Practices (ISMP), the manufacturer/labeler, and to the Food and Drug Administration (FDA). **USP may release my identity to: (check boxes that apply)**

❑ ISMP ❑ The manufacturer and/or labeler as listed above ❑ FDA ❑ Other persons requesting a copy of this report ❑ Anonymous to all

Your Name and Title

Your Facility Name, Address, and Zip

Telephone Number (include area code)

Signature

Date

Return to: USP PRN℠ 12601 Twinbrook Parkway, Rockville, Maryland 20852-1790

Call Toll Free: 1-800-23-ERROR (1-800-233-7767) or FAX 1-301-816-8532

Date Received by USP:

File Access Number:

FIGURE 15–1 Form for reporting potential or actual errors in medication administration to the USP Medication Errors Reporting Program (*Reprinted with permission of the United States Pharmacopeia*)

prove accuracy, but they do not eliminate the need for a second person to review the calculations and solution concentrations used.

Another important way to minimize calculation errors is to avoid doing calculations by using the unit-dose system exclusively, by using commercially available unit-dose items such as premixed critical care parenterals, and by standardizing doses and concentrations, especially of critical care drugs. The

TABLE 15–1   **Standard Dosage Chart for a Dopamine Infusion (800 mg/500 mL)**

	Micrograms/Kilogram per Minute						
	2	5	7.5	10	20	25	30
Patient Weight (lb)	Milliliters/Hour to Run Infusion						
90	3	8	12	15	31	38	46
100	3	9	13	17	34	43	51
110	4	9	14	19	38	47	56
120	4	10	15	20	41	51	61
130	4	11	17	22	44	55	66
140	5	12	18	24	48	60	72
150	5	13	19	26	51	64	77
160	5	14	20	27	55	68	82
170	6	14	22	29	58	72	87
180	6	15	23	31	61	77	92
190	6	16	24	32	65	81	97
200	7	17	26	34	68	85	102
210	7	18	27	36	72	89	107
220	7	19	28	38	75	94	112
230	8	20	29	39	78	98	118
240	8	20	31	41	82	102	123
250	9	21	32	43	85	107	128

Note: From "Cooperative Approaches to Medication Error Management" by M.R. Cohen, *Topics in Hospital Pharmacy Management, 11*(1), p. 60. Copyright 1991 by Aspen Publishers, Inc. Reprinted by permission.

use of standard dosage charts on the floors and standard formulations in the pharmacy minimizes the possibility of error and makes calculations much easier for everyone. For example, in the critical care units, physicians must order only the amount of drug they want infused and list any titration parameters. No one has to perform any calculations, since dosage charts can be made readily available for choosing appropriate flow rates by patient weight and dose ordered (**Table 15–1**).

Standard concentrations for frequently prepared formulations should be recorded and be readily accessible for reference in the parenteral preparation area in the pharmacy. Of course, all calculations must be double-checked and documented by the pharmacist. Diluents and active drugs must be checked. The stock container of each additive with its accompanying syringe should be arranged in the order it appears on the container label to facilitate the checking procedure. The final edge of the plunger piston should be aligned with the calibration marks on the syringe barrel indicating the amount used.

In many hospitals, automated compounders are being used for admixing both large- and small-volume parenterals. Automated equipment has been known to fail occasionally. Also, some accidents have occurred in which solutions were placed on the wrong additive channel. In either case the result could be a serious medication error. Therefore, it is important that the pharmacy have an ongoing quality assurance program for the use of automated compounding equipment. This program should include double checks and documentation of solution placement within the compounder, final weighing or refractometer testing of the solution to ensure that proper concentrations have been compounded, and ongoing sampling of electrolyte concentrations. Pharmacists that batch-prepare special parenteral solutions (e.g., total parenteral nutrition base solutions and cardioplegic solutions) should have additional quality assurance procedures in place, including sterility testing and quarantine until confirmation.

All drug-dispensing procedures must be examined regularly, and the cause of breakdowns discovered, so that prevention measures can be designed. Pharmacy technicians need to communicate clearly to their pharmacist supervisors what it takes to do the job correctly in terms of personnel, training programs, facilities design, equipment, drug products and supplies, computer systems, and quality assurance programs.

Multidisciplinary educational programs should be developed for health care personnel about medication error prevention. Because many errors happen when procedures are not followed, this is one area on which to focus through newsletters and in-service training. It is also important for institutions to focus not only on their own internal errors, but also to look at other institutions' errors and methods of prevention, and to learn from these. ISMP provides ongoing features to facilitate these reviews in *ASHP Newsletter, ASHP Homecare Newsletter, Hospital Pharmacy, American Pharmacy,* and *Pharmacy Today.* ISMP also publishes its own biweekly *ISMP Medication Safety Alert!* which reports on current medication safety issues and offers recommendations for changes.

Summary

Pharmacists and other members of the pharmacy department should lead the multidisciplinary effort in examining where errors arise in the drug-use process (see **Table 15–2**). Pharmacists and pharmacy technicians need to work together in designing quality assurance programs to obtain information that helps establish priorities and make changes. For example, joint reviews of the accuracy of unit-dose cartfills are of great help in detecting reasons for missing or inaccurate doses and changing the drug-dispensing system accordingly. Programs can be established to monitor the accuracy of pharmacy computer order entry. Quality assurance efforts that include a review of medication error reports help to develop a better understanding of the kinds of system or behavioral defects being experienced, so that necessary corrections can be identified. The medication error problem will never go away, but pharmacists and pharmacy technicians can pool their expertise to address issues of safety and thus ensure the safest environment possible.

TABLE 15–2 **The Drugs and Dosage Forms Frequently Implicated in Medication Error Deaths**

Heparin injection (all forms)

Insulin injection

I.V. narcotic injections, especially hydromorphone and morphine and dosing via patient-controlled analgesia

Lidocaine injection in vials containing more than 300mg

Cisplatin

Magnesium sulfate injection (vials greater than 10 mL)

Potassium chloride injection (all forms)

Potassium acetate and phosphate injection

Sodium chloride injection 14.6 percent and 23.4 percent in small-volume parenteral containers

Sodium chloride injection in 5 percent large-volume parenteral containers

Vincristine injection in vials containing more than 2 mg

Other critical care drugs such as dopamine, nitroprusside sodium, nitroglycerin, neuromuscular blockers such as pancuronium, and cancer chemotherapeutics

Note: Adapted from "Cooperative Approaches to Medication Error Management" by M.R. Cohen, *Topics in Hospital Pharmacy Management, 11*(1), p. 62. Copyright 1991 by Aspen Publishers, Inc. Reprinted by permission.

ASSESSMENT

Multiple Choice Questions

1. Medication errors are a growing concern in hospitals because of
   a. increased numbers of critically ill patients
   b. development of more potent medications
   c. increased media awareness
   d. all of the above

2. Pharmacy technicians can help prevent medication errors by
   a. calling physicians to change orders
   b. making known to supervisors what is needed to do their job
   c. both a and b
   d. neither a nor b

3. According to Allan and Barker, medication errors are estimated to occur at a rate of
   a. one per patient per day
   b. one per hospital per day
   c. one per health care personnel per day
   d. one per nursing unit per day

4. The "five rights" of medication prescribing, dispensing, and administering include all but the
   a. right medication
   b. right dose
   c. right prescriber
   d. right time
   e. right patient

5. To minimize the chance of misinterpretation, physicians with poor handwriting should
   a. print their orders in block letters
   b. review the orders with nursing before leaving the floor
   c. use direct order entry if possible
   d. all of the above.

6. Experienced pharmacy technicians can review and interpret prescription orders without a doublecheck by the pharmacist.
   a. True
   b. False

7. An order for a drug whose strength is a whole number should never be followed by a zero (e.g., 10.0 mg), because
   a. the patient could be underdosed tenfold
   b. the patient could be overdosed tenfold
   c. the patient could be underdosed 100-fold
   d. the patient could be overdosed 100-fold

8. Which order below is most clearly written and least ambiguous?
   a. " Synthroid 100mcg daily"   c. "Synthroid 0.1 mg daily"
   b. "Synthroid 1 tablet daily"   d. "Synthroid 100 mcg daily"

9. Which order below is most clearly written and least ambiguous?
   a. "Phenobarbital elixir 15 mg/5 mL: Give 15 mg = 5 mL at bedtime."
   b. "Phenobarbital elixir: Give 5 mL at bedtime."
   c. "Phenobarbital elixir 15 mg/5 mL: Give 5.0 mL at bedtime."
   d. "Phenobarbital elixir: Give one teaspoonful at bedtime."
   e. "Phenobarbiral elixir 15 mg/5 mL: Give 5 cc at bedtime."

10. When you see an order for "AZT" written, it could stand for
    a. azidothymidine
    b. azathioprine
    c. aztreonam
    d. all of the above—better check with prescriber before filling

11. Computerized order entry enhances routine drug dispensing activities by
    a. serving as a double check of the patient's medication for physicians, nurses, and pharmacists
    b. eliminating pharmacists from having to check technicians' bin filling
    c. eliminating technicians from having to restock floor stock items
    d. none of the above

12. Confirmation bias occurs when
    a. a physician orders medication for the wrong patient
    b. an item is chosen once you confirm what you think you are looking for on the label
    c. a nurse confirms the identity of a patient before administering medication
    d. a pharmacist does a clinical screening of a patient's medication profile

13. Medication errors can be reported to the USP-ISMP MERP by
    a. pharmacists   d. both a and b
    b. pharmacy technicians   e. all of the above
    c. the public

Bibliography

Allan, E.L., & Barker, K.N. (1990). Fundamentals of medication error research. *American Journal of Health System Pharmacy, 47,* 555–571.

ASHP. (1993). Guidelines on preventing medication errors in hospitals. *American Journal of Health System Pharmacy, 50,* 305–314.

ASHP. Medication errors: A closer look (videotape production for ASHP with the co-operation and support of Lederle Laboratories).

Center for Proper Medication Use (Pennsylvania Society of Hospital Pharmacists). Preventing medication errors through failure mode and effects analysis (videotape production for the Center for Proper Medication Use with the cooperation and support of Burroughs Wellcome Company).

Cohen, M.R. (1991). Cooperative approaches to medication error management. *Top Hospital Pharmacy Management, 11*(1), 53–65.

Davis, N.M., & Cohen, M.R. (1983). *Medication errors: Causes and prevention.* Philadelphia: George F. Stickley Company.

Davis, N.M., Cohen, M.R., & Teplitsky, B. (1992). Look-alike and sound-alike drug names: The problem and the solution. *Hospital Pharmacy, 27,* 95–98, 102–105, 108–110.

PART

IV

Professional Aspects of Pharmacy Technology

16 Pharmaceutical Terminology and Medical Abbreviations

COMPETENCIES

Upon completion and review of this chapter, the student should be able to

1. Recognize word elements and be able to define and be aware of word element combinations in medical terminology.
2. Define commonly used medical terminology and abbreviations.
3. Graphically illustrate apothecary symbols.
4. Identify drugs by both the brand/trade names and generic names.
5. Differentiate "look-alike" and "sound-alike" drugs.

Introduction

Pharmacists and technicians both are exposed to a myriad of terms and abbreviations in the daily practice of institutional pharmacy. Not all of the terms, symbols, or abbreviations included in this chapter pertain solely to pharmacy, but technicians should be acquainted with these and other terms to carry out their duties effectively.

This chapter is divided as follows:

1. common word elements
2. common medical terms
3. abbreviations
4. commonly used apothecary symbols
5. brand/trade names and generic names
6. look-alike and sound-alike drugs

Common Word Elements

Medical terminology is a combination of word elements. For example, bradycardia means a slowing of the heartbeat. The word was created by combining the word elements of the prefix "brady-", which means slow, and the suffix "-cardia", which means heart. This list of commonly used word elements should enable the technician to understand and create many acceptable medical terms. (*Note:* Elements followed by a hyphen are prefixes; elements preceded by a hyphen are suffixes.)

a(n)-	an absence, not	micr(o)-	small
aden(o)-	gland	morph(o)-	shape, form
adipo-	fat	my(o)-	muscle
-algia	pain	myel(o)-	bone marrow, spinal cord
ante-	before		
anti-	against	nas(o)-	nose
arthro-	joint	necr(o)-	dead
aur(i)-	ear	nephr(o)-	kidney
brady-	slow	-oma	tumor
-cardi(a)	heart action	ophthalm(o)-	eye
-cele	tumor, hernia	os, oste(o)-	bone
chole-	bile, gall	-osis	disease process
-cid(e)	kill	-ostomy	surgical opening
col(i), (o)-	colon	ot(o)-	ear
cop(o)-	vagina	path(o)-	disease
cyst(i), (o)-	sac, bladder	phleb(o)-	vein
dermat-	skin	-plasty	forming, shaping
-ectomy	excision	-plegia	paralysis
eu-	well, normal	pneum(o)-	lung, air
gluc(o)-	sweet, sugar	pod(o)-	foot
hem(o)-, hema-,		poly-	many
hemat(o)-	blood	post-	after
hemi-	half	procto(o)-	anus, rectum
hepat(o)-	liver	pulm(o)-	lung
hyper-	above	recto-	backward, behind
hypo-	below	rhin(o)-	nose
infra-	beneath	-rrhea	flow
inter-	between	super-	over, above (amount)
intra-	within		
-itis	inflammation	supra-	above (position)
lith(o)-	stone	tachy-	rapid
macr(o)-	large, long	thora(o)-	chest
mal-	abnormal	ur(o)-	urine, urological
mast(o)-	breast	vesic(o)-	bladder

Common Medical Terms

accelerated care unit (ACU) Separate unit in the hospital where patients are prepared to better care for themselves and their condition after being discharged from the hospital.

acidosis Acid/base imbalance causing the blood and body tissues to become excessively acidic.

acute A severe condition, rising rapidly to a peak and then subsiding.

additive (parenteral) An addition of an active ingredient to a solution that is intended for intravenous administration or irrigation.

alkalosis Acid/base imbalance causing the blood and body tissues to become excessively alkaline (basic).

allergen An agent that provokes the symptoms of an allergy.

allergy An abnormal reaction to a substance, situation, or physical state.

ambulatory patient A patient who is able to walk and is not restricted to bed.

amphetamine A stimulant drug; also known as uppers, bam, bennies, browns, bumblebee, butterflies.

anabolic agent A substance that builds up tissue protein.

anabolism The body process during which proteins are synthesized and tissues are formed.

analgesic A substance that relieves pain.

anaphylaxis A hypersensitivity reaction that is immediate, shocklike, and possibly fatal.

anesthetic A drug used to decrease sensation.

aneurysm A dilation or bulging out of a blood vessel wall.

antepartum Before the onset of childbirth.

antibiotic A substance that is able to kill or inhibit the growth of bacteria or other microorganisms.

anticoagulant A drug that prevents or delays coagulation or clotting of blood; a "blood thinner."

antiflatulent A drug that facilitates expulsion of gas from the GI tract.

antigen An agent that stimulates antibody formation.

antineoplastic A substance that prevents the development or spread of tumor cells.

antipruritic A drug that relieves itch.

antipyretic A drug that reduces fever.

antiseptic An agent that inhibits the growth of microorganisms but does not necessarily kill them.

antitoxin A specific agent neutralizing a poison or toxin.

antitussive A drug used for the relief of cough.

arrhythmia An abnormal, irregular heartbeat.

arteriosclerosis Hardening of the arteries.

arthritis Inflammation of joints.

ascites Accumulation of fluid within the abdominal cavity.

aseptic technique A method of preparation that will prevent contamination of a site (e.g., wound) or product (e.g., I.V. admixture).

atherosclerosis Lipid (fat) deposits in large and medium size arteries.

atonic Weak tone or absence of tone.

bactericide An agent capable of killing bacterias.

bacteriostat An agent that inhibits the growth of bacteria.

benign Not malignant or invasive.

biopsy Excision of a small piece of tissue for diagnostic purposes.

blood urea nitrogen (BUN) An indication of kidney function.

bradycardia Slow heart rate.

buccal Between the gum and cheek.

callibration A method of standardizing a measuring device.

carcinogen Any substance that causes cancer.

catabolism The breakdown of body proteins.

cathartic A drug used to produce evacuation of the bowel.

central service An area in the hospital where general sterilization procedures are performed; serves as a storage facility for various types of equipment.

chemotherapy Treatment of a condition with drugs. Currently used in reference to the treatment of cancer.

chronic Of long duration or frequent recurrence.

coagulation Blood-clotting process.

cocaine A topical anesthetic, also known as coke, crack, snow, blow, white horse, 8-ball.

colostomy Creation of an opening into the colon through the abdominal wall.

compliance Act of adhering to prescribed directions.

congestive heart failure (CHF) Failure or diminished ability of the heart to pump an adequate blood supply to the rest of the body.

crack An illicit, pure form of cocaine, usually smoked in a pipe.

creatinine clearance A measure of renal function.

decongestant A drug used to open the air passages of the nose and lungs.

decubitus ulcer A bedsore.

deoxyribonucleic acid (DNA) A double-stranded structure that is the molecular basis of heredity.

diabetes mellitus A chronic disease affecting carbohydrate metabolism.

diagnosis The identification of a disease from its signs and symptoms.

disastolic pressure The force exerted by the blood on the blood vessels when the ventricles of the heart are in a state of rest before systole.

diluent An agent that dilutes or reconstitutes a solution or mixture.

diuretic A drug used to increase urinary output; "water pill."

electrocardiogram A graphic record of the heart's action by electronic measurement.

electroencephalogram A tracing or electronic recording of brain waves.

embolism A traveling blood clot that may deposit in a vessel and obstruct flow through that vessel.

emergency room A hospital unit where patients are treated for conditions that require immediate attention.

equivalent weight The gram molecular weight divided by the highest valent ion in the molecule.

erythrocyte A red blood cell.

estrogen A hormone that produces secondary sex characteristics in the female.

etiology The cause(s) of a disease.

expectorant A drug that promotes the secretion and excretion of mucus from the lungs and trachea.

febrile Body temperature above normal.

fibrillation Rapid, ineffectual heartbeat.

floor stock Medications that are routinely kept on the nursing unit.

gastric Pertaining to the stomach.

generic drug name The nonproprietary (non-brand) name of a drug.

glucose tolerance test A test for diabetes, based on the ability of the liver to store glycogen.

hemorrhage Severe bleeding.

hemostat An agent used to arrest hemorrhage.

hepatitis Inflammation of the liver.

heroin An illicit drug derived from morphine; also known as brown sugar, salt, horse.

hyperalimentation Intravenous feeding; total parenteral nutrition (TPN), literally.

hypertension High blood pressure.

hypnotic A drug used to induce sleep.

hypotension Low blood pressure.

immunity Resistance to infection.

incubation The period between exposure to an infective disease process and the symptoms of infection.

infection The successful invasion of the body by pathogenic organisms.

inflammation The condition characterized by pain, heat, redness, and swelling.

infusion The slow injection of a solution into a vein, subcutaneous tissue, or other tissue.

injection The act of forcing a liquid medication into the blood or body.

inpatient A patient who requires the use of a hospital bed and is registered in the hospital to receive medical or surgical care.

intensive care unit (ICU) A hospital where the patient receives constant and vigilant attention.

intradermal Situated or applied within the skin.

intrathecal Within the subdural space of the spinal cord.

intramuscular Within the muscle.

iontophoresis Introduction of medication into the tissue by means of an electric current.

jaundice Yellow appearance of skin and mucous membranes resulting from the deposition of bile pigment.

laboratory A hospital department where chemical and/or biological testing is performed for the purpose of aiding diagnosis.

leukemia A disease characterized by an extremely high white blood cell count.

lozenge A small, medicated or flavored disk intended to be dissolved in the mouth.

LSD **Lys**ergic acid **d**iethylamide, a hallucinogen; also known as beast, black sunshine, the chief.

MAO inhibitors A class of drugs that act as antidepressants by inhibiting the enzyme **m**ono**a**mine **o**xidase.

malignant A type of tumor that invades healthy tissue and becomes progressively worse.

marijuana Substance, from hemp, that has an effect on mood, perception, and psychomotor coordination; also known as sinse, weed, herb, grass, dope, reefer, maryjane.

mastectomy Removal of the breast.

medication administration record (MAR) A record maintained by the nursing staff containing information about the patient's medication and its frequency of administration.

meninges The membrane that surrounds the brain and spinal cord.

meningitis Inflammation of the meninges.

metabolism The process by which an organism converts food to energy needed for anabolism.

metastasis The spread of disease from one organ to another.

milliequivalent (mEq) One-thousandth of an equivalent weight.

miotic A drug that causes constriction of the pupil.

mnemonic code An abbreviation used in computerized medication order entry.

morgue A place where a corpse is kept until released for burial.

mucolytic A substance that liquifies, dissolves, or digests mucus.

mydriatic An agent that dilates the pupil of the eye.

myocardial infarction (MI) Injury to the heart muscle (myocardium), due to inadequate oxygen supply caused by the occlusion of a coronary artery.

narcotic A drug that is habit forming and addictive and produces relief from pain.

nephritis Inflammation of the nephron.

nephron Functional unit of the kidney.

obstructive jaundice Jaundice that results from an impediment to the flow of bile from the liver to the duodenum.

occlusion Blockage of a blood vessel.

operating room A unit in the hospital where major surgical procedures are performed.

outpatient department An area of the hospital where various medical services are provided to patients who do not require a hospital bed (outpatients).

oxytocic An agent that causes uterine contractions.

palliative A treatment that provides relief but no cure for a condition.

parenteral solution Sterile solutions intended for subcutaneous, intramuscular, or intravenous injection.

pathogen Any disease-producing organism.

pathology That branch of medicine concerned with the essential nature of disease, especially the structural and functional changes in tissues caused by the disease process.

patient medication profile A record kept in the pharmacy of patient data and current drug therapy. It contains such information as initiation and discontinuation of medication orders and dosage form and strength. It also indicates any allergies, diagnosis, or other information pertinent to drug therapy.

PCP Phencyclidine, a hallucinogen; also known as busy bee, buzz, zombie.

pertussis Whooping cough; an acute infectious disease of the respiratory tract.

pH A measurement of acidity or alkalinity.

pharmaceutics The science of drug-delivery systems.

pharmacist A person licensed to dispense medication and to counsel on drug therapy.

pharmacogenetics The study of the relationship between heredity and response to drugs.

pharmacognosy The study of therapeutic agents derived from natural sources, e.g., plants.

pharmacokinetics The study of bodily absorption, distribution, metabolism, and excretion of drugs.

pharmacology The study of the action of drugs on the body.

pharmacotherapeutics Pertaining to the use of drugs in the prevention and/or treatment of disease.

pharmacy, contemporary A health service concerning itself with the knowledge of drugs and their effects on the body.

pharmacy intern A person obtaining practical experience and training in pharmacy to meet the requirements of the state board of pharmacy for licensure as a pharmacist.

pharmacy resident A graduate from an accredited pharmacy school enrolled in a program designed to develop expert skills in pharmacy practice.

pharmacy technician Support personnel with education and training that allows performance of select tasks as delegated by the supervising pharmacist.

pharmacy, traditional The art and science of compounding and dispensing medications.

phlebitis Inflammation of the veins.

physical therapy (PT) Physical manipulation for the purpose of rehabilitation.

plasma The fluid portion of the blood in which the blood cells are suspended.

postpartum Occuring after childbirth, or delivery.

prognosis The expected outcome of the course of the disease.

pulmonary Pertaining to the lungs.

purified protein derivative (PPD) Product used as a skin test for tuberculosis antibodies.

radiation therapy The use of X rays in the treatment of a disease.

radiology (X-ray) department An area of the hospital where diagnosis and treatment are performed using X rays, radioisotopes, and other similar methods.

radiopharmacy A branch of pharmacy dealing with radioactive diagnostics.

recovery room (RR) Area in the hospital where patients are monitored and treated immediately after leaving the operating room.

renal Pertaining to the kidney.

respiration The breathing process.

ribonucleic acid (RNA) A single-stranded structure that is the molecular basis for protein synthesis.

rubella German measles.

sedative A drug used to allay anxiety and excitement; often used to help a patient sleep.

serum The clear fluid of the blood separated from solid parts.

signs Objective bodily evidence of distress found by physical examination.

solvent A substance used to dissolve another substance.

sterilization The act or process of rendering sterile; the complete destruction of microorganisms by heat or bactericidal compounds.

styptic An agent that stops or slows bleeding by contracting blood vessels when applied locally.

subcutaneous Under the skin.

sublingual Under the tongue.

symptom Subjective evidence of a disease; evidence of disease as perceived by the patient.

syncope Fainting; a transient loss of consciousness due to inadequate blood flow to the brain.

syndrome A group of signs and symptoms that characterize a particular abnormality.

synergism A joint action of agents in which the total effect of the combination is greater than the sum of their individual independent effects.

systolic The force exerted by the blood when the ventricles are in a state of contraction.

tachycardia Rapid heart rate.

telephone order An order for a drug or other form of treatment that is given over the phone to an authorized receiver by an authorized prescriber.

testosterone A hormone that produces secondary sex characteristics in the male.

toxic A toxin that has been detoxified by moderate heat and chemical treatment that retains its antigenicity.

toxin, bacterial A noxious or poisonous product that causes the formation of antibodies called antitoxins.

trachea Windpipe.

tracheotomy An incision into the trachea.

tranquilizer A drug to relieve anxiety or agitation.

urticaria Eruption or rash associated with severe itching.

vaccine Any material that produces active immunization in the formation of antibodies.

valence Those electrons that are associated with bonds between elements.

vasconstriction Narrowing of blood vessels.

vasodilation Relaxation of smooth muscles of the vascular system that produces dilation of the blood vessel.

ventricular fibrillation Rapid ineffectual action of the ventricle of the heart.

verbal order An order for a drug or other treatment that is given verbally to an authorized receiver by an authorized prescriber.

vertigo A sensation the patient experiences that the external world is revolving around the patient; dizziness.

virus A submicroscopic agent of infectious disease that is capable of reproduction.

viscosity An expression of the resistance of a fluid to flow.

vitamin A general term for a number of organic substances that occur in many foods in small amounts required for normal growth and maintenance of life.

written order An order for a drug or other form of treatment that is written on the appropriate form by an authorized prescriber.

Common Medical/Pharmacy Abbreviations

a, ante	before		aq	aqueous
aa	of equal parts		a.s.	left ear
ac	before meals		ASA	aspirin
a.d.	right ear		ASHP	American Society of Health-Systems Pharmacists
ad lib	as much as desired			
ADI	American Drug Index		a.u.	both ears
adm	admission		AZT	azidothymidine, zidovidine
ADR	adverse drug reaction		BBVD	blood-borne viral disease
AHFS	American Hospital Formulary Service		bid	twice daily
AIDS	acquired immune deficiency syndrome		biw	twice weekly
			BM	bowel movement
alb.	albumin		BMR	basal metabolic rate
am	morning		BP	blood pressure
amb	ambulatory		BUN	blood urea nitrogen
amt	amount		c̄	with
anes.	anesthesia		Ca	calcium
ANDA	Abbreviated New Drug Application		CAD	coronary artery disease
AP	appendectomy		caps	capsules
APAP	acetaminophen		CAT	computerized axial tomography
APT	Association of Pharmacy Technicians		cath	catheter
APhA	American Pharmaceutical Association		CBC	complete blood count
ARC	AIDS-related complex		CC	chief complaint

cc	cubic centimeter (milliliter)		H2O	water
CCU	coronary care unit		Hct	hematocrit
CDC	Centers for Disease Control		Hgb	hemoglobin
CHF	congestive heart failure		HIV	human immunodeficiency virus
Cl	chloride		H&P	history and physical
cm	centimeter		hs	hour of sleep
CNS	central nervous system		hx	history
CO2	carbon dioxide		ICU	intensive care unit
COPD	chronic obstructive pulmonary disease		im	intramuscular
			IND	investigational new drug
CPR	cardiopulmonary resuscitation		INH	isoniazid
C&S	culture and sensitivity		I & O	intake and output
CQI	continuing quality improvement		IV	intravenous
CSF	cerebrospinal fluid		IVPB	intravenous piggyback
CTU	cardiac transition unit		IVSS	intravenous soluset
CV	cardiovascular		JCAHO	Joint Commission on Accreditation of Healthcare Organizations
CVA	cerebral vascular accident (stroke)			
CVP	central venous pressure		K	potassium
dc	discontinue		KCl	potassium chloride
DEA	Drug Enforcement Agency		kg	kilogram
DIC	Drug Information Center		kvo	keep vein open
diag	diagnosis		l	liter
Disp	dispense		lb	pound
DTD	let such doses be given		LPN	licensed practical nurse
DM	diabetes mellitus		LR	lactated Ringer's solution
DME	durable medical equipment		mcg	microgram
DNA	deoxyribonucleic acid		MD	Medical Doctor
DO	Doctor of Osteopathy		mEq	milliequivalent
DPT	diphtheria, pertussis, tetanus vaccine		Mg	magnesium
DRG	diagnosis-related group		MI	myocardial infarction
D5W	dextrose 5% in water		ml	milliliter
D5/0.33	dextrose 5% in 0.33% sodium chloride		MOM	milk of magnesia
D5/0.45	dextrose 5% in 0.45% sodium chloride		ms	morphine sulfate, multiple sclerosis
D5/0.9	dextrose 5% in 0.9% sodium chloride		mvi	multivitamin
DRL	dextrose 5% in Ringer's lactate		NARD	National Association of Retail Druggists
DR	delivery room			
DUE	drug utilization evaluation		Na	sodium
dx	diagnosis		NDA	new drug application
ECG or EKG	electrocardiogram		NF	National Formulary
ECT or EST	electroconvulsive therapy		ngt	nasogastric tube
EEG	electroencephalogram		non rep (nr)	do not repeat
ENT	ear, nose, and throat		NPH	neutral protamine hagerdorn insulin
ER	emergency room		npo	nothing by mouth
FBS	fasting blood sugar		NS	normal saline, 0.9% sodium chloride
FDA	Food and Drug Administration		NSAID	nonsteroidal antiinflammatory drug
fuo	fever of unknown origin		NTG	nitroglycerin
g, gm	gram		n/v	nausea/vomiting
GI	gastrointestinal		O2	oxygen
gr.	grain		OB	obstetrics
gtt	drop		o.d.	right eye
GU	genitourinary		oob	out of bed
GYN	gynecology		OPD	outpatient department
h, hr	hour		OR	operating room

o.s.	left eye		r/o	rule out
o.u.	both eyes		rt, R	right
p	after		Rx	prescription
PA	physician's assistant		s̄	without
PACU	post anesthesia care unit (recovery room)		sc, sub Q	subcutaneous
			SDS	same day surgery
pb	piggyback		sig	let it be imprinted, label
pc	after meals		sl	sublingual
PDR	*Physician's Desk Reference*		sos	if necessary
pH	hydrogen ion concentration		s̄s̄	half
Pharm D.	Doctor of Pharmacy		SSE	soap suds enema
PID	pelvic inflammatory disease		SSKI	saturated solution of potassium iodide
pm	afternoon, evening			
PMU	pain management unit		stat	immediately and once only
po	by mouth		STD	sexually transmitted disease
PPD	purified protein derivative		tab(s)	tablet(s)
premi	premature		TB	tuberculosis
prep	prepare for		tid	three times daily
prn	as needed		tiw	three time weekly
PT	physical therapy, prothrombin time		t.o.	telephone order
PVC	premature ventricular contraction		TPN	total parenteral nutrition
PZI	protamine zinc insulin		tr	tincture
q	each, every		TWE	tap water enema
QA	quality assurance		ung	ointment
qam	every morning		USP	United States Pharmacopoeia
qd	daily		USPDI	United States Pharmacopoeia Drug Information
q_h	every _ hour(s)			
qhs	every bedtime		ut dict, ud	as directed
qid	four times daily		UTI	urinary tract infection
qod	every other day		VA	Veterans Administration
qs	quantity sufficient		vs	vital signs
rbc	red blood cell		vss	vital signs stable
RL	Ringer's lactate		WBC	white blood cell count
RN	registered nurse		WDWN	well developed, well nourished
RNA	ribonucleic acid			

Commonly Used Apothecary Symbols

ℨ	drachm, teaspoonful
℥	ounce
℥ss	half ounce, tablespoon
m	minim
=	equal
♀	female
♂	male
>	greater than
<	less than

Not all symbols and abbreviations are absolute; many of them have more than one meaning when used in different contexts. When in doubt, the technician should consult the registered pharmacist on duty.

Brand/Trade Names and Generic Names

The following section lists the brand/trade names of commonly used medications and their corresponding generic names. This list does not contain every drug available. The technician is advised to become familiar with the appropriate texts that contain this information.

Brand	**Generic**
Achromycin	tetracycline
Actifed	triprolidine/pseudoephedrine
Activase	alteplase, t-PA
Adalat	nifedipine
Advil	ibuprofen
Afrin	oxymetazoline
Aldomet	methyldopa
Alternagel	concentrated aluminum hydroxide
Amoxil	amoxicillin
Amphojel	aluminum hydroxide
Ancef	cefazolin
Antivert	meclizine
Apresoline	hydralazine
Aricept	donepezil
Artane	trihexyphenidyl
Atarax	hydroxyzine
Ativan	lorazepam
Auralgan	antipyrine/benzocaine
Axid	nizatidine
Bactrim	trimethoprim/sulfamethoxazole
Benadryl	diphenhydramine
Bentyl	dicyclomine
Brethine	terbutaline
Biaxin	clarithromycin
Buspar	buspirone
Calan	verapamil
Capoten	captopril
Carafate	sucralfate
Cardizem	diltiazem
Cardura	doxazosin
Catapres	clonidine
Ceclor	cefaclor
Cefotan	cefotetan
Chlor-Trimeton	chlorpheniramine
Cipro	ciprofloxacin
Claritin	loratadine
Cleocin	clindamycin
Cogentin	benztropine
Colace	docusate sodium
Compazine	prochlorperazine
Corgard	nadolol
Coumadin	warfarin
Cozaar	losartan

Brand	Generic
Cytotec	misoprostol
Decadron	dexamethasone
Deltasone	prednisone
Demerol	meperidine
Depakene	valproic acid
Depakote	divalproex sodium
Desyrel	trazodone
Diabinese	chlorpropamide
DiaBeta	glyburide
Diamox	acetazolamide
Dilantin	phenytoin
Diflucan	fluconazole
Dimetapp	brompheniramine/phenylpropanolamine
Ditropan	oxybutynin
Dramamine	dimenhydrinate
Dulcolax	bisacodyl
Duragesic	fentanyl
Dyazide	triamterene/hydrochlorothiazide
E.E.S.	erythromycin ethylsuccinate
Effexor	venlafaxine
Elavil	amitriptyline
Ery-Tab	erythromycin base
Flagyl	metronidazole
Floxin	ofloxacin
Fortaz	ceftazidime
Fragmin	dalteparin
Fungizone	amphotericin B
Garamycin	gentamicin
Glucotrol	glipizide
Halcion	triazolam
Haldol	haloperidol
Hexadrol	dexamethasone
Hytrin	terazosin
Hydrodiuril	hydrochlorothiazide
Ilosone	erythromycin estolate
Ilotycin	erythromycin base
Imdur	isosorbide mononitrate
Inderal	propranolol
Indocin	indomethacin
Isoptin	verapamil
Keflex	cephalexin
Kefzol	cefazolin
Kenalog	triamcinolone
Klonopin	clonazepam
Kwell	lindane
Lanoxin	digoxin
Lasix	furosemide
Levaquin	levofloxacin
Levothroid	levothyroxine
Lipitor	atorvastatin
Lopid	gemfibrozil

Brand	Generic
Lopressor	metoprolol
Lotrimin	clotrimazole
Lovenox	enoxaparin
Luvox	fluvoxamine
Mefoxin	cefoxitin
Mellaril	thioridazine
Micronase	glyburide
Minipress	prazosin
Motrin	ibuprofen
Mycelex	clotrimazole
Mycostatin	nystatin
Mylicon	simethicone
Naprosyn	naproxen sodium
Nebcin	tobramycin
Neurontin	gabapentin
Nizoral	ketoconazole
Norvasc	amlodipine
Oretic	hydrochlorthiazide
Paxil	paroxetine
Pepcid	famotidine
Phenergan	promethazine
Plavix	clopidogrel
Prilosec	omeprazole
Prinivil	lisinopril
Procan SR	procainamide sustained release
Procardia	nifedipine
Pronestyl	procainamide
Propulsid	cisapride
Prozac	fluoxetine
Proventyl	albuterol
Reglan	metoclopramide
Retrovir	zidovidine
Robinul	glycopyrrolate
Robitussin	guaifenesin
Rocephin	ceftriaxone
Rufen	ibuprofen
Septra	trimethoprim/sulfamethoxazole
Sorbitrate	isosorbide dinitrate
Stadol	butorphanol
Synthroid	levothyroxine
Tagamet	cimetidine
Tazicef	ceftazidime
Tazidime	ceftazidime
Tegretol	carbamazepine
Tenormin	atenolol
Theo-Dur	theophylline sustained release
Thorazine	chlorpromazine
Tobrex	tobramycin
Tofranil	imipramine
Toprol XL	metoprolol extended release
Trental	pentoxifylline

Brand	Generic
Trovan	trovafloxacin
Trilafon	perphenazine
Tylenol	acetaminophen
Ultram	tramadol
Vanceril	beclomethasone
Vasotec	enalapril
Ventolin	albuterol
Vibramycin	doxycycline
Vistaril	hydroxyzine
Xanax	alprazolam
Zantac	ranitidine
Zestril	lisinopril
Zithromax	azithromycin
Zocor	simvastatin
Zoloft	sertraline
Zovirax	acyclovir
Zyloprim	allopurinol

Common Look-Alike and Sound-Alike Drug Names

The following list contains names of some drugs that are easily mistaken for each other due to similar pronunciation or spelling. This list serves as a warning. It cannot replace proper care in reading medication orders.

acetazolamide	acetohexamide	diphenhydramine	dimenhydrinate
albuterol	atenolol	enalapril	Anafranil
Aldomet	Aldoril	flurbiprofen	fenoprofen
alprazolam	lorazepam	Gantrisin	Gantanol
Alupent	Atrovent	glipizide	glyburide
amiodarone	amrinone	Hycodan	Hycomine
amitriptyline	nortriptyline	Hycodan	Vicodin
Amoxil	Amcill	Hydralazine	hydroxyzine
Apresazide	Apresoline	Inderal	Isordil
Atarax	Ativan	Indocin	Minocin
atenolol	timolol	Lioresal	lisinopril
bacitracin	Bactroban	Lovenox	Luvox
Catapres	Cataflam	Orinase	Ornade
cefotaxime	cefoxitin	Prilosec	Prozac
chlorpromazine	promethazine	quinine	quinidine
clonidine	Klonopin	terbutaline	tolbutamide
Cordarone	Corvert	tolazamide	tolbutamide
desipramine	imipramine	Trimox	Diamox
digitoxin	digoxin	Vasosulf	Velosef
Dynapen	Dynacin	Xanax	Zantac

Adapted from: "Look-Alike and Sound-Alike Drug Names" by N.M. Davis, M.R. Cohen, and B. Teplisky, 1992, *Hospital Pharmacy, 27,* pp. 96–106.

ASSESSMENT

Multiple Choice Questions

1. An erythrocyte is
   a. a red blood cell
   b. a white blood cell
   c. a platelet
   d. a thrombocyte
   e. a leucocyte

2. Fibrillation is a synonym for
   a. a flutter of the left ventricle
   b. a spasm of the myocardium
   c. rapid ineffectual heartbeat
   d. trembling of the fingers
   e. difficulty in breathing

3. A test for kidney function is
   a. CBC
   b. CHF
   c. KFT
   d. BUN
   e. EKG

4. Diabetes mellitus affects
   a. protein metabolism
   b. carbohydrate metabolism
   c. purine metabolism
   d. lipid metabolism
   e. all of the above

5. A bedsore is known as
   a. an abscess
   b. a bulus
   c. a decubitus ulcer
   d. a laceration
   e. dermatitis

6. A traveling blood clot is
   a. an embolism
   b. a thrombus
   c. a hematoid
   d. all of the above
   e. none of the above

7. A pathogen is
   a. a bacillus
   b. a virus
   c. a carcinogen
   d. a septic substance
   e. any disease-producing organism

8. Syncope is a synonym for
   a. fainting
   b. ataxia
   c. dizziness
   d. fatigue
   e. coma

9. Vertigo is another name for
   a. fainting
   b. ataxia
   c. dizziness
   d. fatigue
   e. coma

10. An ostomy is
    a. a disease process
    b. an excision
    c. a surgical opening
    d. an incision
    e. a plastic repair

Matching I

11. __c__ anaphylaxis
12. __a__ anabolism
13. __e__ antitussive
14. __b__ immunity
15. __d__ febrile

a.   protein synthesis
b.   resistant to infection
c.   hypersensitivity reaction
d.   temperature above normal
e.   cough reliever

Matching II

16. __c__ AZT
17. __d__ K
18. __b__ PCP
19. __a__ Na
20. __e__ TPN

a.   sodium
b.   hallucinogen
c.   zidovidine
d.   potassium
e.   hyperalimentation solution

Bibliography

Davis, N. M., Cohen, M. R., & Teplisky, B. Look-alike and sound-alike drug names. *Hospital Pharmacy,* 27, 96–106.

Dorland's Illustrated Medical Dictionary. (1985). Philadelphia: W.B. Saunders Co.

Mason, R. (1978). Medical terminology. In Durgin, Hanan, & Ward (Eds.), *Pharmacy Technician's Manual* (2nd ed.). St. Louis: C.V. Mosby Co.

17 Pharmaceutical Dosage Forms

COMPETENCIES

Upon completion and review of this chapter, the student should be able to

1. Explain the different interpretations of "dosage form" by the patient, by members of the health care team, and by pharmacists.
2. List four physiochemical properties of a drug.
3. Name four formulation aids used in the preparation of a given dosage form.
4. Describe the advantages and disadvantages of the major classes of pharmaceutical dosage forms—namely liquids, solids, and aerosols.
5. Differentiate the characteristics of a solution and a suspension.
6. List five desirable qualities for an external suspension.
7. Name and define four solid dosage forms currently in use.
8. Explain the differences between compressed tablets, sublingual or buccal tablets, and multiple compressed tablets.
9. Describe an oral osmotic (OROS) drug dosage design and give an example.
10. Outline five advantages of the transdermal patch.

Introduction

A **dosage form** is a system or device for delivering a drug to the biological system. Drugs are defined as chemicals of synthetic, semisynthetic, natural, or biological origin that interact with human or animal biological systems resulting in an action that may either be intended to prevent, cure, or reduce ill effects in the human or animal body or to detect disease-causing manifestations. In actual practice a pure drug is seldom used. What is generally administered to obtain the desired effect is the drug product, that is, the active ingredient (drug) combined with the so-called inert or physiologically inactive materials to produce a dosage form.

The term "dosage form" means different things to different people. To a patient, for instance, the term signifies the gross physical or pharmaceutical form in which the drug is made available for administration or use (tablet, capsule, **solution,** injection, **ointment**). To the members of the health care team the dosage form of a drug is a drug-delivery system. Any alteration in the system will be expected to alter the delivery rate and the total amount of drug delivered to the site of action.

The pharmacist, however, uses the term "dosage form" in a more comprehensive manner to include (1) the physiochemical properties of the drug itself (e.g., particle size, salt form, **polymorphic state,** dissolution characteristics) and (2) the nature and quantities of various formulation aids used in the preparation of the given dosage form (e.g., diluents, excipients, additives, and preservatives).

Classification

Because of the diverse nature, mode of action, and route of administration, dosage forms may be classified in several different ways. The major classes of pharmaceutical dosage forms may be broadly categorized as liquid, solid, and miscellaneous.

Liquid Dosage Forms

It is well known that biological responses are elicited by the **molecular form** of the drug. Thus, no matter in what dosage form (solid, liquid, or gas) a drug is administered, the action at the molecular level involves interaction of biological constituents with the individual molecules of the drug. Therefore, for a drug to elicit the desired response, it has to be present in the form of a molecular dispersion (solution) at the site of action. Thus, liquid dosage forms are often the dosage form of choice for the following reasons:

1. They are more quickly effective than a solid dosage form, because the solid form will have to undergo **dissolution** after administration.
2. They are easier to swallow (especially for pediatric and geriatric patients) than solid dosage forms.
3. Certain substances can be given only in a liquid form because either the character of the remedy or the large dose makes administration in any other form inconvenient.
4. Certain chemical substances may cause pain (e.g., potassium iodide and bromide) or gastric irritation (e.g., aspirin) when administered in a solid state.
5. Uniformity and flexibility of dosage are easily obtained in liquid dosage forms.
6. Liquid forms are the dosage forms of choice in certain types of pathological conditions in which absorption of particular ions is dependent on dissolution and the absorption environment is deficient in effecting dissolution. For example, a liquid dosage form provides calcium ions in an absorbable form in patients who lack acidity to dissolve calcium carbonate powder.

Liquid dosage forms also have the following disadvantages:

1. They are liable to undergo deterioration and loss of potency much faster than solid dosage forms.
2. They present many flavoring and sweetening problems.
3. Many instances of incompatibility arise because of interaction between dissolved substances.
4. In the absence of proper **preservatives,** liquids provide excellent media for bacterial and mold growth.
5. The presence of preservatives may present problems of diverse nature.
6. Inaccuracy in various doses may arise due to the patient measuring the dose with a household device (e.g., a teaspoon).

7. Oral liquid dosage forms are bulkier to carry than oral solid dosage forms and necessitate the use of a measuring device (e.g., a teaspoon).

8. Many interactions arise because of changes in solubility produced by solvent alterations.

The major classes of liquid pharmaceutical dosage forms are (1) those containing soluble matter, and (2) those containing insoluble matter.

Liquid dosage forms containing soluble matter

Liquid dosage forms containing soluble matter—true solutions—consist of one or several soluble substances (solute) dissolved in a solvent (usually water). The solute may be solid, liquid, or gas and the solvent may be any water-miscible (**hydrophilic**) liquid. Hydrophilic solvents are preferred because such a solvent system is miscible with body fluids.

Some of the potential problems that one should be aware of in dealing with the solution dosage forms are described next.

Solvent system. Most drugs, being weak organic acids or weak organic bases, possess sufficient solubility in organic solvents (e.g., alcohol) but lack adequate water solubility. Solutions of such drugs are generally made using a blend (mixture) of solvents. Products intended for oral administration usually utilize a **hydroalcoholic** solvent system, sometimes containing more than 20 percent alcohol (e.g., elixirs). A mixture of such a product with another product utilizing only water as the solvent or dilution of the product with water is likely to cause precipitation of the poorly water-soluble compound.

pH change. In some instances it is desirable not to use a hydroalcoholic solvent system. In such cases the manufacturer uses a salt form of the drug that, unlike the drug itself, possesses good water solubility. For acidic drugs the salt form is generally the sodium salt; for basic drugs the commonly used forms are the hydrochloride or the sulfate. Since the conjugate entity of these salts is a strong acid or strong base, the pH of the resulting solution is far removed from neutrality. Although dilution of these solutions with water does not pose any problems, one must be careful if two such solutions are mixed. For example, a solution containing the hydrochloride of one drug when mixed with a solution containing the sodium salt of another drug is likely to result in the precipitation of both drugs, because the hydrochloride and sodium moieties of the two drugs will neutralize each other, resulting in poorly water-soluble, weakly basic, and weakly acidic drugs.

Buffer system. A number of drug solutions are stable within a given pH range. To ensure maximum stability and a longer shelf life of such solutions, a **buffer** system is used to maintain the pH of such solutions within the range of optimal stability. Dilution of a drug product's solution that has been formulated with a buffer system is likely to alter the pH of the solution and possibly reduce the buffer capacity.

Liquid dosage forms containing insoluble matter

To derive some or all of the advantages of administering a liquid dosage form, insoluble solutes may be suspended in a vehicle. Two common dosage forms are **suspensions** and **emulsions.**

Suspensions. Suspensions consist of a two-phase system in which the internal (dispersed) phase is solid and the external phase is liquid. The dispersed solid is generally in a state of fine subdivision, having a particle size that may approach colloidal dimensions. The liquid phase in most pharmaceutical suspensions is aqueous. A suspension formulation may be preferred over the administration of the solute as a solid dosage form because the solid may have poor solubility. When formulated as a suspension, the solid will generally show a better rate of solubility because of improved wetting of the drug particles and increased surface area.

Pharmaceutical suspensions may be classified into three groups: orally administered mixtures, externally applied lotions, and injectable preparations.

Orally administered mixtures may supply insoluble and often distasteful substances in a pleasant-tasting form. Examples of oral suspensions are the oral antibiotic syrups, which normally contain 250–500 mg of the solid material per 5 mL of suspension. The concentration of the suspended material may be greater in the case of pediatric drops or in antacid and **radiopaque** suspensions.

Externally applied **lotions** provide dermatological materials in a form that is convenient and suitable for application to the skin. The concentration of the dispersed phase in such formulations may exceed 20 percent (e.g., calamine lotion).

Injectable preparations provide an insoluble drug in a form suitable for intramuscular administration. Such preparations contain from 0.5 percent to 30 percent of solid particles and are generally of low viscosity, since viscosity affects the ease of injection. Particle size is another significant factor since it affects the availability of the drug, especially in depot therapy (e.g., Procaine Penicillin G). However, injectable preparations are formulated with a relatively minute particle size of the solute so as to enable the suspension to pass through the needle of the syringe.

An acceptable suspension possesses the following desirable qualities:

1. The suspended material should not settle rapidly. The particles that do settle down must be readily redispersed into a uniform mixture (suspension) when the container is shaken.
2. The suspension must not be too viscous, but should pour freely from the orifice of the bottle or through a syringe needle.
3. In the case of suspensions intended for external application (e.g., a lotion), the product
   a. must be fluid enough to spread easily over the affected area;
   b. must not be so mobile that it runs off the surface of application;
   c. should dry quickly after application to the affected area;
   d. should provide an elastic protective film that will not rub off easily; and
   e. should have an acceptable color and odor.

Gels and jellies. Gels and jellies are also two-phase systems of a solid and a liquid. However, they differ from true suspensions because in these preparations it is difficult to distinguish between the external phase and the internal phase. The particles of the solid phase are interlinked like irregular meshwork; thus, the liquid partly surrounds the interconnected solid particles and is partly occluded by them (e.g., lidocaine gel).

Emulsions. Emulsions consist of a heterogenous system of at least one immiscible liquid intimately dispersed in another in the form of droplets, whose diameters, in general, range from about 0.1 to 10 micrometers. The system is stabilized by the presence of an **emulsifying agent,** the choice of which is governed by the composition of the emulsion and the route of administration of the emulsion. Either the dispersed phase or the continuous phase may range in consistency from that of a mobile liquid (emulsions and lotions of relatively low viscosity) to a semisolid.

Emulsions are considered to be dispersions of oil or water. When an oil or any oily substance is the dispersed phase, the emulsion is called an oil-in-water (o/w) emulsion. When water is the dispersed phase, the emulsion is called a water-in-oil (w/o) emulsion. More recent in its origin is a third type of emulsion, described as a microemulsion or transparent emulsion. The transparent emulsions possess the property of transparency because of the very small particle size (generally 0.05 micrometer or less) of the dispersed phase (e.g., Haley's M.O.).

Medicinal emulsions for oral administration are usually of the o/w type and require the use of o/w emulsifying agents (e.g., synthetic nonionic surface active agents, acacia, tragacanth, and gelatin). An o/w emulsion is a convenient means of orally administering water-insoluble liquids, especially those that have an unpleasant taste and/or odor. Because the oil globules are completely surrounded by an aqueous **medium,** the taste of the oil is almost completely masked and the odor is also markedly suppressed. Also, it has been observed that some oil-soluble compounds (e.g., some of the vitamins) are absorbed more completely when emulsified than when administered orally as an oily solution, because in an emulsion a large surface area of the oily solution (provided by the oil droplets) is made available for contact at the absorption site. Similarly, the use of intravenous emulsions has been studied as a means of maintaining debilitated patients who are unable to assimilate materials administered orally. Radiopaque emulsions have found application as diagnostic agents in X-ray examinations.

Emulsions intended for external application may be o/w or w/o type. Oil-in-water emulsions for external use offer the advantage of being water-washable and non-staining. In the preparation of such emulsions the following emulsifying agents (in addition to the ones already mentioned) are used: triethanolamine stearate, sodium lauryl sulfate, and monovalent soaps, such as sodium oleate. The water-in-oil emulsions, which are used almost exclusively for external application, contain one or several of the following emulsifying agents: polyvalent soaps, such as calcium palmitate; synthetic nonionic sorbitan esters; wool fat; and cholesterol. In the pharmaceutical and cosmetic products for external use, emulsification is widely used to formulate dermatological and cosmetic lotions and creams that have a better patient acceptability.

For example, in the formulation of foam-producing aerosol products, the **propellent** forms the dispersed liquid phase within the container, which vaporizes when the emulsion is discharged from the container.

Because emulsions are heterogeneous in nature, they present stability problems. An improper selection of the emulsifying agent, either in quality or in quantity, may lead to separation of the emulsion on storage. On shaking the container, the emulsion may reform (creaming) or not reform at all (breaking). Caution must be exercised when an emulsion is to be diluted or mixed with another liquid. An emulsion may be diluted only with a liquid that is miscible with the external phase. Also, dilution of an emulsion may dilute the concentration of the emulsifying agent leading to creaming or breaking of the emulsion. If the dilution is done with a liquid that possesses characteristics different from those of the external phase of the emulsion, the emulsion can break. The same is true when an emulsion is mixed with another liquid. When two emulsions are mixed, another factor that must be considered is the nature of the emulsifying agent in the two emulsions. If one emulsion contains an **anionic** emulsifying agent and the other contains a **cationic** agent, the mixture will tend to produce interaction between the emulsifying agents and both emulsions may break.

A simple method to determine the type of emulsion (o/w or w/o) is to dilute the emulsion with an equal quantity of water and shake the container. An o/w emulsion will dilute with water, but a w/o emulsion will not dilute.

Solid Dosage Forms

Solid dosage forms in current use include powders, granules, capsules, and tablets. Powders and granules constitute a very small portion of the solid dosage forms dispensed today. Capsules and tablets have gained popularity because they are

- easy to package, transport, store, and dispense
- convenient for self-medication

- largely devoid of taste and/or odor
- more stable than other solid dosage forms
- predivided dosage forms, and therefore provide an accurate dose
- especially suited for those drugs that are not stable in liquid form and, therefore, provide a longer shelf life for such drugs
- more suited for the formulation of sustained and delayed release of medication because controlled-release techniques are generally more applicable to solid than to liquid dosage forms

Powders

Powders have certain inherent advantages. For example, they give the physician free choice of drugs, dose, and bulk; they permit the administration of large "bulk" of medicinals; and they may be administered as a suspension if the patient has difficulty swallowing a tablet or capsule. However, powders are not the dosage form of choice for drugs that have an unpleasant taste or are not stable when exposed to the atmosphere.

Powders are prescribed for both internal and external use. When intended for internal use, powders may be prescribed as bulk, dispersible, or divided powders. Powders prescribed for external use are dispensed as dusting powders.

Bulk powders are supplied as multidose preparations, the dose being measured by the patient. This dosage form is used for drugs having a large dose and low toxicity because of the variation in dose weight inherent in domestic methods of measurement (e.g., with a household teaspoon). Also, such measurements are volumetric and the dose weight will vary with the bulk **density** of the powder and the degree of fill, depending on whether level or heaped measures are used.

Antacids are frequently prescribed in this manner. They contain substances such as aluminum hydroxide, calcium or magnesium carbonate, magnesium trisilicate, and sodium bicarbonate.

Bulk powders may also be used as antiseptics or cleansing agents for a body cavity. For example, dentifrices generally contain a soap or detergent and a mild abrasive. Similarly, douche powders are products that are completely soluble and are most commonly intended for vaginal use, although they may be formulated for nasal, otic, or ophthalmic use.

Dispersible powders are readily wetted by water to form an extemporaneous suspension for oral administration. The quantity contained in a dispersible powder may be enough for a single dose or may contain a sufficient amount to last 2 to 3 days. It is important that the formulation is such that the powder settles slowly and that foam is not produced. If a wetting agent is used, it must be relatively free from any toxicity.

Dispersible powders are used for substances that are unstable in the presence of water and therefore cannot be formulated as liquid dosage forms.

Divided powders are dispensed in individual doses. To achieve accuracy, each dose is individually weighed, transferred to a powder paper, and the powder paper is folded. Divided powders containing **hygroscopic** and **volatile** drugs are stored in waxed paper, then double wrapped with a bond paper to improve the appearance of the completed powder. They may also be dispensed in metal foils, small heat-seal plastic bags, or other containers.

Dusting powders are locally applied nontoxic preparations that are intended to have no **systemic** action. They are dispensed in a very fine state of subdivision to enhance effectiveness and minimize irritation. Commercial dusting powders are available in sifter-top cans, sterile envelopes, or pressure aerosols. Foot powders, talcum powders, and antiperspirants available as pressure aerosols are generally more expensive than those marketed in other containers, but they offer the advantage of protection from air, moisture, and contamination, as well as convenience of application.

Absorbent powders are intended to absorb excretions on the surface of the skin from superficial infections. They usually contain starch, often with zinc oxide, kaolin, or talc.

Antifungal substances, such as salicylic acid and zinc undecylenate, are applied as powders diluted with starch, kaolin, or talc. Insecticides, such as chlorophenothan and benzene hexachloride, are incorporated in dusting powders for the destruction of lice, fleas, ticks, and so forth.

Granules

Granules are small, irregular particles. They are used as effervescent granules or they may be marketed for therapeutic purposes.

The effervescent granules contain sodium bicarbonate and either citric acid, tartaric acid, or sodium biphosphate in addition to the active ingredients. On solution in water, carbon dioxide is released as a result of the acid-base reaction causing effervescence, which serves to mask the taste of salty and bitter medications. Laxative salts, such as magnesium and sodium sulfate, are frequently formulated as effervescent granules.

Capsules

Capsules are solid dosage forms in which the drug is enclosed in a "shell" of a suitable form of gelatin. On administration the gelatin shell dissolves in 10 to 20 minutes, releasing the drug. Since the shell usually does not dissolve completely, capsules should not be used for very soluble compounds such as potassium or calcium chloride, potassium bromide, or ammonium chloride. In these cases when the partly dissolved capsule comes in contact with the stomach wall, the concentrated solution may cause localized irritation and gastric distress.

Capsules may be made of hard or soft gelatin. Hard capsules are generally used for dry powders. The contents may range from 50 mg to 1 gm per capsule. Some manufacturers prefer to seal their capsules to prevent the loss of drug because of accidental opening and/or to discourage easy removal of the contents. Soft capsules, also known as "soft shell" or "soluble elastic" capsules, are a one-piece construction with the liquid fill material literally wrapped inside a sealed, gelatin matrix. The contents of the soft capsule range from 1 to 480 minims. The capsule may be spherical (pearls) or ovoid (globules) in shape.

Hard capsules are two-piece capsules, manufactured as empty shells. The contents are filled in the capsules mechanically or manually after the capsule shells are manufactured. Soft capsules are filled with the contents during their manufacture. They cannot be filled after the soft capsules have been manufactured.

Tablets

Tablets are solid pharmaceutical dosage forms prepared either by compressing or by molding. They are the most popular of all the medicinal preparations intended for oral use. They offer the advantages of accuracy and compactness of dosage, portability, convenience of administration, and blandness of taste.

Although most frequently discoid in form, tablets may be round, oval, oblong, cylindrical, or triangular. Manufacturers generally add a colorant to a tablet formulation either for identification or for aesthetic purposes. Some tablets are scored so that they may be easily broken in halves or quarters. However, sustained-action tablets should never be broken or crushed unless directed by the manufacturer because the technology used in such tablets may not warrant their breaking or crushing. A majority of tablet dosage forms are embossed with the name of the manufacturer and/or tablet code number. Depending on whether they are made by molding or by compression, tablets are classified as molded or compressed.

Molded tablets were originally made from moist materials on a triturate mold but are now usually made by compression on a tablet machine. Such tablets must be completely and rapidly soluble. Three types are common:

- *Hypodermic tablet (HT).* These were meant to be placed in the barrel of the hypodermic syringe where they must dissolve in less than 10 seconds. They are not presently used in clinical practice.
- *Dispensing tablets (DT).* These are designed solely to provide an accurate quantity of a potent drug for use in compounding another form, such as capsules, powders, and solutions. They are never intended for administration in their original form.
- *Tablet triturates (TT).* These contain a potent drug (usually one part) and a suitable diluent (usually nine parts), such as lactose.

Compressed tablets are formed by compression and are made from powdered, crystalline, or granular material, alone or in combination with binders, disintegrants, lubricants, and fillers.

The three major methods of preparing compressed tablets are described as wet granulation, dry granulation, and direct compression. For those materials that do not lend themselves to direct compression, the formulation is first granulated (wet or dry) and then compressed. The basic steps involved in the preparation of tablets by granulation are as follows:

Wet Granulation	Dry Granulation
Weighing	Weighing
Preblending	Preblending
Granulation	**Milling**
Drying	Blending
Milling	Compression
Blending	
Compression	

Whereas wet granulation is the most common method of preparing compressed tablets, dry granulation is preferred for heat- and moisture-sensitive drugs.

Among the various types of compressed tablets available in the market, the following are more common:

- *Standard compressed tablets (CT).* These are the conventional tablets we are all familiar with and are compressed on a tablet machine.
- *Enteric-coated tablets (ECT).* These are compressed tablets coated with substances that resist solution in gastric fluid but release the medication in the intestinal tract.
- *Sugar-coated tablets (SCT).* These are tablets containing a sugar coating. Sugar coating is used to cover the objectionable taste and/or odor of medicinals and to protect sensitive materials subject to deterioration due to light, air, oxygen,

etc. However, sugar is a hygroscopic substance and the coating operation is very time consuming.

■ *Film-coated tablets (FCT).* These are tablets covered with a thin film of a water-soluble material. Such coverings impart the same general characteristics as a sugar coating and the coating operation is relatively simple, less time consuming, and economical.

■ *Sublingual or buccal tablets (ST).* These are tablets intended to be inserted below the tongue or in the buccal pouch where the active ingredient may be directly absorbed through the mucosa.

■ *Multiple compressed tablets (MCT).* These are tablets made by more than one compression cycle. Layered tablets are prepared by compressing additional tablet granulation on a previously compressed tablet. Press-coated tablets are prepared by compressing another layer around a preformed compressed tablet.

Miscellaneous tablets are those that are specially formulated and/or intended for a specific function. Common types include the following:

■ *Chewable tablets.* These are compressed tablets that are to be chewed rather than swallowed.

■ *Delayed- and/or sustained-action tablets.* These are special formulations of tablets in which the active ingredient is either released at a constant rate for prolonged periods or the release is delayed. These products are also variously described as "timed release," "long acting," "prolonged action," or some similar term implying an extended period of action for a given drug. **Table 17–1** lists some of the terms that have been used synonymously in recent years.

It should be mentioned that the U.S.P. recognizes and defines the term "modified release" to embody the terms in common use today. The definition of "modified release" includes those dosage forms for which the drug-release characteristics (i.e., time and location of release) are chosen to accomplish convenience or therapeutic objectives that are not offered by conventional dosage forms such as solutions, ointments, or dissolving dosage forms. The two types of modified-release dosage forms are (1) extended release—one that allows at least a twofold reduction in dosing frequency as compared with conventional dosage forms—and (2) delayed release—one that releases the drug at a time other than promptly after administration.

■ *Lozenges.* Also known as troches or pastilles, these are discoid-shaped solids containing the medicinal agent in a suitable flavored base, meant to be placed in the mouth where they slowly dissolve, liberating the active ingredient.

■ *Pellets.* As used now, the term signifies small cylinders meant to be implanted, usually **subcutaneously,** for prolonged and continuous absorption of potent hormones, such as testosterone or estradol.

Miscellaneous Dosage Forms

The dosage forms considered under this section have been classified miscellaneous for the sake of convenience. The properties associated with these dosage forms are either unique to themselves or represent a combination of the properties of solid and liquid dosage forms.

Aerosols

Aerosols are systems consisting of a suspension of fine solid or liquid particles in air or gas. Aerosols may be classified as either pharmaceutical aerosols or medicinal aerosols.

TABLE 17–1

Alphabetical Listing of Some Names Associated with Oral Sustained-Release Dosage Forms

Constant release	Prolonged action
Continuous action	Prolonged release
Continuous release	Protracted release
Controlled action	Repeat action
Controlled release	Repository
Delayed absorption	Retard
Delayed action	Slow acting
Delayed release	Slowly acting
Depot	Slow release
Extended action	Sustained action
Extended release	Sustained release
Gradual release	Sustained release depot
Long acting	Timed coat
Long lasting	Timed disintegration
Long-term release	Timed release
Programmed release	

Pharmaceutical aerosols are intended for topical administration or for administration into one of the body cavities, such as ear, eye, rectum, or vagina.

Medicinal aerosols are intended both for local action in the nasal areas, the throat, and the lungs and for prompt systemic effect when absorbed into the bloodstream (e.g., from lungs—inhalation or aerosol therapy).

Aerosols offer convenience and ease of application. If the product is packaged under sterile conditions, sterility can be maintained without danger of contamination. The use of aerosols eliminates the irritation produced by the mechanical application of a medicinal, especially over an abraded area. Medication can also be applied to areas that are difficult to reach otherwise.

Inhalation therapy avoids the trauma of injections and the decomposition of orally administered drugs in the gastrointestinal tract.

Because the particle size of therapeutic aerosols affects their clinical usefulness, it is essential that the aerosol dosage form be formulated with most effective particle size. For example, particles larger than 30 nm are most likely to be deposited in the trachea; those 10–30 nm may reach the terminal bronchiole; those 3–10 nm may reach the alveolar duct; those 1–3 nm may reach the alveolar sac; and particles less than 0.5 nm in size may reach the alveolar sac and be exhaled.

Isotonic solutions

Body fluids, including blood and **lacrimal fluids,** have an osmotic pressure identical to that of a 0.9 percent solution of sodium chloride. Thus, a 0.9 percent solution of sodium chloride is said to be **iso-osmotic** with physiological fluids. The term *iso-osmotic,* which is a physical term comparing the osmotic pressure, is used interchangeably with the term **isotonic,** which means "having the same tone." A solution is isotonic with a living cell if there is no net gain or loss of water by the cell, or other change in the cell, when in contact with that solution. A solution that is iso-osmotic may not necessarily be isotonic. For example, a solution of boric acid is iso-osmotic with blood and lacrimal fluid but is isotonic only with lacrimal fluids.

It causes hemolysis of red blood cells because the molecules of boric acid pass freely through the erythrocyte membrane regardless of concentration.

When dealing with isotonic solutions, caution must be exercised because any alteration in the composition of the solution (e.g., dilution) may affect the tonicity of the solution.

Ointments and pastes

Ointments and pastes are semisolid preparations used mainly for local application to skin or mucous membrane. They may be classified according to the relationship of water to the composition of the base used to prepare the ointment or paste.

Absorption bases, although essentially **anhydrous** in nature, absorb water. However, they are insoluble in water and are not water washable.

Emulsion bases are of two types. Water-in-oil emulsion bases contain water in the internal phase and oil in the external phase. Thus, they are insoluble in water. They absorb water but are not water washable. Oil-in-water emulsion bases contain oil in the internal phase and water in the external phase. Thus, they are water washable.

Oleaginous bases are insoluble in water, do not contain or absorb water, and are not water washable.

Water-soluble bases may be essentially anhydrous or they may contain water. In either case they absorb water to the point of solubility. Thus, they are water soluble and water washable.

Suppositories

Suppositories are solid unit dosage forms intended for the application of medication to any of several body orifices, namely the rectum, vagina, or urethra. These dosage forms may exhibit their therapeutic activity locally or systematically, either by melting at body temperature or by dissolving in the aqueous secretions of the mucous membrane. Suppositories intended for administration via the vagina or the urethra are sometimes referred to as "inserts," particularly when made by compression as a specially shaped tablet. Melting or dissolution of suppositories in the secretions of the cavity usually releases the medication over a prolonged period. Commonly used suppository bases can be oleaginous (e.g., cocoa butter or theobroma oil and synthetic triglyceride mixtures), water soluble (e.g., glycerinated gelatin and polyethylene glycol polymers), or hydrophilic (e.g., polyethylene sorbitan monostearate and polyoxyl 40 stearate).

Rectal suppositories for adults are usually 2.5–3.5 cm long, weigh about 2 gm each, and have a tapered shape. The largest diameter is 1.2–1.3 cm, usually tapered to about 6–7 mm. For pediatric use, the diameter and the length is less, with reduction of weight to about 1 gm.

Vaginal suppositories vary in shape from globular or ovoid to modified conical shapes. They weigh from 3–5 gm and are used primarily for local effects.

Urethral suppositories, like vaginal suppositories, are primarily used for local action. These are slender rods, from 3–5 mm in diameter, and range in length from 60–75 mm for the female urethra and from 100–150 mm for the male urethra. Although somewhat flexible, urethral suppositories are firm enough for insertion.

Gastrointestinal System

The gastrointestinal therapeutic system (GITS) is based on Alza Corporation's OROS (oralosmosis) design. This dosage form resembles an ordinary tablet, but the characteristics of drug release and drug delivery are very different.

The system consists of an osmotic drug-containing core surrounded by a semi-permeable polymer membrane that is pierced by a small, laser-drilled delivery orifice. Upon ingestion of the dosage form, water is osmotically drawn through the membrane from the gastrointestinal tract at a constant and controlled rate, thereby creating a drug solution inside the tablet. The influx of water pushes the drug solution out of the orifice at a constant rate.

The first product marketed in this country based on this technology is Ciba-Geigy's Acutrim, an over-the-counter appetite suppressant. Administered once daily, this dosage form delivers 20 mg of phenylpropanolamine initially and then 55 mg released osmotically for approximately 16 hours.

Ocular System

Topical application of drugs to the eye is common for eye disorders. The most prescribed ocular dosage form is the traditional eyedrop solution. But the eyedrop is not an efficient drug-delivery system, because the greater part of the 1 to 2 drops (50–100 microliters) is squeezed out of the eye by the first blink following administration. The residual volume mixes with the lacrimal fluid (about 7–8 microliters), becomes diluted, and is drained away by the nasolacrimal drainage system until the solution volume returns to the normal tear volume of 7–8 microliters. The initial drainage results in the loss of about 75 to 80 percent of the administered dose within 5 minutes of instillation. Then drainage stops and the residual dose declines slowly.

The efficiency of an ophthalmic drug delivery system can be greatly improved by prolonging its contact with the corneal surface. To achieve this purpose, suspensions of drug particles in pharmaceutical vehicles are prepared, viscosity-enhancing agents such as methylcellulose are added to the eyedrop preparation, or the drug is provided as an ointment.

Recently, drug-presoaked hydrogel-type contact lenses have been shown to prolong the drug-eye contact time. The Bionite lens, for example, is inserted into the eye after being presoaked in the drug solution. Similarly, sauflon hydrophilic contact lenses are manufactured from a vinyl pyrrolidone acrylic copolymer of high water content. These contact lenses have been shown to improve the delivery of fluorescein, phenylephrine, pilocarpine, chloramphenicol, and tetracycline.

The new generation of drug-dispersing ocular inserts consists of a medicated core matrix confined within a pair of flexible, transparent, biocompatible, and tear-insoluble polymer membranes that provide the required degree of permeability for the drug. When the insert is placed in the conjunctival cul-de-sac between the sclera of the eyeball and the lower lid, the drug is continuously released by diffusion through the membrane as a result of solvation in the lacrimal fluid.

Alza Corporation's Ocusert System is a pilocarpine core reservoir sandwiched between two sheets of transparent, **lipophilic,** rate-controlling membranes. When placed in the cul-de-sac, the pilocarpine molecules penetrate through the rate-controlling membranes. This controlled pilocarpine-releasing therapeutic system has several advantages over the conventional eyedrop solution. It provides better patient compliance, less-frequent dosing, around-the-clock protection for 4 to 7 days, fewer ocular and systemic side effects, possible delay in the **refractory** state, and a significantly smaller dose of pilocarpine for the effective management of **intraocular** pressure in the treatment of glaucoma. The administration of one Ocusert Pilo-20 insert, for example, delivers a daily dose of only 0.4–0.5 mg compared with the 4–8 mg provided by the instillation of 1 to 2 drops of the conventional 2 percent pilocarpine solution administered four times a day.

Transdermal System

The **transdermal** system is an innovation that employs the skin as a portal of drug entry into the systemic circulation. Using the **percutaneous** route instead of the more conventional oral, parenteral, pulmonary, or rectal routes, this technique is designed to provide systemic therapy for acute or chronic conditions that do not involve the skin.

Among the most popular and intriguing percutaneously administered drug-delivery systems is the transdermal patch. The advantages of this system include convenience, uninterrupted therapy, better patient compliance, accurate drug dosage, and regulation of drug concentration. The patch is formulated to deliver a constant, controlled dose of the drug through the intact skin, where it enters directly into the bloodstream. These delivery systems have a backing layer, a drug reservoir, a membrane, and an adhesive layer that incorporates a priming dose of the drug.

Nitroglycerin is available in various forms—sublingual, oral, intravenous injection, topical ointment, and transdermal preparations **(Table 17–2)**. The popular transdermal preparations of nitroglycerin are Ciba-Geigy's Transderm-Nitro, Searle's Nitrodisc, and Key's Nitro-Dur.

All nitroglycerin transdermal patches are designed to be applied to the upper arm or chest to provide the drug for 24 hours. Although these patches can be applied anywhere on the body except the distal parts of the extremities, most patients have a tendency to apply these near the thorax, perhaps on the assumption that the medication for the heart should be placed near the heart. Manufacturers do recommend, however, that each patch should be applied at a site different from that used the previous day to avoid irritation.

Transderm-Scop, a scopolamine-containing transdermal delivery system marketed by Ciba-Geigy, is a circular, flat, tan disc, about 2 mm thick and the size of a dime. Each disc contains 1–5 mg of scopolamine and is programmed to deliver 0.5 mg of scopolamine over 3 days. According to Ciba, this delivery system is more effective than the conventional oral dose, which has been reported to cause excessively rapid heartbeat, confusion, and hallucination. The patch works best when placed behind the ear on a hairless site, delivering scopolamine through intact skin directly into the bloodstream for 3 days.

Other drugs available as transdermal patches include hormone preparations and nicotine (for smoking cessation).

TABLE 17–2   **Comparison of Nitroglycerine Dosage Forms**

Dosage Form	Dose	Antianginal Effect	
		Onset	Duration
Intravenous	Variable	Minutes	Minutes
Sublingual	0.15–0.6 mg every 30 min	2 minutes	up to 30 minutes
Oral, timed release	2.5–9.0 mg twice daily	1/2–1 hour	8–9 hours
Topical ointment (2%, 15 mg/in.)	1–2 in. every 4 hours	30 minutes	3 hours
Transdermal	1 patch every 12–24 hours	30 minutes	20–24 hours

Summary

In recent years the pharmaceutical industry has made significant progress in the development and manufacture of dosage forms. The new concepts of bioavailability have made it possible to prepare more efficient delivery systems. The latest developments include such dosage forms as the transdermal delivery system (TDS) popularly known as the "patch," the osmotic pump, and the insulin pump. In the future, one can expect dosage forms containing optimal amounts of active ingredients to provide maximal therapeutic benefits, thus markedly reducing or completely eliminating the side effects of therapeutic agents.

ASSESSMENT

Multiple Choice Questions

1. Drugs are defined as chemicals of
   a. natural origin
   b. synthetic origin
   c. semisynthetic origin
   d. biological origin
   e. all of above

2. Which of the following is not a drug dosage form?
   a. brew
   b. tablet
   c. solution
   d. injection
   e. ointment

3. Drug formulation aides include
   a. diluents
   b. excipients
   c. additives
   d. preservatives
   e. all of the above

4. For a drug to elicit the desired response, it is required at the site of action to be in the form of
   a. a hydrosolvent
   b. a molecular dispersion
   c. an isotonic solution
   d. a soluble gel
   e. an acidic vehicle

5. A soluble substance is called
   a. a solvent
   b. a solubilizer
   c. a solute
   d. a solution
   e. none of the above

6. Medicinal emulsions for oral administration are usually
   a. o/w type
   b. w/o type

7. Which of the following is not a solid dosage form?
   a. powder
   b. capsule
   c. gel
   d. granule
   e. tablet

8. Antifungal substances are applied as powders that may be diluted with
   a. starch
   b. kaolin
   c. talc
   d. a and c
   e. a, b, and c ✓

9. The most prescribed ocular dosage form is
   a. eyedrop solution ✓
   b. ophthalmic ointments
   c. drug-presoaked hydrogel-type contact lens
   d. ocular inserts
   e. core reservoirs in lipophilic membranes

10. Advantage(s) of transdermal patches include
    a. convenience
    b. uninterrupted therapy
    c. better patient compliance
    d. regulation of drug concentration
    e. all of the above ✓

True/False Questions

11. __T__   In actual practice a "pure" drug is seldom used.

12. __F__   Liquid dosage forms are rarely the drug of choice.

13. __T__   In an acceptable suspension the particles never settle down.

14. __T__   Emulsions contain at least one immiscible liquid.

15. _____   Tablets should never be chewed before swallowing. *unless chewable or directed too.*

Matching

16. __c__   medicinal aerosols

17. __d__   transdermal patches

18. __e__   bionite lens

19. __a__   lozenges

20. __b__   pellets

a. slowly dissolved in the mouth

b. implanted subcutaneously

c. inhaled through nose or mouth

d. applied to the skin

e. inserted into the eye

COMPETENCIES

Upon completion and review of this chapter, the student should be able to

1. Interpret a medication order accurately.

2. Convert quantities stated in apothecary units to their equivalent units in the metric system.

3. Convert quantities stated in metric or apothecary units to other units within those systems (e.g., g to mg).

4. Set up valid proportions to perform calculations required in administering medications.

5. Calculate quantities to be administered when ordered in fractional doses.

6. Calculate safe dosages for infants and children.

7. Calculate dosages for individual patients given the patient's weight and/or height and the recommended dose.

8. Perform calculations necessary for the infusion of I.V. medications.

9. List five steps to decrease errors in interpreting the strength of drugs from the written order.

Introduction

It is common practice in hospitals today for the pharmacist to calculate and prepare the drug dosage form for administration to the patient. Often the drug is provided in a unit-dose package. However, this practice does not relieve the nurse from the legal and professional responsibility of ensuring that the patient receives the right dose of the right medication at the right time in the right manner. This chapter will review the necessary calculations involved in the safe administration of drugs to the patient.

Interpreting the Drug Order

The welfare of the patient necessitates proper interpretation of the medication order. If any doubt exists, or if a particular order appears unusual, it is the nurse's responsibility to check with the physician or the pharmacist.

Abbreviations derived from Latin are often used by physicians and pharmacists in writing and preparing drug orders. Refer to **Tables 18–1 through 18–5** for common abbreviations. The technician must be able to interpret these abbreviations correctly when they are encountered in the drug order. Some examples of drug orders encountered in practice include the following:

EXAMPLE 1

Caps. Diphenhydramine (Benadryl) 25 mg q4h po
Interpretation: "Give the patient one 25 mg capsule by mouth every 4 hours."

TABLE 18–1

Amount/Dosage

Abbreviation	Latin Derivation	English
C	congius	gallon
cc		cubic centimeter
g	gramma	gram
gr	granum	grain
gtt	gutta	drop
lb	libra	pound
m	minimum	minim
mL		milliliter
no	numerus	number
qs	quatum sufficit	quantity sufficient
ss	semis	one-half
3	drachma	dram
℥	unica	ounce

TABLE 18–2

Preparations

Abbreviation	Latin Derivation	English
cap	capsula	capsule
elix	elixir	elixir
EC		enteric coated
ext	extractum	extract
fl	fluidus	fluid
pil	pilula	pill
sol	solutio	solution
supp	suppositorium	suppository
susp		suspension
syr	syrupus	syrup
tab	tabella	tablet
tr	tinctura	tincture
ung	unguentum	ointment

EXAMPLE 2

Elixir Acetaminophen (Elixir Tylenol) gtts 20 tid pc and hs po
Interpretation: "Give 20 drops of elixir acetaminophen by mouth three times a day after meals and 20 drops by mouth at bedtime.

EXAMPLE 3

100 mg Demerol IM stat. 50 mg q4h prn pain
Interpretation: "Give 100 mg of Demerol intramuscularly immediately, then give 50 mg of Demerol intramuscularly not more often than every 4 hours prn."

The abbreviation "prn" can often be a source of trouble if not interpreted carefully. In the order described in the last example, the medication (Demerol) can be administered if the dosing interval of at least 4 hours is maintained. The nurse as-

TABLE 18–3

Routes

Abbreviation	Latin Derivation	English
ID		intradermal
IM		intramuscular
IV		intravenous
IVPB		intravenous piggyback
OD	oculus dexter	right eye
OS	oculus sinister	left eye
OU	oculo utro	both eyes
AD	auricula dexter	right ear
AS	auricula sinister	left ear
AU	auriculi utro	both ears
po	per os	by mouth
sc	sub cutis	subcutaneous
sl	sub lingual	sublingual
GT		gastrostomy
NG		nasogastric
NJ		nasojejunal

TABLE 18–4

Special Instructions

Abbreviation	Latin Derivation	English
aa	ana	of each
ad lib	ad libitum	as desired
c̄	cum	with
dil	dilutus	dilute
per	per	through or by
Rx	recipe	take
s̄	sine	without
stat	statim	immediately

TABLE 18–5 **Times**

Abbreviation	Latin Derivation	English
ā	ante	before
ac	ante cibum	before meals
am	ante meridian	before noon
bid	bis in die	twice a day
h	hora	hour
hs	hora somni	hour of sleep or at bedtime
noct	noctis	night
o	omnis	every
od	omni die	every day
oh	omni hora	every hour
p	post	after
pc	post cibum	after meals
pm	post meridian	after noon
prn	pro re nata	whenever necessary
q	quaque	every
qd	quaque die	every day
qh (q3h, etc.)	quaque hora	every hour (3, 4, etc.)
qid	quarter in die	4 times a day
sos	si opus sit	if necessary (one dose only)
tid	ter in die	3 times a day

TABLE 18–6 **Values of Single Roman Numbers**

Roman Numerals		Value
$\overline{ss}$	=	½
I or i	=	1
V or v	=	5
X or x	=	10
L or l	=	50
C or c	=	100
D or d	=	500
M or m	=	1000

sesses the patient's need for the Demerol to control pain or the patient requests the medication, and it may be administered if it has been 4 hours or more since the previous injection.

Most prescriptions are written in the metric system; however, the apothecary system using Roman numerals is still used by some prescribers through force of habit. A few of the most common Roman numerals are shown in **Table 18–6.**

Ratio and Proportion

Nearly every problem that arises in calculations involving medication can be broken down to simple ratio and proportion. Developing skill in setting up ratios and proportions will be an invaluable aid to the nurse in solving medication problems quickly and accurately.

Ratio

A ratio is the relationship of two quantities. It may be expressed in the form 1:10 or 1:2500, or it may be expressed as a fraction—1/10 or 1/2500. The ratio expression 1:10 or 1/10 can be read as one in ten, or one-tenth, or one part in ten parts.

EXAMPLE 4

For every twenty students there is one teacher. The ratio of teachers to students is 1 in 20 or 1:20 or 1/20.

Proportion

A proportion is formed by using two ratios which are equal. For example, $1/2 = 5/10$. When two ratios or fractions are equal, their cross product is also equal. The cross product is obtained by multiplying the denominator of one ratio by the numerator of the other, as follows:

$$\frac{1}{2} \diagup\!\!\!\!\!\diagdown \frac{5}{10} = 2 \times 5 = 10 \times 1$$

The cross products are equal: $10 = 10$. Therefore, the ratio 1/2 is equal to the ratio 5/10.

Does $1/4 = 3/12$?

$$\frac{1}{4} \diagup\!\!\!\!\!\diagdown \frac{3}{12} = \frac{12}{12}$$

The cross products are equal: $12 = 12$. Therefore, 1/4 is equal to 3/12.

This characteristic of proportions is very useful in solving problems that arise in drug administration. If any three of the values of a proportion are known, the fourth value can be determined.

EXAMPLE 5

The prescriber orders 20 mg I.M. of a drug for a patient. The drug is available in a 10 mL vial which contains 50 mg of drug. How many milliliters will be needed to supply the dose of 20 mg?

SOLUTION

Three things are known from the statement of the problem.

1. 10 mL vial on hand
2. 50 mg of drug in the 10 mL vial
3. 20 mg is the desired dose

A ratio can be stated for the drug on hand.

$$\frac{10 \text{ mL}}{50 \text{ mg}} \text{ reduced to lowest terms} = \frac{1 \text{ mL}}{5 \text{ mg}}$$

A ratio can also be stated for the required dosage.

$$\frac{x \text{ mL}}{20 \text{ mg}}$$

Thus, the proportion is

$$\frac{1 \text{ mL}}{5 \text{ mg}} = \frac{x \text{ mL}}{20 \text{ mg}}$$

Note in the proportion that the units are labeled and like units are located in the same position in each fraction or ratio (1 mL is opposite $\times$ mL and 5 mg is opposite 20 mg). It is important to label the parts of the proportion correctly. Note that the answer label is always the label with the "x."

Important: Three conditions must be met when using ratio and proportion.

1. The numerators must have the same units.
2. The denominators must have the same units.
3. Three of the four parts must be known.

To solve the last example, simply find the cross product and solve for the unknown (x).

$$\frac{1\text{mL}}{5 \text{ mg}} = \frac{x \text{ mL}}{20 \text{ mg}}$$

$$5 \times x; = 1 \times 20$$

$$5x = 20$$

$$x = 4 \text{ mL (20 divided by 5)}$$

[handwritten: $5x = 20$ $\frac{1}{5} \cdot 5x = 20 \cdot \frac{1}{5}$ $x = 4$]

Therefore, 4 mL of the solution contains 20 mg of drug.

It is helpful to note that a proportion is similar to the way we think logically: If this is so, then that will follow. Problems can be analyzed with the if-then approach.

In the last example, we could say IF we have 10 mL containing 50 mg of drug, THEN x mL of solution will contain 20 mg of drug.

$$\frac{10 \text{ mL}}{50 \text{ mg}} \text{ or } \frac{1 \text{ mL}}{5 \text{ mg}} = \frac{x \text{ mL}}{20 \text{ mg}}$$

| IF | THEN |

Remember that the first ratio of a proportion is always formed from the quantity and strength (concentration) of the drug on hand.

EXAMPLE 6

Ampicillin oral suspension contains 250 mg of the drug in each 5 mL. How many milliliters would be measured into a medication syringe to obtain a dose of 75 mg of **ampicillin?**

SOLUTION

1. Set up the proportion beginning with the drug on hand.

$$\frac{5 \text{ mL}}{250 \text{ mg}} = \frac{x \text{ mL}}{75 \text{ mg}}$$

| IF | THEN |

[handwritten: $250 \times x = 5 \times 75$]

2. Then cross multiply.

$250(x) = 375$

$$250(x) = 5(75)$$
$$250(x) = 375$$
$$x = 1.5 \text{ mL}$$

PRACTICE PROBLEMS

Solve the following problems by setting up the proportion and finding the unknown quantity. Answers are at the end of the chapter.

1. Elixir of digoxin contains 50 micrograms (mcg) of digoxin in each milliliter. How many micrograms of the drug are in 0.3 mL of the elixir?
2. Lugol's solution contains 50 mg of iodine per milliliter. How many milligrams of iodine are in 0.3 mL of the solution?
3. Elixir of diphenhydramine (elixir of Benadryl) contains 12.5 mg per 5 mL (tea-spoonful). How many milliliters are needed to provide 30 mg of the drug?
4. The physician orders 2.5 mg of theophylline to be administered orally to a pe-diatric patient. If elixir of theophylline contains 80 mg of theophylline per ta-blespoonful (15 mL), how many milliliters of the elixir should be administered?
5. A vial contains 250 mg of tetracycline HCl in a total of 2 mL of solution. How many milligrams of tetracycline HCl are contained in 0.6 mL of this solution?

Conversion between Systems of Measurement

Before reviewing the types of calculations used in determining medication dosages, it is necessary to examine conversions between systems of measurement. It was mentioned previously that nearly all medication orders today are written using the metric system. However, some orders will be written using apothecary notation. The technician must be able to convert from the apothecary system to the metric system, and from one unit to another unit within both systems.

Conversion between systems requires the use of approximate weight and measure equivalents. The key word here is "approximate." The approximate values are not *exact* equivalents. For example, 1 g = 15 gr approximately = 15.432 gr exactly. The pharmacist uses the exact equivalents in compounding medications. In calculations involving dosages, however, it is not necessary to use exact equivalents. In fact, since the exact equivalents involve many decimal places and fractional numbers, their use could lead to awkward calculations with an increase in errors. Thus, the approximate equivalents are used in calculations for medication dosages. Approximate equivalents are used in the examples and problems in the remainder of this chapter. For example, 30 milliliters (mL) = 1 fluid ounce (fl oz) in all calcu-lations. Similarly, 1 gram (g) = 15 grains (gr).

Review of the Metric System

The three basic units of the metric system are the meter (length), the gram (weight), and the liter (volume). Only the units of weight and volume are consid-ered in this chapter. Multiples or parts of these basic units are named by adding a prefix. Each prefix has a numerical value, as shown in **Table 18–7.**

TABLE 18–7

Metric Prefixes

Small Units	Large Units
deci = 0.1	deka = 10
centi = 0.01	hecto = 100
milli = 0.001	kilo = 1,000
micro = 0.000001	mega = 1,000,000
nano = 0.000000001	

TABLE 18–8

Common Metric Abbreviations

Measure	Abbreviation
nanogram	ng
microgram	mcg
milligram	mg
gram	g
kilogram	kg
milliliter	mL
deciliter	dL
liter	L
millimeter	mm
centimeter	cm
meter	m
kilometer	km

Examples of the use of the metric prefixes are as follows:

- 1 milliliter (mL) = 1/1000 liter = 0.001 L
- 1 milligram (mg) = 1/1000 gram = 0.001 g
- 1 microgram (mcg) = 1/1,000,000 gram = 0.000001 g
- 1 nanogram (ng) = 1/1,000,000,000 gram = 0.000000001 g
- 1 kilogram (kg) = 1000 times 1 gram = 1000 g
- 1 deciliter (dL) = 1/10 liter = 0.1 L

Table 18–8 shows examples of common metric abbreviations.

Liter
The liter is the basic unit of volume used to measure liquids in the metric system. It is equal to 1000 cubic centimeters of water. One cubic centimeter is considered equivalent to one milliliter (mL); thus 1 liter (L) = 1000 milliliters (mL).

Gram
The gram is the basic unit of weight in the metric system. The gram is defined as the weight of one cubic centimeter of distilled water at 4°C.

Conversions

Using Table 18–7, the following values can be determined:

- 1000 g   = 1 kg
- 1000 mg = 1 g
- 1000 ng   = 1 mcg
- 1000 mcg = 1 mg
- 1000 mL = 1 L
- 100 mL   = 1 dL

Two rules apply to conversions within the metric system.

- *Rule 1.* To convert a quantity in the metric system to a larger denomination, move the decimal point to the left.
  —Smaller to larger (S to L) = Right to left (R to L)
      Smaller ⟶ Larger
      Right ⟶ Left
      Example:
      0.001 ⟶ 0.1
- *Rule 2.* To convert a quantity to a smaller denomination, move the decimal point to the right.
  —Larger to smaller (L to S) = Left to right (L to R)
      Larger ⟶ Smaller
      Left ⟶ Right
      Example:
      89.5 ⟶ 0.895

Note that the two Ls are on the same side in each rule.

EXAMPLE 7

Convert 22 g to milligrams.

SOLUTION

The change is from larger to smaller with a difference of 1000 between the units. The rule in this case is: Larger to smaller (L to S) = Left to right (L to R).

Because the difference is 1000 between grams and milligrams, the decimal point is moved three places to the right. Thus, 22 g = 22,000 mg.

EXAMPLE 8

Convert 150 mL to liters.

SOLUTION

In changing from milliliters to liters, the change is from smaller to larger (S to L), with a difference of 1000 between the units (1000 mL = 1 L). Therefore, move the decimal point from right to left (R to L). Because there is a difference of 1000 between the units, move the decimal point three places to the left. Thus, 150 mL = 0.15 L.

PRACTICE PROBLEMS

6. 2000 mg = _____ g
7. 50 g   = _____ mg
8. 2 L   = _____ mL
9. 230 ng = _____ mcg

10. 250 mg = _____ g
11. 2.5 kg = _____ g
12. 0.5 L   = _____ mL
13. 1.5 L   = _____ dL
14. 20 mg   = _____ g
15. 0.7 mg = _____ mcg

Apothecary System of Weights

The apothecary system of weights is based upon the grain (gr), which is the smallest unit in the system. The origin of the grain is uncertain, but it is believed that at one time solids were measured by using grains of wheat as the standard.

In practice, the technician will seldom see apothecary units of weight with the exception of the grain, which is still commonly used in ordering medications such as nitroglycerin (1/100 gr, 1/150 gr), atropine sulfate (1/200 gr, 1/150 gr), codeine sulfate (1/8 gr, 1/4 gr, 1/2 gr, 1 gr), and morphine sulfate (1/6 gr, 1/8 gr, 1/2 gr). To convert grains to metric units, the following approximate equivalent is used:

$$15 \text{ grains} = 1 \text{ gram}$$

EXAMPLE 9

Convert 4 grains to grams.

SOLUTION

$$\frac{15 gr}{1 g} = \frac{4 \ gr}{xg}$$

$$x = 0.27 \text{ g}$$

Apothecary System of Volume (Liquid) Measure

The apothecary liquid measures are the same as the avoirdupois measures which we use daily, such as ounces, pints, and quarts. The smallest unit of volume in the apothecary system is the minim (m). The minim should *not* be confused with the drop as they are not equivalent. The size of a drop varies with the properties of the liquid being dispensed or measured. **Table 18–9** shows the common units of liquid measure in the apothecary system.

Apothecary System Notation

In the apothecary system, the unit is written first, followed by the quantity. For small numbers, lowercase Roman numerals are used. Arabic numbers are commonly used for large numbers (i.e., greater than 40). **Table 18–10** shows examples of apothecary system notation.

Converting from the Apothecary System to the Metric System

The use of tabular information is helpful in converting between the systems of weights and measures. Many conversions, however, can be made readily by use of two important equivalents and the ratio and proportion method.

The equivalents are:

$$15 \text{ gr} = 1 \text{ g}$$

$$m \ 16 = 1 \text{ mL}$$

TABLE 18–9

Liquid Measure in the Apothecary System

Measure		Equivalent
60 minims (m)	=	1 fluid dram (fl dr or fl ʒ)*
8 fluid drams (fl dr)	=	1 fluid ounce (fl oz or fl ʒ) = 480 minims (m)
16 fluid ounces	=	1 pint (pt)
2 pints	=	1 quart (qt) = 32 fluid ounces (fl oz)
4 quarts	=	1 gallon = 128 fluid ounces

*The fluid dram sign (ʒ) is often used by physicians to represent 1 teaspoonful or 5 mL. The apothecary symbol for one-half fluid ounce or 1 tablespoonful is ʒ s̄s̄. When this appears in the directions for use (Signa), it is read as 1 tablespoonful or 15 mL.

TABLE 18–10

Apothecary Notation

Quantity	Notation
1/10 grain	gr 1/10
1 grain	gr i
1½ grains	gr is̄s̄
10 grains	gr x
15 minims	m XV
150 minims	m 150
2½ ounces	ʒ iis̄s̄

EXAMPLE 10

The physician orders 7 1/2 grains of aminophylline p.o. for a patient. On hand are aminophylline tablets 500 mg. How many tablets are required for one dose?

SOLUTION

First the physician's order must be converted to a metric unit, or the strength of the tablets on hand must be converted to an apothecary unit. It is preferable to convert to metric units in all cases.

Setting up the proportion gives:

$$\underset{\displaystyle \frac{1 \text{ g}}{15 \text{ gr}}}{\text{IF}} = \underset{\displaystyle \frac{x \text{ g}}{7.5 \text{ gr}}}{\text{THEN}}$$

Cross multiplying:

$$15\,x = 7.5$$
$$x = 0.5 \text{ g (500 mg)}$$

Thus, the 7 1/2 gr ordered by the physician is equal to one of the 500 mg tablets on hand. The dose is 1 tablet of 500 mg aminophylline (7 1/2 gr aminophylline).

EXAMPLE 11

How many milligrams of nitroglycerin are in one 1/150 gr tablet of the drug?

SOLUTION

This problem requires conversion from the apothecary system to the metric system. Use the equivalent 1 g = 15 gr. The proportion is:

$$\text{IF} \qquad \text{THEN}$$

$$\frac{1\text{ g}}{15\text{ gr}} = \frac{x\text{ g}}{1/150\text{ gr}}$$

Cross multiplying:

$$15\,x = 1/150 = .0067$$
$$x = 0.0004\text{ g} = 0.4\text{ mg}$$

Remember, when converting in the metric form from larger to smaller, the decimal point moves left to right.

PRACTICE PROBLEMS

16. 6 pints   = _____ fluid ounces
17. 17 g   = _____ gr
18. 26 quarts   = _____ gallons
19. 200 minims   = _____ fluid ounces
20. 65 grains   = _____ g
21. 3 gallons   = _____ pints

Calculation of Fractional Doses

Nurses encounter fractional or partial medication dosages frequently as physicians often order medication for a patient in a strength that differs from the strength of the preparation on hand.

The ratio and proportion method can be used to solve all problems of fractional dosages. The concentration of the medication on hand forms the IF ratio of the proportion.

EXAMPLE 12

The physician orders 1 million units of penicillin G for a patient. The penicillin G on hand is available as a solution containing 250,000 units/mL.

SOLUTION

Find the strength of the product on hand. This expression forms the IF ratio of the proportion:

$$\text{IF} \qquad\qquad \text{THEN}$$

$$\frac{250,000\text{ units}}{1\text{ mL}} = \underline{\qquad\qquad}$$

Place the number of units wanted in the THEN ratio and solve for the unknown x.

$$\text{IF} \qquad\qquad \text{THEN}$$

$$\frac{250{,}000 \text{ units}}{1 \text{ mL}} = \frac{1{,}000{,}000 \text{ units}}{x \text{ mL}}$$

$$250{,}000x = 1{,}000{,}000$$

$$x = 4 \text{ mL}$$

Remember to label all parts of the proportion carefully with the appropriate units.

EXAMPLE 13

The physician orders 250 mcg of cyanocobalamin (vitamin B_{12}) I.M. daily. The vitamin B_{12} on hand is labeled 1000 mcg/mL. How many milliliters should be given to the patient?

SOLUTION

The concentration of B_{12} on hand is 1000 mcg/mL. Therefore, the IF ratio is:

$$\frac{1000 \text{ mcg}}{1 \text{ mL}}$$

Placing the number of micrograms needed opposite the micrograms of the IF ratio results in:

$$\text{IF} \qquad\qquad \text{THEN}$$

$$\frac{1000 \text{ mcg}}{1 \text{ mL}} = \frac{250 \text{ mcg}}{x \text{ ML}}$$

Solving for x yields:

$$x = 0.25 \text{ mL}$$

To supply 250 mcg of vitamin B_{12} requires 0.25 mL.

EXAMPLE 14

A patient is to be given 25 mg of diphenhydramine (Benadryl) p.o. The Benadryl is available as elixir of Benadryl 12.5 mg/5 mL. How many milliliters should be given to the patient?

SOLUTION

$$\text{IF} \qquad\qquad \text{THEN}$$

$$\frac{12.05 \text{ mg}}{5 \text{ mL}} = \frac{25 \text{ mg}}{x \text{ mL}}$$

$$x = \frac{125}{12.5}$$

$$x = 10 \text{ mL}$$

EXAMPLE 15

A medication order calls for 750 mg of calcium lactate to be given tid po. On hand are tablets of calcium lactate 0.5 g. How many tablets should be given for each dose?

SOLUTION

Note: When using ratio and proportion the units must be alike. Grams cannot be used in a proportion with milligrams. Therefore, in this example the grams must be converted to milligrams or the 750 mg converted to grams. Changing the grams to milligrams yields:

$$0.5 \text{ g} = 500 \text{ mg}$$

Remember: Larger to smaller = Left to right. A 1000 difference means moving the decimal point three places to the right.

$$\underset{\text{IF}}{\frac{500 \text{ mg}}{1 \text{ tab}}} = \underset{\text{THEN}}{\frac{750 \text{ mg}}{\text{x tab}}}$$

$$x = 1.5 \text{ or } 1\frac{1}{2} \text{ tablets}$$

PRACTICE PROBLEMS

22. A patient is to receive a 100 mg dose of gentamicin. On hand is a vial containing 80 mg/mL of the drug. How many milliliters should be given to the patient?
23. A multiple dose vial of a penicillin G potassium solution contains 100,000 units per milliliter. How many milliliters of this solution must be administered to a patient who requires a 750,000 unit dose?
24. A physician orders 30 mg of Demerol I.M. for a patient. How many milliliters of a Demerol solution containing 100 mg/mL must be given to the patient?
25. The nurse is asked to administer an intramuscular dose of 45 mcg of an investigational drug. How many milliliters must be withdrawn from a vial containing 20 mcg/mL of the drug?
26. A pediatric patient is to be given a 70 mg dose of Dilantin by administering an oral suspension containing 50 mg of Dilantin per 5 mL. How many milliliters of the suspension must be administered?

Calculation of Dosages Based on Weight

The recommended dosages of drugs are often expressed in the literature as a number of milligrams per unit of body weight per unit of time (refer to package inserts or the *Physician's Desk Reference*). Such dosage expressions are commonly used in depicting pediatric doses. For example, the recommended dose for a drug might be 5 mg/kg/24 hours. This information can be utilized by the pharmacist to

1. calculate the dose for a given patient; and
2. check on doses ordered that are suspected to be significant over- or under-doses.

EXAMPLE 16

The physician orders Mintezol tablets for a 110-pound child. The recommended dosage for Mintezol is 20 mg/kg per dose. How many 500 mg tablets of Mintezol should be given to this patient for each dose?

SOLUTION

1. Since the dose provided is based on a kilogram weight, convert the patient's weight to kilograms by proportion.

$$1 \text{ kg} = 2.2 \text{ lb}$$

$$\frac{1 \text{ kg}}{2.2 \text{ lb}} = \frac{x \text{ kg}}{110 \text{ lb}}$$

$$x = 50 \text{ kg}$$

2. Calculate the total daily dose using the recommended dosage information: 20 mg/kg. This is interpreted as, "For each kilogram of body weight, give 20 mg of the drug."

$$\frac{20 \text{ mg}}{1 \text{ kg}} = \frac{x \text{ mg}}{50 \text{ kg}}$$

$$x = 1000 \text{ mg}$$

3. Calculate the number of tablets needed to supply 1000 mg per dose. The concentration of tablets on hand = 500 mg/tablet.

$$\frac{500 \text{ mg}}{1 \text{ tab}} = \frac{1000 \text{ mg}}{x \text{ tab}}$$

$$x = 2 \text{ tablets per dose}$$

EXAMPLE 17

The recommended dose of meperidine (Demerol) is 6 mg/kg/24 h for pain. It is given in divided doses every 4 to 6 hours. How many milliliters of Demerol injection (50 mg/mL) should be administered to a 33-pound child as a single dose every 6 hours?

SOLUTION

1. Calculate the daily dose for a 33-pound child.

$$\frac{6 \text{ mg}}{1 \text{ kg } (2.2 \text{ lb})} = \frac{x \text{ mg}}{33 \text{ lb}}$$

By inserting the conversion unit 2.2 lb for 1 kg in the ratio, there is no need to do a separate calculation of the number of kilograms in 33 pounds.

$$x = 90 \text{ mg of Demerol per day (24 hours)}$$

2. Calculate the number of milliliters of Demerol injection (50 mg/mL) needed for the total daily dose.

$$\frac{50 \text{ mg}}{1 \text{ mL}} = \frac{90 \text{ mg}}{x \text{ mL}}$$

$$50x = 90$$

$$x = 1.8 \text{ mL every 24 hours}$$

3. Calculate the number of milliliters to be given every 6 hours.

$$\frac{1.8 \text{ mL}}{24 \text{ h}} = \frac{x \text{ mL}}{6 \text{ h}}$$

$$24x = 10.8$$

$$x = 0.45 \text{ mL}$$

PRACTICE PROBLEMS

27. The recommended dose of cefamandole nafate (Mandol) for a pediatric patient is 50 mg/kg/day. How many milligrams must be given daily to a 60-pound child?

28. Acyclovir (Zovirax) is administered in a dose of 15 mg/kg/day. How many milligrams of the drug must be administered daily to a 175-pound adult?

29. The recommended dose for methotrexate is 2.5 mg/kg every 14 days. How many milligrams of this drug must be administered to a 125-pound adult for each dose?

30. Chlorpromazine HCl is to be administered in a dose of 0.25 mg/lb. How many milligrams of this drug must be administered to an 85-kilogram patient?

31. A recommended dose for the administration of streptomycin sulfate is 10 mg/lb/day. How many milligrams of this drug must be administered daily to a 63-kilogram adult?

Pediatric Dosage Calculations

When the manufacturer's recommended dosage is not available to determine dosages for children, the nomogram is the most accurate method to use. The nomogram is a chart that uses the weight and height (size) of the patient to estimate his or her body surface area (BSA) in square meters (m^2). This body surface area is then placed in a ratio with the body surface area of an average adult ($1.73m^2$). The formula used with the nomogram method is:

$$\frac{\text{Child's}}{\text{dose}} = \frac{\text{Child's body surface area in } m^2}{1.73 \; m^2 \; (\text{BSA of average adult})} \times \frac{\text{Adult}}{\text{dose}}$$

To determine the child's BSA, the weight and height of the child must be known. The nomogram scales contain both metric (kg, cm) and avoirdupois (lb, inches) values for height and weight. Thus, the BSA can be determined for pounds and inches or kilograms and centimeters without making conversions.

Appendix H of this text contains the nomogram "Body Surface Area of Children." Note the three columns labeled height, body surface area, and weight. Also note that the height and weight scales show both metric and avoirdupois values.

To determine the body surface area, a ruler or straightedge is needed. (A piece of paper or cardboard can be used if there is at least one even, straight edge.) The following steps demonstrate the use of the nomogram.

1. Determine the height and weight of the patient. This information may be given in metric values (e.g., height = 84 cm, weight = 12 kg) or in avoirdupois values: height = 33.5 inches, weight = 26.5 pounds. Mixed values can also be used: height = 85 cm, weight = 26.5 pounds.

2. Place the straightedge on the nomogram connecting the two points on the height and weight scales that represent the patient's values. Assume the patient is a child weighing 26.5 pounds and standing 33.5 inches tall. Then, 26.5 pounds on the weight scale and 33.5 inches on the height scale are connected using the straightedge.

3. Where the straightedge crosses the center column (body surface area) a reading is taken. This value is the body surface area in square meters for the patient. In our example, BSA = 0.52 m^2.

Note: The three scales are divided into five divisions between the major numbered sections, which vary in value as the scales are ascended. To interpret the value of the divisions, take the difference between the two numbers and divide by 5.

For example, on the kg scale between 5 kg and 6 kg there is a difference of 1, so each division between 5 and 6 is 0.2 kg (1 divided by 5). Between 1.5 kg and 2 kg, the difference is 0.5. Therefore, each division between 1.5 and 2 kg is 0.1 kg (0.5 divided by 5).

4. Substitute the BSA value in the formula to calculate the dosage for the child. For example, if the dose of aminophylline is 500 mg for an adult, what is the dose for a child with a calculated BSA of 0.52 m²?

$$\frac{\text{Child's}}{\text{dose}} = \frac{\text{BSA of child in m}^2}{1.73 \text{ m}^2 \text{ (BSA of average child)}} \times \frac{\text{Adult}}{\text{dose}}$$

Therefore,

$$= \frac{0.52 \text{ m}^2}{1.73 \text{ m}^2} \times 500 \ mg$$

$$= 0.3 \times 500 \text{ mg}$$

$$= 150 \text{ mg of aminophylline}$$

With practice, the nurse can become proficient in using the nomogram and will find it a useful tool for calculating dosages.

PRACTICE PROBLEMS

Solve the following problems using the nomogram in Appendix H.

32. Find the BSA for the following children.
    a. 9 pounds, 23 inches BSA = _____ m²
    b. 3.2 kg, 50 cm BSA = _____ m²
    c. 15 kg, 40 inches BSA = _____ m²
33. The adult dose of methyldopa (Aldomet) is 250 mg. What is the dose for the child in problem 32-c?
34. If the adult dose of furosemide (Lasix) is 40 mg, what is the dose for a child whose BSA is 0.53 m²?
35. An adult dose of theophylline is 400 mg. What is the dose for a child who weighs 25 kg and who has a height of 105 cm?
36. If the adult dose of diazepam (Valium) is 10 mg, what is the dose for an 18-pound child with a height of 27 inches?

Calculations Involving Intravenous Administration

Pharmacists are often required to determine the flow rates for intravenous infusions, to calculate the volume of fluids administered over a period of time, and to control the total volume of fluids administered to the patient during a stated period of time. The calculations necessary to perform these tasks can all be accomplished by the use of ratio and proportion.

Chapter 20 provided information on the techniques involved in I.V. administration, the equipment used, and the documentation to be prepared by the nurse administering I.V. solutions. The calculations required for I.V. administration are detailed in the following sections.

Calculating the Rate of I.V. Administration

When the physician orders intravenous solutions to run for a stated number of hours, the pharmacist may have to compute the number of drops per minute to comply with the order.

To calculate the flow rate using the ratio and proportion method, three steps are required. One must determine

1. the number of milliliters the patient will receive per hour;
2. the number of milliliters the patient will receive per minute; and
3. the number of drops per minute that will equal the number of milliliters computed in step 2. The drop rate specified for the I.V. set being used must be considered in this step. The drop rate is expressed as a ratio of drops per mL (gtt/mL).

EXAMPLE 18

The physician orders 3000 mL of dextrose 5% in water (D5W) I.V. over a 24-hour period. If the I.V. set is calibrated to deliver 15 drops per milliliter, how many drops must be administered per minute?

SOLUTION

1. Calculate mL/hr.

$$\frac{3000 \text{ mL}}{24 \text{ hr}} = \frac{x \text{ mL}}{1 \text{ hr}}$$

$$x = 125 \text{ mL/hr or}$$
$$= 125 \text{ mL/60 min}$$

2. Calculate mL/min.

$$\frac{125 \text{ mL}}{60 \text{ min}} = \frac{x \text{ mL}}{1 \text{ min}}$$

$$x = 2 \text{ mL/min}$$

3. Calculate gtt/min using the drop rate per minute of the I.V. set.
   I.V. set drop rate = 15 drops/mL

$$\frac{15 \text{ gtt}}{1 \text{ mL}} = \frac{x \text{ gtt}}{2 \text{ mL (amt needed /min)}}$$

$$x = 30 \text{ gtt/min}$$

EXAMPLE 19

The physician orders 1.5 L of lactated Ringer's solution to be administered over a 12-hour period. The I.V. set is calibrated to deliver 10 gtt/mL. How many drops per minute should the patient receive?

SOLUTION

1. Determine the number of milliliters to be administered in 1 hour. Since the answer requested is in milliliter units, first convert liter quantity to milliliters.

$$1.5 \text{ L} = 1500 \text{ mL}$$

$$\frac{1500 \text{ mL}}{12 \text{ hr}} = \frac{x \text{ mL}}{1 \text{ hr}}$$

$$x = 125 \text{ mL/hr or}$$
$$= 125 \text{ mL/60 min}$$

2. Calculate the number of milliliters per minute.

$$\frac{125mL}{60\ min} = \frac{x\ mL}{1\ min}$$

$$x = 2\ mL/min\ (approx.)$$

3. Calculate the number of drops per minute.

I.V. set drop rate = 10 gtt/mL

$$\frac{10\ gtt}{1\ mL} = \frac{x\ gtt}{2\ mL}$$

$$x = 20\ gtt/min$$

The following example shows how to calculate the time required to administer an I.V. solution when the volume and flow rate are known.

EXAMPLE 20

How long will it take to complete an I.V. infusion of 1.5 L of D5W being administered at the rate of 45 drops/minute? The I.V. set is calibrated to deliver 15 drops/mL. This problem is a variation of the flow rate problem considered earlier.

SOLUTION

1. Determine the number of milliliters/minute being infused.

$$Drop\ rate\ of\ I.V.\ set = \frac{15\ gtt}{1\ mL} = \frac{45\ gtt}{x\ mL}$$

$$15x = 45$$

$$x = 3\ mL/min$$

2. Calculate the number of milliliters/hour.

$$3\ mL/min \times 60\ min/hr = 180\ mL/hr$$

3. Calculate the number of hours required to administer the total volume of the solution. If 180 mL are delivered each hour, then how many hours are required to administer 1500 mL (1.5 L)?

$$\frac{180\ mL}{1\ hr} = \frac{1500\ mL}{x\ hr}$$

$$180x = 1500$$

$$x = 8.3\ hours,\ or\ 8\ hours\ 20\ minutes$$

PRACTICE PROBLEMS

37. The physician orders 1200 mL of D5W solution to be administered over a 10-hour period. The I.V. set is calibrated to deliver 18 gtt/mL. How many drops per minute should the patient receive?

38. A patient is to receive 150 mL of an I.V. infusion over a period of 4 hours. The I.V. set is calibrated to deliver 15 gtt/mL. How many drops per minute should the patient receive? (Round off answer to nearest whole drop.)

39. An I.V. infusion containing 750 mL is to be administered at a drop rate of 40 gtt/min. The I.V. set is calibrated to deliver 20 gtt/mL. How long will it take to administer the entire infusion?

40. A nurse wishes to administer 1200 mL of an I.V. infusion at a rate of 45 gtt/min. The I.V. set is calibrated to deliver 15 gtt/mL. How long will it take to administer the entire infusion?

41. The physician orders 100 mL of a drug solution to be administered at a rate of 20 gtt/min. The I.V. set is calibrated to deliver 12 gtt/mL. How long will it take to administer the entire infusion?

Calculations Involving Piggyback I.V. Infusion

The physician may order medications to be run piggyback with the I.V. electrolyte fluids. The medications are usually dissolved in 50 or 100 mL of an I.V. solution and run for 1 hour through the open I.V. line. The flow rate for these piggyback infusions is calibrated the same way as the rate for the regular I.V. solutions.

EXAMPLE 21

An I.V. piggyback of cefazolin sodium (Ancef, Kefzol) 500 mg in 100 mL/hour is ordered. The piggyback I.V. set is calibrated to deliver 10 gtt/mL. How many drops/minute should be administered?

SOLUTION

1. The entire 100 mL is to be infused in 1 hour. Calculate the number of milliliters/minute.

$$\frac{100 \text{ mL}}{60 \text{ min}} = \frac{x \text{ mL}}{1 \text{ min}}$$
$$60x = 100$$
$$x = 1.7 \text{ mL/min}$$

2. Calculate the flow rate.

$$\text{Drop rate} = \frac{10 \text{ gtt}}{1 \text{ min}} = \frac{x \text{ gtt}}{1.7 \text{ mL}}$$
$$x = 17 \text{ gtt/min}$$

The volume of the piggyback and the time of its administration must be accounted for in calculating the daily fluid requirements of the patient. In Example 21, assume that the patient is to have a total of 2000 mL of electrolyte solution administered in 24 hours, and that cefazolin sodium 500 mg in 100 mL/hr is ordered q.i.d. The number of milliliters per day and the times of the piggyback infusion must be subtracted from the daily fluid requirement.

$$\text{cefazolin 100 mL q.i.d.} = 100 \times 4 = 400 \text{ mL}$$
$$\text{Run 1 hour} \times 4 = 4 \text{ hr}$$
$$\text{Daily requirement} = 2000 \text{ mL in 24 hours}$$
$$\text{Subtract piggyback} = -400 \text{ mL in 4 hours}$$
$$= 1600 \text{ mL in 20 hours}$$

Calculate the flow rate based on 1600 mL over a 20-hour period to administer the correct amount of fluid to the patient.

EXAMPLE 22

The medication order indicates that the patient is to have a maximum of 2000 mL of I.V. fluids in 24 hours. In addition, the patient is to receive **gentamicin** 50 mg in 100 mL

D5W over 30 minutes q8h. The I.V. set is calibrated to deliver 10 gtt/mL. How many drops/minute should the piggybacks be run and how many drops/minute should the I.V. solution D5W be administered between piggybacks to keep the vein open?

SOLUTION

1. Calculate the total volume of the piggyback solutions and the total hours they run. Order calls for 100 mL over 30 minutes q8h (q8h = 3 doses in 24 hours).

$$100 \text{ mL} \times 3 = 300 \text{ mL total}$$
$$30 \text{ min} \times 3 = 90 \text{ min or } 1.5 \text{ hr}$$

2. Subtract these totals from the daily total of I.V. fluid.

$$2000 \text{ mL} - 300 \text{ mL} = 1700 \text{ mL}$$
$$24 \text{ hr} - 1.5 \text{ hr} = 22.5 \text{ hr}$$

3. Calculate the flow rate for the D5W to be used between the three piggybacks using the adjusted totals.

$$\frac{1700 \text{ mL}}{22.5 \text{ hr}} = \frac{75 \times \text{mL/hr}}{1 \text{ hr}}$$
$$75 \text{ mL hr} \div 60 = 1.25 \text{ mL/min}$$

Using a drop rate of 10 gtt/mL, we have

$$\frac{10 \text{ gtt}}{1 \text{ mL}} = \frac{\times \text{ gtt}}{1.25 \text{ mL}}$$

$$x = 12.5 \text{ or } 12 \text{ drops/min}$$

4. The piggyback calculation is as follows:

$$100 \text{ mL} = 30 \text{ min}$$
$$100 \text{ mL} \div 30 = 3.3 \text{ mL/min}$$
$$\text{Drop set calibration} = 10 \text{ gtt/mL}$$
$$\frac{10 \text{ gtt}}{1 \text{ mL}} = \frac{\times \text{ gtt}}{3.3 \text{ mL}}$$
$$x = 33 \text{ drops/minute}$$

Will deliver 100 mL of gentamicin solution in 30 minutes.

PRACTICE PROBLEMS

42. An I.V. piggyback of lincomycin containing 1 g of drug in 100 mL is to be infused over 1 hour. The I.V. set is calibrated to deliver 15 gtt/mL. How many drops/minute should be administered?

43. An I.V. piggyback of pentamidine isethionate (Pentam-300) containing 300 mg of drug in 150 mL of D5W is to be infused over 1 hour. The I.V. set is calibrated to deliver 20 gtt/mL. How many drops/minute should be administered?

44. An I.V. piggyback of enalapril maleate (Vasotec I.V.) containing 10 mg of drug in 50 mL of 0.9% sodium chloride injection is to be infused over 30 minutes. The I.V. set is calibrated to deliver 15 gtt/mL. How many drops/minute should be administered?

Calculations Related to Solutions

Solutions are formed in two ways: (1) by dissolving a solid called the *solute* in a liquid called the *solvent,* or (2) by mixing two liquids together to form a solution. An example of the first way is adding salt to water to make a normal saline solution. Mixing Zephiran Chloride solution with water to make an antiseptic wash is an example of the second way.

Percentage Solutions

Many solutions are available in or are prepared to a specified percentage strength. To produce a solution of the desired strength, it is necessary to calculate the exact amount of drug to be added to a specific volume of liquid. Although most solutions are prepared by the pharmacist if they are not commercially available, the nurse must understand the concept of percentage to interpret medication labels.

Percentage is defined as the number of parts per hundred and is expressed as follows:

$$\frac{\text{No. of parts} \times 100}{100 \text{ parts}} = \text{Percentage (\%)}$$

To calculate the percentage of active ingredient in a solution, the amount of active ingredient in grams is divided by the total volume of the solution. To convert the result to a percentage, it is multiplied by 100.

Problems in percentage solutions generally are concerned with three types of percentages: weight to volume, weight to weight, and volume to volume. Weight to volume percentage (W/V%) is defined as the number of grams of solute in 100 mL of solution. Typical W/V% examples include the following:

■ 1 L of D5W, which contains 5 g of dextrose in each 100 mL of solution
■ a 1/4% solution of pilocarpine HCl, which contains 1/4 g (0.25 g) of pilocarpine HCl in each 100 mL of solution

EXAMPLE 23

What is the weight to volume percentage (W/V%) of sodium chloride (solid solute) in normal saline solution if 9 g of the salt are dissolved in 1000 mL of water?

SOLUTION

$$\frac{\text{Amount of salt in grams: 9 g}}{\text{Total volume of solution: 1000 mL}} \times 100 + 0.9\%$$

Weight to weight percentage (W/W%) is defined as the number of grams of solute in 100 g of a solid preparation. *Note:* Some W/W% solutions are used primarily in laboratory work. Concentrated hydrochloric and sulfuric acids are two examples of weight to weight percentage solutions. Typical W/W% examples include the following:

■ a 10% ointment of zinc oxide, which contains 10 g of zinc oxide in each 100 g of ointment
■ hydrocortisone cream 1/2%, which has 1/2 g (0.5 g) of hydrocortisone in each 100 g of cream

The third form of percentage is volume to volume (V/V%), which is defined as the number of milliliters of solute in each 100 mL of solution. Examples of this form include the following:

- rubbing alcohol 70%, which contains 70 mL of absolute alcohol in each 100 mL of the solution
- a 2% solution of phenol, which contains 2 mL of liquified phenol in each 100 mL of solution

When the type of percentage is not stated, assume that for solutions of a solid in a liquid the percentage is W/V; for solutions of a liquid in a liquid the percentage is V/V; and for mixtures of two solids the percentage is W/W.

Prevention of Medication Errors

Medication errors fall into several categories, such as omitting the dose, administering the wrong dose, administering an extra dose, administering an unordered drug, administering by the wrong route, and administering at the wrong time. Here we will consider the errors that occur when the drug order is misinterpreted. Very often, the way the amounts are expressed in the original order for weights, volumes, and units can cause interpretational errors.

For instance, writing .5 instead of 0.5 can result in a tenfold error if the decimal point is missed. In general, the following rules should be followed in transcribing orders.

- Never leave a decimal point naked. Always place a zero before a decimal expression less than one. Example: 0.2, 0.5.
- Never place a decimal point and zero after a whole number, as the decimal may not be seen and result in a tenfold overdose. Example: 2.0 mg read as 20 mg by mistake. The correct way is to write 2 mg.
- Avoid using decimals when whole numbers can be used as alternatives. Example: 0.5 g should be expressed as 500 mg and 0.4 mg should be expressed as 400 mcg.
- When possible use the metric system rather than grains, drams, or minims.
- Always spell out the word *units*. The abbreviation "U" for unit can be mistaken for a zero. Example: 10 U interpreted as 100 units. The better way is to write out 10 units.

SUGGESTED ACTIVITIES

- Visit a pharmacy, ask to see the prescription balance and examine the apothecary and metric weights. Compare the 1 g weight with the 1 gr weight. Check the size of the 10 mg, 50 mg, and 500 mg weights.
- Examine a number of medication orders from past weeks. See how many orders violated the principles listed in the section on prevention of medication errors.
- Examine the labels of some foodstuffs for sodium content (usually listed in milligrams). Calculate the percentage of sodium in the products.
- Using the manufacturer's suggested dosage information found in the package insert for a drug, calculate the dose for several patients who have been taking the drug. Compare the prescribed dose with the calculated dose.

- Prepare a chart of flow rates for the most commonly ordered I.V. volumes and times of administration. Use the calibrated flow rate of your institution's I.V. sets.
- Using the information on the label, compare the alcohol content of various cough syrups by calculating the number of milliliters of alcohol present in 5 mL of each preparation.

ANSWERS TO PRACTICE PROBLEMS

1.	15 mcg	13.	15 dL	25.	2.25 mL	35.	190 mg (BSA = 0.82)
2.	15 mg	14.	0.02 g	26.	7 mL	36.	2.14 mg (BSA = 0.37)
3.	12 mL	15.	700 mcg	27.	1364 mg	37.	36 drops/minute
4.	0.46 mL	16.	96 fluid ounces	28.	1193 mg	38.	9 drops/minute
5.	75 mg	17.	255 gr	29.	142 mg	39.	6.25 hr (375 min)
6.	2.0 g	18.	6.5 gal	30.	47 mg	40.	6.67 hr (400 min)
7.	50,000 mg	19.	0.42 fluid ounces	31.	1386 mg	41.	1 hr (60 min)
8.	2000 mL	20.	4.33 g	32. a.	0.25 m^2	42.	25 drops/minute
9	0.23 mg	21.	24 pints	b.	0.198 m^2	43.	50 drops/minute
10.	0.25 g	22.	1.25 mL	c.	0.65 m^2	44.	25 drops/minute
11.	2,500 g	23.	7.5 mL	33.	94 mg		
12.	500 mL	24.	0.3 mL	34.	12.25 mg		

Summary

Accuracy in pharmaceutical calculations is one of the most critical and most important functions in the profession of pharmacy. Every dosage calculation should always be doublechecked by a pharmacist. Pharmacists frequently doublecheck each other in this important matter. Life and death can hinge on a proper or improper dose being administered. Emergency situations or other life-threatening situations are never an excuse for undue haste and lack of sufficient doublechecks. Care and vigilance are required whenever drug doses or formulations are calculated.

Bibliography

Carr, D. S. (1989). New strategies for avoiding medication errors. *Nursing 89, 19* (8), 39–45.

Daniels, J. M., & Smith, L. M. (1990). Clinical calculations. *Nursing 90, 20* (7), 78–79.

Davis, N. M., & Cohen, M. R. (1981). *Medication errors.* Philadelphia: G. F. Stockley.

Deglin, J., & Mull, V. L. (1989). Dosage calculations. *Nursing 89, 19* (9), 100–102.

Hyams, P. A. (1990). Hospital drug quiz. *Nursing 90, 20* (1), 77.

McCaffery, M., & Beebe, A. (1989). Giving narcotics for pain: The secrets to giving equianalgesic doses. *Nursing 89, 19* (10), 161–165.

Morris, L. L. (1989). Dosage calculation charts. *Critical Care Nurse, 9* (5), 92–94.

Richardson, L. I., & Knight Richardson, J. (1985). *The mathematics of drugs and solutions with clinical applications* (3rd ed.). New York: McGraw-Hill.

Stoklosa, M. J., & Ansel, H. C. (1991). *Pharmaceutical calculations* (9th ed.). Philadelphia: Lea and Febiger.

Wolf, Z. R. (1989). Medication errors and nursing responsibility. *Holistic Nursing Practice, 4* (1), 8–17.

Extemporaneous Compounding

COMPETENCIES

Upon completion and review of this chapter, the student should be able to

1. Define a Class A prescription balance, a counter balance, and a solution balance.
2. Describe what is meant by extemporaneous compounding.
3. Explain the circumstances that may require the extemporaneous compounding of a drug dosage form.
4. Outline the steps required to accurately weigh a pharmaceutical ingredient.
5. Describe the meaning of the term "geometric dilution."
6. Explain the difference between a solution and a suspension; an ointment and a cream.
7. Describe the process of levigation.
8. List the steps involved in the process of compounding suppositories.
9. Give an example of the ingredients found in an enteral solution.
10. List the essential equipment used in the compounding process.

Introduction

This chapter will familiarize the student with terminology, equipment, and principles of **extemporaneous compounding** and their role in providing this service. The student should understand this to be an introduction to compounding; experience is needed to develop this valuable skill. While it is beyond the scope of this chapter to review all types of compounding, the most common and relevant practices are reviewed. The student is referred to compounding textbooks for more detailed knowledge.

Extemporaneous compounding is a true pharmaceutical service, not simply the redistribution of a commercially available commodity. This service requires a specialized knowledge of physical and chemical properties of drugs and their vehicles. This knowledge is based on sound scientific principles; however, the practice is closer to an art.

Extemporaneous compounding may be defined as the timely preparation of a drug product according to a physician's prescription, a drug formula, or a recipe in which the amounts of the ingredients are calculated to meet the needs of a particular patient or group of patients.

The need for extemporaneous compounding has decreased due to the availability of standardized commercial drug products. There are fewer situations in which physicians prescribe their own personal remedies. Sometimes a product that was originally extemporaneously compounded is replaced by a commercially available product. For example, Brompton's Cocktail (a potent oral analgesic) has been replaced by the commercially available morphine sulfate oral solution. Other prescription ingredients used in the past to prepare the so-called "elegant preparation," such as strychnine and bromides, are now considered either potentially toxic or only marginally effective.

Although demand is less, the need for extemporaneous preparations continues. When dispensing pediatric medications, it may be necessary to dilute standard adult strengths of drugs to obtain measurable doses. There may be a need to convert oral solid and even injectable dose forms to oral solutions or suspensions that can be tolerated by children. Because doses in children are often based on body surface area or weight, standard doses and standard dosage forms may not be appropriate. These orphanlike dosage requirements are often extemporaneously prepared.

The combination of topical products for use in dermatology remains a steady need. The use of a certain antibiotic with a specific anti-inflammatory agent is often desired, although the combination may not be marketed. The fortification or dilution of commercially available topical products is often required.

Many commercially prepared pharmaceuticals contain dyes, preservatives, or flavoring agents to which a patient may be allergic. In such a situation it may be necessary for a nonallergenic preparation to be extemporaneously compounded in the pharmacy.

In practice a pharmacist may find the stock of a particular dose form or strength depleted with no alternative source readily available. For the resourceful pharmacist, the compounding of the desired product is an available alternative as long as the raw materials are available. Alternately a pharmacist may elect to limit the number of permutations of similar products and to manufacture the products that have only occasional use. An example may be the addition of codeine phosphate powder to a readily available nonnarcotic expectorant syrup.

The recent development of pharmacokinetic parameters to obtain optimum dosage schedules will require an increase in individualized drug dosage formulations that will depend upon available expertise in extemporaneous compounding.

Equipment

The tools of pharmaceutical practice are those used to measure, transfer, transform, and handle medications in any way desired. Those involved in nonsterile compounding are classic and every pharmacy technician should be familiar with their proper handling.

Every pharmacy is required to have a **Class A prescription balance (Figure 19–1).** Class A balances have a sensitivity requirement of 6 mg. A scale sensitivity is the smallest weight required to move the indicator at least one degree. A typical Class A torsion balance can weigh quantities up to 120 g.

A **solution balance** is a single pan instrument with an unequal arm that acts as a compound lever. These balances are less accurate than Class A balances but are useful for measuring large masses with a weighing capacity of about 20 kg.

Counter balances (Figure 19–2) are double-pan balances also capable of weighing large quantities, but again are not intended for small weights having a sensitivity of 100 mg and a limit of about 5 kg.

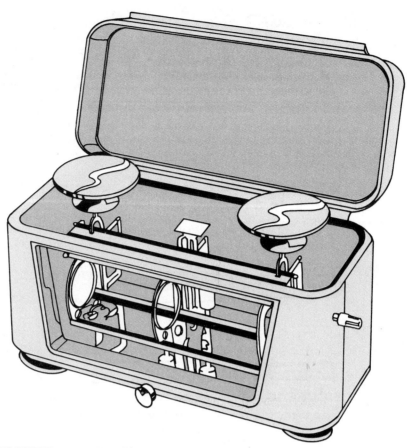

FIGURE 19–1 The Class A prescription balance, required in every pharmacy, has a scale sensitivity of 6 mg to 120 g.

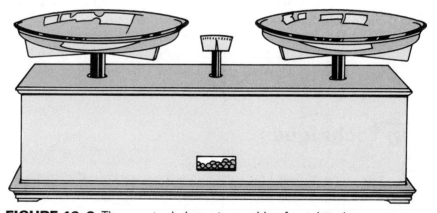

FIGURE 19–2 The counter balance is capable of weighing large quantities.

Weights used should be of good quality and stored well. These are preferred in corrosion-resistant metals such as brass (**Figure 19–3**). Metric weight sets commonly are available in a range of from less than 1 g to 50 g. Always use forceps to transfer the weights and take care not to drop them. Keep the weights covered in their original case when not in use.

Spatulas (**Figure 19–4**) are used to transfer solid ingredients to weighing pans. They are the preferred mixing instruments with semisolid dosage forms, such as ointments and creams. These are available in stainless steel and hard rubber or

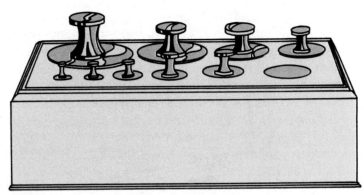

FIGURE 19–3 Pharmaceutical weights should be corrosion resistant and handled with forceps.

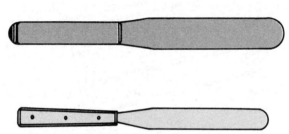

FIGURE 19–4 Spatulas, available in stainless steel and hard rubber or plastic, are used to transfer solid ingredients to weighing pans.

plastic. Care must be used with materials that corrode metals such as iodine, salts of mercury, or tannins. Use rubber spatulas for these agents. Check that spatulas are clean and have indented edges.

Weighing papers, preferably nonabsorbable paraffined glassine paper, should always be used to weigh powders and other solid and semisolid pharmaceuticals to prevent contamination or damage to the weighing pans. For small amounts of powders the paper should be creased diagonally from each corner and then flattened and placed on the pans. This ensures a collection trough in the paper. Discard the paper after each product to prevent contamination.

Weighing Techniques

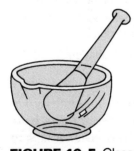

FIGURE 19–5 Glass mortar and pestle is preferable for mixing liquids and semisoft dosage forms.

The critical first step in any pharmaceutical dispensing is the selection of the proper drug and dose. Qualitative and quantitative accuracy is the hallmark of our profession. Technicians given the responsibilities of compounding must learn the skills and work carefully under the supervision of a pharmacist.

Prior to weighing with a Class A balance, the technician should gather and organize all materials in a level, well-lighted, draft-free area. The balance should be leveled by adjusting the thumbscrew at the base of the legs until the pointer rests at zero. Place weighing papers on each pan and adjust balance again if necessary. The beam weight should be all the way to the left and set at zero. When equilibrium is reached, the balance is arrested in place by a lock screw. The desired weights are placed in the right pan using forceps. The desired material is placed on the left pan using a spatula. When weighing less than a gram, one may wish to shift the weight beam to the appropriate weight. The balance is carefully unlocked to observe the

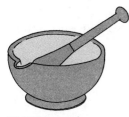

FIGURE 19–6

Porcelain mortar and pestle is used for trituration of crystals and large particles.

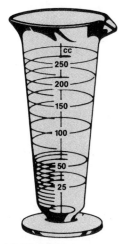

FIGURE 19–7

Conical graduates have a wide mouth and a wide base.

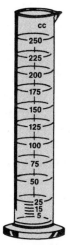

FIGURE 19–8

Cylindrical graduates provide greater accuracy for measuring.

movement of the pointer, which will shift to the side with the greater weight. Relock the balance and use a spatula to subtract or add material being weighed. This process is repeated until equilibrium is reached and the indicator is at the zero point. The balance is then locked, the lid closed, and the lock released one final time to verify the equilibrium. The weight should be checked by a pharmacist. If it is correct, the material can be removed from the balance in the cradle of the folded weighing paper. Weights should be checked three times: when selected, when resting on the pan, and when returned to the kit.

When weighing, we must keep in mind the sensitivities and limitations of the balance used.

Essential equipment that technicians must be familiar with include the mortar and pestle, commonly available in three types: glass (**Figure 19–5**); wedgewood; and porcelain (**Figure 19–6**), which is quite similar to wedgewood in use and appearance. Wedgewood and porcelain mortars are relatively coarse and are used to grind (**triturate**) crystals and large particles into fine powders. Both are earthenware and are somewhat porous and will easily stain. Glass mortars are preferable for mixing liquids and semisoft dosage forms.

When mixing ingredients always place the most potent drug, which is usually the smallest amount, into the mortar first. Then add an equal amount of the next most potent ingredient and mix thoroughly. This process is repeated until all ingredients are added. Because each addition is approximately equal to the amount in the mortar, the process is called geometric dilution.

Ointment slabs are ground glass plates, often square or rectangular, that provide a hard nonabsorbable surface for mixing compounds. When combining creams and ointments, we use the spatula to spread the material, using a shearing force to mix ingredients. Some pharmacists use disposable, nonabsorbent parchment paper to cover the work area, which is not as durable as the ointment slabs but saves time in cleaning.

Accurately measuring liquids is an essential skill technicians must master. Equipment consists of conical **graduates** (**Figure 19–7**); cylindrical graduates (**Figure 19–8**); and syringes. Beakers are generally not accurate enough for prescription work.

Conical graduates are the easiest to use with wide mouths, and bases and are the easiest to clean. Liquids may be stirred in them with the aid of a stirring rod. As the diameter of the graduate increases, the accuracy of the measurement decreases. This design makes the narrow-diameter cylindrical graduates preferable when greater accuracy is desired. Graduates are available in sizes ranging from 10 mL to 4000 mL. When selecting a graduate, always choose the smallest graduate capable of containing the volume to be measured. Avoid measurements of volumes that are below 20 percent of the capacity of the graduate because the accuracy is unacceptable. For example a 100 mL graduate cannot accurately measure volumes below 20 mL. When measuring small volumes, such as 30 mL and less, it is often preferable to use a syringe. Disposable plastic injectable and oral syringes are readily available in all pharmacies and have essentially replaced the use of smaller-sized graduates.

When measuring liquids in a graduate, it is important that the reading be done at eye level. The surface of the liquid has a concave or crescent shape that bulges downward, called the **meniscus.** When measuring liquids, the correct reading is the mark at the bottom of the meniscus.

Most graduates are marked "TD" (to deliver). They are calibrated to compensate for the excess of fluid that adheres to the surface after emptying the graduate. Caution must be used to differentiate this from older glassware marked "TC" (to contain), or errors in accuracy will result. Keep in mind that even "TD" glassware will retain excessive amounts of viscous liquids if not drained completely. Essentially no liquid should remain in the graduate after emptying.

Compounding Principles

Liquids

Liquids are probably the most common form of compounded medications. Extemporaneous nonsterile compounds most often involve solutions and suspensions, whereas emulsions and lotions are less popular. Solutions are clear liquids in which the drug is completely dissolved. The simplest compound solution involves the addition of a drug in liquid form to a vehicle such as water or syrup. This involves careful liquid measurement of the drug, using graduates or syringes, and then dilution to the final volume desired. Gentle shaking effects thorough dispersion of additives.

Solids

When solids are required in solution, they must be carefully weighed, using a prescription balance. Most solids dissolve readily in the solvent but others require intervention. Some solids may be reduced in size by grinding in a mortar to increase dissolution rates. Other times the vehicle is heated to enhance dissolution, but care must be used as some drugs decompose at higher temperatures. Dissolution of solute may require vigorous shaking or stirring.

Suspensions

Suspensions are liquid preparations of drugs containing finely divided drug particles distributed uniformly throughout the vehicle. Suspensions appear cloudy in nature and shaking is often required to resuspend drug particles that have settled. Depending on particle size, some suspensions settle so rapidly that a uniform dispersion cannot be maintained long enough for an accurate dose to be withdrawn. Such preparations require a **suspending agent,** a thickening agent that gives some structure to a suspension. Typical agents are carboxymethylcellulose, methylcellulose, bentonite, tragacanth, and others. Some suspending agents may bind the drug, limiting availability, so these agents should not be used indiscriminately. While some solid drugs may be added directly to a suspending vehicle, some agents need to be "wetted" first. That is, the powder to be added is first mixed with a wetting agent such as alcohol or glycerin in a mortar with pestle. This displaces the air from the particles of the solid and allows them to mix more readily with a suspending vehicle. Next the vehicle is added in portions and mixed with mortar and pestle until a uniform mixture results. This mixture is then blended into the remaining vehicle. The mortar and pestle can be rinsed with small portions of the vehicle and added until the final volume is reached. Suspensions should be dispensed in tight, light-resistant containers that contain enough air space for adequate shaking. The bottle should contain the auxiliary label "Shake well." Refrigeration may be used to slow separation.

Ointments and Creams

These two semisolid external dosage forms are still popular choices for extemporaneous compounds and share common preparation techniques. Ointments are oil based in nature, whereas creams are water based. Given the commercial availability of unmedicated cream and ointment bases, their preparation is more of historic interest, but we will focus on the addition of drugs to these bases. In the simplest cases physicians often desire the combined effects of two or more ointments or creams in a specified proportion. This usually involves the thorough mechanical mixing of the weighed bases on an ointment slab, using a spatula until a uniform preparation has been obtained. Using the spatula, transfer the material into an ointment jar just big enough for the final volume. When filling the ointment jar, use the spatula to bleed out air pockets. Tapping the jar on the countertop will settle the contents. Wipe any excess material from the outside of the jar, including the cap screw threads. Cover the jar and label appropriately.

Drugs in powder or crystal form—such as salicylic acid, precipitated sulfur, or hydrocortisone—are often prescribed to be mixed into cream or ointment bases. Large particles should be reduced to fine powder with a mortar and pestle. The ointment base may be placed on one side of the working area, with the powders to be incorporated on the other. Using a spatula, mix a small portion of powder with a portion of the base on an ointment slab. Repeat this until all powder is incorporated into the base and a uniform product is produced.

Occasionally the direct mixture method results in a gritty product with poorly dispensed clumps of powder that fail to blend in despite vigorous mixing. Here it is desirable first to reduce the particle size of the powder by levigating it. **Levigation** is the mixing of powder with a vehicle in which it is insoluble to produce a smooth dispersion of the drug. The dispersion is then mixed with the base. When using ointments, mineral oil is a good levigating agent. When working with creams, glycerin or water can often be used.

Suppositories

Suppositories are solid dosage forms intended for insertion into body orifices, predominantly rectal or vaginal, where they melt or dissolve to release their active ingredients. Extemporaneous manufacture of suppositories remains a vital art today for several reasons. Industrial manufacturers market relatively few products in suppository form in this country, in part because rectal administration is not socially popular. So although the products are limited, there is a subgroup of patients who cannot tolerate oral medications but who also are not candidates for parenteral drug therapy.

Suppositories must be manufactured so that they remain solid at room or refrigerated temperatures, yet melt readily at body temperature—a fine line indeed. This process is accomplished by using special bases, such as cocoa butter or polyethylene glycol. Polyethylene glycols are available in various molecular weight ranges. Those of 200, 400, or 600 are liquids; those over 1000 are solid and waxlike. Often combinations of liquid (low molecular weight) and solid polyethylene glycol are used to achieve a suppository that melts as desired. By increasing the waxy portion of the blend, we gain a suppository that melts more slowly and provides more sustained action.

To prepare suppositories, the base material is melted and the active ingredients are added. The material is poured into molds and chilled until congealed. Then they are removed from the mold.

The first step in preparing suppositories is the selection of a proper mold, commonly made of steel or aluminum and containing from 12 to 100 cavities (**Figure 19–9**). If the prescription does not follow a previously determined master formula, we then must calibrate the mold. Molds vary in capacity, and suppository bases vary in density. To calibrate the mold, melt a quantity of base material and pour it into the mold. Fill each cavity to capacity and chill to congeal. Unmold and weigh the suppositories to arrive at an average weight. Melt the suppositories in

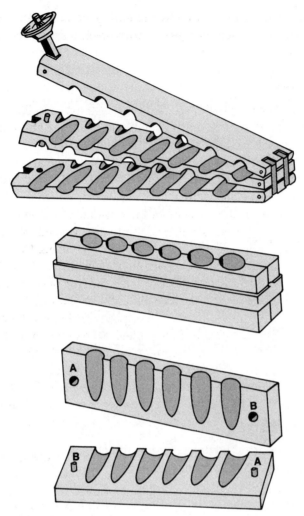

FIGURE 19–9 Suppository mold

a calibrated beaker to arrive at a volume. If the amount of medication is negligible, we need not deduct the volume. If the amount of added medication is significant, we can use the following method. Multiply the determined volume of each suppository by the number of suppositories desired. Place medications in a calibrated beaker and pour the melted base into the drugs until the desired volume is reached.

The base material is melted with the least possible heat, often over a water bath in a beaker or porcelain casserole with a lip to facilitate pouring into the mold. The drug additive is often incorporated into a portion of the melted base on an ointment slab and mixed well with a spatula. This mixture is then added to the melted base material (which has been allowed to cool almost to the point of congealing) and thoroughly stirred.

The material is then poured into a chilled mold and promptly placed in a refrigerator or freezer. Rapid congealing is desired to prevent settling of added drugs. When solid, any excess material is scraped off the top of the mold with a spatula. Unmold the suppositories and place into labeled jars. Refrigeration is required for suppositories made with cocoa butter base. Those made of polyethylene glycol may be stored at room temperature.

Suppositories (both commercial and extemporaneous sources) are still commonly used to deliver analgesics, hormones, antiemetics, laxatives, and vaginal anti-infectives.

Capsules

Extemporaneous capsule manufacturing remains a popular means of providing unusual (and often low) doses of oral medication. The student may recall that commercially available capsules cannot be divided. Tablets can only be reliably broken in quarters at best and usually only halves. A typical situation for capsule compounding may be when a drug is only available in 50 mg tablets or capsules, but the prescribing physician desires 12.5 mg doses, or what would amount to a one-quarter dose. If crushed, the resulting powder would be too small to handle accurately. To facilitate measuring, first dilute the crushed tablet (or emptied capsule) with inactive filler and measure a portion containing the desired amount. Select empty, hard gelatin capsules available in eight sizes, with 000 the largest and 5 the smallest. In general, the smallest capsule capable of containing the final volume is used because patients often have difficulty swallowing large capsules. To fill each capsule, place the powder on a tile or paper and press the body of the capsule repeatedly into the powder until it is filled. Be careful not to touch the powder with your fingers. This is called the punch method of capsule filling. Place the cap onto the body and weigh the result, using an empty capsule the same size as the **tare.** Adjust the weight, if needed, by adding or removing powder. To keep the capsule clean during the process, the compounder may wear rubber gloves or finger cots. Since some material is lost in the process, always calculate a little extra material to compensate for this loss.

In this example we select a #3 capsule and set the final weight at 200 mg. To make ten capsules, we need three 50 mg tablets, which would produce twelve doses in theory. Twelve doses of 200 mg requires 2400 mg of final powder. Three tablets might weigh 700 mg, to which we would add 1700 mg of diluent, such as lactose powder, by trituration. We would pack 200 mg of this powder into each capsule to yield the 12.5 mg dose.

Lotions

Lotions are liquid preparations intended for external application. The most common lotions are "shake" lotions in which insoluble substances are dispersed by agitation. Often gums or other agents are used as suspending agents to prevent rapid settling of suspended particles. To prepare shake lotions, place the measured powders of the formula into a mortar and triturate until well blended. Slowly add a liquid levigating agent and triturate to form a smooth paste, free of gritty particles. Add the vehicle in small portions with continued trituration. After roughly two-thirds of the vehicle has been added, transfer the solution to a graduated vessel and rinse the mortar with remaining vehicle to bring the lotion to its final volume. Transfer this to a well-sealed bottle and label "Shake well."

Enteral Preparations

Pharmacy departments may also prepare enteral nutrition products. Although enteral literally means "in the intestine," the term is commonly used to mean a refined liquid diet often administered by nasogastric tube to patients unable to eat solid foods. Preparation of enteral products usually involves simple dissolution of powdered material in a blender, following package directions. But at times there is a need for varied dilutions of feedings to match a patient's clinical state. We use pharmaceutical calculations to prepare a ⅔- or ¾-strength formula. For example, suppose a package of powdered dietary supplement is normally diluted to 500 mL. To prepare a ⅔-strength enteral formula, we divide 500 mL by ⅔ to yield 750 mL. Each packet should be dissolved to 750 mL to yield the more diluted ⅔ mixture required.

At times these oral feedings are supplemented with additional electrolytes, such as sodium chloride or potassium chloride. The student may be required to convert weight in milligrams to milliequivalents (mEq).

It is important to use clean equipment, precise measurement, and proper packaging, labeling, and storage of these products. They often require refrigeration after preparation and each product has a recommended expiration period.

As the student readily learns, there are quite a few pharmaceutical skills involved in the proper preparation and dispensing of enteral products.

Labeling of Finished Products and Record Keeping

Extemporaneous products should be labeled with neat, well-designed labels, in accordance with hospital policy. Outpatient prescription labels must contain all information required by state and local laws. Labels should be typed and affixed with adhesive tape to protect the label. Auxiliary labels should be affixed if applicable.

The label should contain the ingredients and proportions of the compounded prescription. If a master compounding form was used, the internally assigned lot number should appear on the label.

In general no specific expiration date can be assigned to an extemporaneous compound unless the institution has a policy for assigning reasonable expiration dates. Even with such a policy some judgment is needed on the part of the supervising pharmacist. It may suffice to list the date of preparation on the label.

Accurate record keeping is essential in extemporaneous compounding. Master formula records (**Figure 19–10**) are excellent sources for both directions for compounding and uniform record keeping. When using a master form, record all lot number information on the form and use the internal lot number on the prescription label. These master records also contain the amount of ingredients used, initials of the preparer and the pharmacist who checked the finished product, and all measurements. All work sheets should be filed as permanent records.

With single extemporaneous compounds without master records, such as those involving outpatient prescriptions, the lot numbers and manufacturers of the ingredients can be recorded on the prescription.

Cleaning Equipment

Cleaning the equipment is as important as the preparation and labeling of the product. It should not be overlooked. Improperly cleaned equipment can contaminate the next preparation and be dangerous to the patient. Cleaning is sometimes not as simple as washing dishes because oily residues, such as ointments, often must be dissolved. Proper cleaning may require a rinse with organic solvents such as alcohols or acetate to facilitate removal. When working with these volatile solvents, the student must be aware of their flammable nature as well as the risk of inhaling fumes. Although these fumes are generally safe for limited exposure, care must be taken to wash solvents down the drain with cold water to limit exposure. Occupational safety data sheets should be available in every pharmacy, outlining the hazards of each substance.

EXTEMPORANEOUS PREPARATION
GENTIAN VIOLET 10%

MATERIALS
- 1 glass flask 600ml
- Absolute alcohol 300ml
- Gentian Violet 30gm
- Stirring rod
- 1 oz. amber dropper bottle

LABEL
- Gentian violet solution
- 10% W/V
- In 95% absolute alcohol
- Volume: 300 ml
- Control # _____
- Tech/R.Ph. _____ Exp. date _____

Procedure
1. Clean all materials to be used and rinse with absolute alcohol.
2. Weigh out 30 gram gentian violet and have pharmacist check it.
3. Measure out 300ml absolute alcohol and have pharmacist check it.
4. In glass flask, dissolve the gentian violet in the absolute alcohol. Stir well until in solution.
5. Measure out 30ml and put in 1 oz. glass amber dropper bottle.
6. Have pharmacist check label.
7. Put label on product.
8. Have pharmacist check final product.

Date Prepared	Control #	Ingredients	Mft. & Lot #	Amt. Used	Check by R.Ph	Expiration Date of Prod. Made	Quant. Prep.	Sample Label	Tech.

FIGURE 19–10 Master formula record

Summary

Bulk compounding by pharmacy technicians should be viewed as a challenge and a rewarding skill. The student can readily appreciate the necessity of competence in other aspects of pharmacy such as calculation, dose forms, and pharmaceutical terminology. The responsibility of bulk compounding should not and will not be required of technicians who are not trained or not competent with these skills. Any bulk compounding must be done only under close supervision of a licensed pharmacist, and in some states must be done only via master manufacturing records.

Bulk compounding is a difficult art to master but it is one of the most rewarding. It remains one service no other health care profession can provide.

ASSESSMENT

Multiple Choice Questions

1. The concave surface of a liquid in a graduate is called the
   a. sight line
   b. metric point
   (c) meniscus
   d. tare

2. Clear liquids in which drugs are completely dissolved are called
   a. suspensions
   b. emulsions
   c. lotions
   (d.) solutions

3. The hazards of using organic solvents are
   a. their flammability
   b. toxic fumes
   c. their explosive nature
   (d.) a and b
   e. all of the above

4. Which product would yield the greatest volume? A packet of external nutrition supplement diluted to
   a. full strength
   b. 3/4 strength
   (c.) 2/3 strength

5. A master formula record should contain
   a. directions for compounding
   b. a record of lot numbers
   c. the initials of preparer and checking pharmacist
   d. the amount of ingredients used
   (e.) all of the above

True/False Questions

6. ___F___ Extemporaneous compounding has increased in demand in modern pharmaceutical practice.

7. ___F___ Class A prescription balances, solution balances, and counter balances are quite similar and can be used interchangeably for any weighing needs of a pharmacy.

8. ___F___ A semisolid external dosage form with an oily base is called a cream.

9. ___F___ A levigating agent would be added to a suspension to reduce the rate of settling.

10. ___F___ Suppositories are only intended for rectal use.

11. ___T___ When selecting capsules, the higher the size number, the smaller the capsule.

12. ___F___ Lotions are most commonly prepared using a mortar and pestle.

Shake solutions

Bibliography

Ansel, H.H. (1972). Introduction to pharmaceutical dosage forms. Philadelphia: Lea and Febiger.

Gennaro, A.R. (Ed.). (1990). *Remington's pharmaceutical sciences* (18th ed.). Easton, PA: Mack Publishing Co.

Lyman, R.A. (1955). *Textbook of pharmaceutical compounding and dispensing.* Philadelphia: J. B. Lippincott Co.

Parrot, E.L. (1970). *Pharmaceutical technology.* Minneapolis, MN: Burgess Publishing Co.

20 Parenteral Admixture Services

COMPETENCIES

After completion and review of this chapter, the student should be able to

1. Outline the major reasons for administering injectable drug products.
2. Define common injectable routes of administration.
3. Describe three characteristics of parenteral products.
4. Define a sterile product.
5. Explain the concept of laminar airflow.
6. Define the technician's role in parenteral admixture services.
7. Describe safety considerations related to handling parenteral products.

Introduction

Parenteral **admixture** services have become an increasingly important aspect of hospital pharmacy practice. Advances in medical technology, new drug products, and other changes in the health care environment all contribute to the need for these services. Parenteral products in the form of injectable drugs have been estimated to account for as much as 40 percent of all drugs administered in hospitals. Additionally there is an increasing use of parenterals in the home health care setting. Many hospitals and home care agencies are providing these services. The pharmacy technician is an integral part of the production of parenteral products, both in hospitals and in the home care industry. This chapter will discuss various aspects of parenteral products and the technician's role in parenteral admixture services.

Background

The term *parenteral* is associated with drugs administered by injection. The discussion of parenteral admixture services in this chapter will emphasize injectable products, but the same general principles apply to all sterile products.

The extent of parenteral admixture services varies considerably among institutions. Nevertheless, all such services share a common goal of providing accurately prepared, sterile products for use by or administration to patients.

Injectable drug products may be administered by several routes and for many reasons. Administration of a drug by injection may be necessary for patients who are unable or unwilling to take medications by mouth. Some drugs, such as insulin, cannot be given orally, because they will be destroyed in the gastrointestinal tract. Others must be given by injection for rapid and/or continued action. Many diagnostic tests involve the injection of dyes or radioactive drugs. These are only a few of the many reasons for administrating injectable drugs.

An extremely important consideration with injectables is that, regardless of the route of administration, all bypass one of the major body defense mechanisms—the skin. When intact, the skin prevents the entry of microorganisms into the circulation. For this reason the necessity of providing a sterile product and using proper techniques in administering it cannot be overemphasized. Quality assurance must be maintained from the point of manufacture, through the pharmacy parenteral admixture service, to the administration of the parenteral product.

Routes of Administration

There are a number of different routes by which injectable drugs can be administered. The route chosen will depend on the characteristics of the drug to be administered, the type of effect desired, and the intended site of action.

Some of the more common routes of administration are outlined here.

- *Intradermal (I.D.)*—injected within the skin, just below the surface, usually used for diagnostic tests and certain vaccines. The volume does not exceed 0.1 ml.
- *Subcutaneous (S.C.)*—injected deeper than I.D. administration, into the loose tissue layer beneath the skin. Volumes of up to 1 ml may be given. This route provides for a more rapid onset of action and shorter duration than intramuscular.
- *Intramuscular (I.M.)*—injected into a muscle mass, usually the deltoid (upper arm) or the gluteus (buttocks). Volumes of up to 5 ml may be given, depending on the size of the muscle mass. I.M. injections have a slower onset of action and a longer duration than S.C. injections.
- *Intravenous (I.V.)*—injected directly into a vein. Large volumes may be given by this route, which is useful for very rapid onset of action or for medications that cannot be given by other routes.
- *Intracardiac (I.C.)*—injected within one of the chambers of the heart, usually used only in emergency situations such as cardiopulmonary resuscitation.
- *Intra-arterial (I.A.)*—injected directly into an artery. This injection is a risky procedure that may result in a spasm of the artery and the stoppage of circulation in the area. This route is sometimes used for cancer chemotherapy to deliver medication directly to the desired site of action (such as the liver).
- *Intrathecal (I.T.)*—injected into the spinal fluid. Preservative-free drugs must be used, because many preservatives can damage the nervous system. Some antibiotics and chemotherapy agents are administered by this route to achieve satisfactory concentrations in the brain or cerebrospinal fluid.

Characteristics of Parenteral Products

All parenteral products must be manufactured or prepared under conditions that ensure sterility and freedom from particulate matter. The word *sterile* indicates there are no living microorganisms present. A product is either sterile or unsterile—there is no in-between. Sterility can be achieved through heat, gas, or filtration methods. The method used will depend on the physical characteristics of the product to be sterilized. The use of moist heat under pressure (autoclaving) is the most commonly used method. The use of gamma radiation to sterilize some empty I.V. containers and other accessories has also been employed. During extemporaneous preparation, the use of proper **aseptic** technique is essential to maintain the sterility of the products being used.

In addition to being sterile, injectable products must also be pyrogen free. Pyrogens are products of microbial metabolism and cause symptoms of fever and chills when injected into a patient. Proper treatment of water and equipment used during manufacturing and the use of nonpyrogenic equipment (such as syringes) are necessary to prevent introduction of pyrogens into the final product.

Parenteral products must also be free from the presence of particulate matter. Particulate matter consists of undissolved substances that are unintentionally present in parenteral solutions. Examples of such substances are glass, rubber, cloth or cotton fibers, metal, and plastic. Undissolved particles may be present in suspensions; however, the particles are active ingredients, not contaminants.

Particulate matter in injectables, especially in I.V. products, could cause inflammation of the vein (phlebitis) or could harm the patient by lodging in small blood vessels and blocking blood flow. For this reason suspensions cannot be administered by the intravenous route. The use of proper techniques and procedures during manufacturing and compounding, and careful visual observation, are essential in preventing particulate contamination.

Intravenous Products

Intravenous products comprise the majority of parenteral preparations in the pharmacy. Because such products are administered directly into the bloodstream, a number of special considerations are involved. Such concerns as drug compatibilities and rates of administration are particularly important.

Drug compatibilities are of concern with I.V. solutions. Incompatibilities often manifest themselves as a precipitation or crystallization, which could have disastrous consequences if either entered the patient's circulation. Not all incompatibilities are visible, however. A drug may be deactivated or lose a significant amount of its potency without being apparent on visual examination. Incompatibilities may occur between two or more drugs or additives or between a drug and the solution in which it is mixed.

The stability of drugs in solution is also an important consideration. As drugs prepared in a parenteral admixture service are usually made in advance of when they are to be administered, the stability must be known and checked. Such information is usually available from several sources, including the package insert. One factor that often affects stability is the concentration of the drug in solution. As a general rule, the more concentrated the solution, the less stable it is.

The pharmacist, using reference sources available, will determine the compatibilities and stabilities of parenteral admixtures. Drugs should never be mixed without knowing and checking this information.

Osmolality is a characteristic that results from the number of dissolved particles in the solution. Blood has an osmolality of approximately 300 milliosmoles (mOsm). Intravenous solutions that have osmolality values of 300 are said to be isotonic. Solutions that have osmolality values of greater (hypertonic) or less than (hypotonic) 300 may cause damage to red blood cells, pain, and tissue irritation. The greater the deviation from 300 mOsm, the more pronounced these reactions will be. At times it may be necessary to administer hypertonic or hypotonic solutions—usually slowly and/or through large, free-flowing veins to minimize the reactions.

Another important characteristic is the pH of the solution. The pH is a measure of the acidity or alkalinity of a product. On the pH scale, which ranges from 1 to 14, a number less than 7 means the product is acidic. A number greater than 7 indicates alkalinity. The farther the number is from 7, the more acidic or alkaline the product is. The pH is important, both from the physiological effects on the patient and for additive compatibilities. Some drugs will be incompatibile in a particular solution due to the effects of pH.

Types of I.V. Solutions

Intravenous solutions are classified as small volume parenterals (SVPs), or large volume parenterals (LVPs). A large volume parenteral is a solution of 100 ml or more. LVPs are primarily used to provide fluid, electrolytes, and/or nutrients to the patient. Small volume parenterals, on the other hand, are usually 100 ml or less and are primarily used as vehicles for delivering medications. I.V. containers are available in plastic or glass (**Figure 20–1**).

Solutions flow from the containers to the patient by means of an I.V. administration set (**Figure 20–2**). For solution to flow from a glass container, air must be able to enter the container as fluid flows out. Air enters through a vent located in the administration set. Flexible plastic containers do not require venting, as the container collapses as fluid flows out of it.

Plastic containers offer many advantages over glass, such as being lightweight and unbreakable. Plastic containers made of polyvinyl chloride (PVC) may sometimes interact with medications. Certain medications have a tendency to adsorb or "stick to" PVC, making less drug available to the patient (e.g., nitroglycerin). In addition, the plasticizer (DEHP) may leach into some products (e.g., fat emulsion). The consequences of such **leaching** to the patient are not clear. Polyolefin and non-DEHP vinyl I.V. containers are available that provide the benefits of flexible plastic without the drawbacks of PVC. There is no plasticizer to leach into solution and less possibility of drug adsorption with these products.

The administration of I.V. medications may be accomplished in one of three ways: I.V. push, infusion, or **piggyback.**

I.V. push involves the injection of a relatively small volume of drug by means of a needle and syringe. This type of injection, sometimes referred to as a bolus, may be administered directly into a vein or into the tubing of a running I.V. solution. This technique is usually used when a very rapid effect is desired.

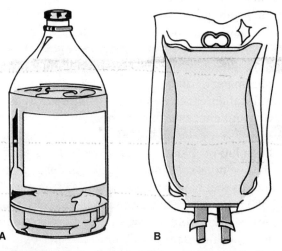

FIGURE 20–1 Types of I.V. containers (A) glass, (B) flexible plastic bag

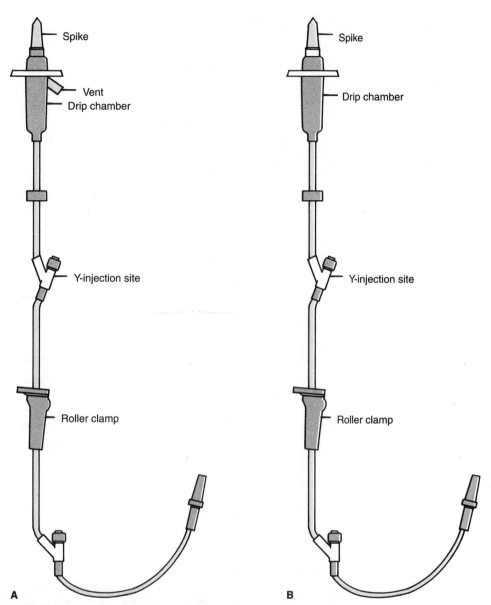

FIGURE 20-2 I.V. administration sets (A) vented, (B) nonvented

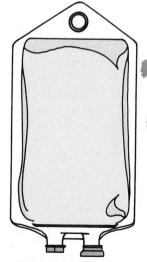

FIGURE 20-3
Plastic piggyback bag

The I.V. administration of a large amount of fluid over a prolonged time period is known as an infusion. Infusions may be used to supply the patient with fluid, nutrients, and medications.

With the piggyback method, medications in small amounts of fluid (usually 50 to 100 ml) are infused into the tubing of a running I.V. solution (primary I.V.). The piggyback solution is contained in a minibag or bottle (see **Figure 20-3**), and is typically infused over a period of 30 to 60 minutes.

Another method of delivering I.V. piggyback medications involves the use of syringes instead of piggyback containers. A syringe containing medication is mounted on a syringe pump, which expels the contents of the syringe over a specific time period.

In some instances a patient may not have a primary I.V. solution, yet must receive piggyback medications. Patients may then receive a heparin lock, which is a short tubing inserted into a vein. When a piggyback is not infusing through it, the heparin lock is filled with a heparin solution or sodium chloride solution so that blood does not clot and block the tube.

Preparation of Parenteral Products

Laminar Airflow Hoods

The preparation of parenteral products requires strict adherence to aseptic technique. Aseptic technique involves the preparation and handling of sterile products in a way that prevents contamination by microorganisms. Contamination can occur from the environment in which the product is prepared, as well as from the person preparing it. The best way to reduce the environmental effects is to control the work area in such a way as to produce a *clean* work area. Laminar airflow hoods, when properly operated, are very effective at providing a clean area; however, using poor technique can easily cancel the benefits of laminar airflow.

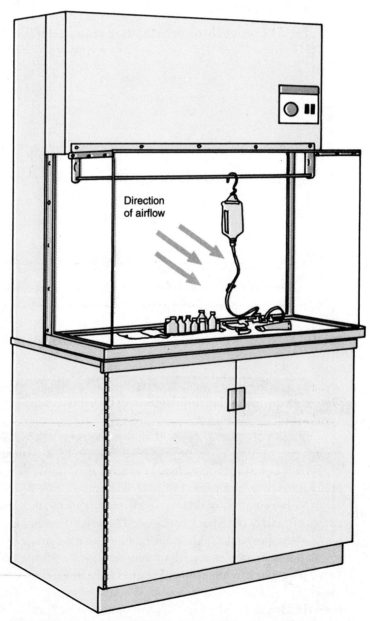

Direction
of airflow

FIGURE 20–4   Horizontal laminar airflow hood

Laminar airflow hoods provide filtered air that flows through the hood in straight, parallel lines. The air is filtered through a **high-efficiency particulate air (HEPA) filter** that removes 99.97 percent of all particles larger than 0.3 μm in size. Essentially this filter is able to remove all microbial contaminants and particulate matter. The air flows at a sufficient velocity to keep a work area free from contamination. The airflow may be in either a vertical or a horizontal direction. In a horizontal hood the HEPA filter is located at the back of the hood, and air flows to the front (as shown in **Figure 20–4**). In a vertical hood, airflow passes through a HEPA filter located at the top, and is drawn out the bottom through grates (**Figure 20–5**). Unlike the horizontal hood, the vertical hood allows protection for the operator, as the airflow is contained within the hood (**Figure 20–6**).

The type of vertical flow hood most commonly used in the pharmacy is the class II hood, divided into the following types:

Type A hoods recirculate a portion of the air (after first passing through a HEPA filter) within the hood and exhaust a portion of this air back into the parenteral's room.

Type B1 hoods exhaust *most* of the contaminated air through a duct to the outside atmosphere. This air first passes through a HEPA filter.

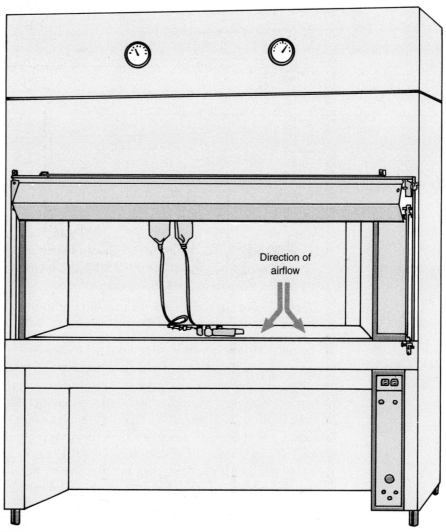

Direction of airflow

FIGURE 20–5 Vertical laminar airflow hood

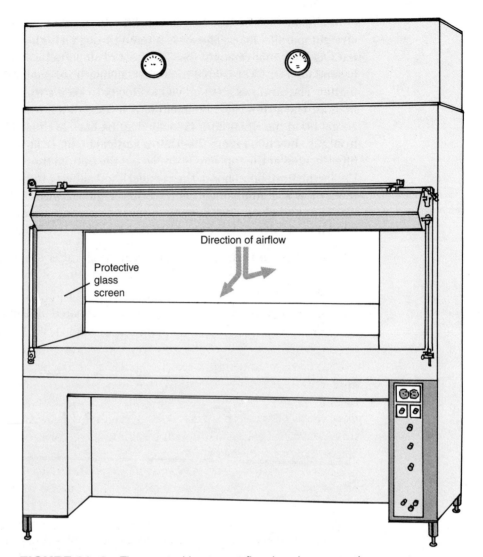

FIGURE 20–6   This vertical laminar airflow hood protects the operators

Type B2 hoods exhaust *all* of the contaminated air to the outside atmosphere after passing through a HEPA filter. Air is not recirculated within the hood or returned to the parenterals room atmosphere.

Type B3 hoods utilize recycled air within the hood. All exhaust air is discharged to the outside atmosphere. Type A hoods may be converted to type B3 hoods.

Laminar airflow hoods of all types need to be properly cleaned and maintained to ensure their ability to provide a clean work area. Hoods are usually cleaned several times during the course of a day. Appropriate antimicrobial solutions such as 70 percent isopropyl alcohol or solutions of povidone iodine are frequently used for disinfection. Care should be taken when cleaning class II hoods with alcohol. Excessive use of alcohol in hoods where the air is recirculated (type A, B1, and B3) may result in a buildup of alcohol vapors in the hood.

Many pharmacies will run their laminar airflow hoods continuously. If the hood has been turned off, it must be allowed to run for 30 minutes before preparing I.V. admixtures. The inside of the hood must be thoroughly cleaned with alcohol or another disinfectant. Cleaning is performed using long, side-to-side motions, starting at the back of the hood and working forward. Cleaning should be done before and after preparing a series of admixtures and if there is a spill in the hood.

Class II hoods that are used in the preparation of hazardous drugs (e.g., cytotoxic drugs) should be decontaminated regularly by using a high pH stainless steel cleaner. The use of aerosol cleaners, although convenient, should be avoided to prevent damage to the HEPA filter and accumulation of aerosol propellants in the hood.

All laminar airflow hoods must be certified on a regular basis to ensure their proper functioning. Inspection occurs annually for horizontal hoods and every 6 months for class II hoods.

Good aseptic technique is essential to maximize the benefits of a laminar airflow hood. It is important to remember, however, that laminar airflow can be easily disrupted. Such disruptions increase the risk of contamination. Sneezing, coughing, and even talking directly into a laminar airflow hood can disrupt the airflow sufficiently to contaminate the work area. Breezes from an open door or window, or sudden, rapid hand movements within the hood, also can disrupt the airflow.

When preparing parenteral products, several steps are critical to follow. First and foremost is proper handwashing with a suitable antimicrobial cleanser, such as chlorhexidine gluconate or povidone-iodine. Careful attention to scrubbing hands and arms up to the elbow is vital. Jewelry should not be worn on the hands and arms. Hands must be rewashed when returning from outside the parenterals area or if there is any possibility that they have been contaminated. Some institutions require gowning and the use of gloves. Unfortunately, gloves may give a false sense of security. It is important to remember that gloves are not a substitute for proper handwashing. In addition, gloves can become contaminated as easily as ungloved hands.

Before preparing any products, all necessary materials should be gathered. Those needed for each product should be placed in the hood in a manner that does not obstruct the clean airflow. Solutions and additives must be checked for expiration dates and freedom from particulate matter. The outer containers should be cleaned of dust and wiped or sprayed with alcohol prior to being placed in the hood. Plastic solution containers should be squeezed to check for leaks.

Work performed in the hood area should be done in the center of it. There must be no obstruction between the HEPA filter and the product being prepared. In a horizontal hood, work must be done at least 6 inches inside it. The airflow at the outer 6 inches of the hood is subject to many disturbances and therefore may be contaminated. With a vertical hood, the viewing screen must be lowered to its proper position, as this acts to contain the airflow within the hood, provides proper laminar airflow, and protects the user.

Ampules and Vials

Drugs and other additives to I.V. solutions are packaged in ampules or vials. They are available either in liquid form or as sterile solids or powders. Sterile solids must be reconstituted with a suitable solution (diluent) before addition to the I.V. fluid. Ampules are sealed glass containers with an elongated neck that must be snapped off. Most ampules are weakened around the base of the neck for easy breaking. Such ampules can be recognized by a colored band around the base of the neck. If the ampule is not weakened it may be necessary to score it with a file to prevent shattering of the top. A filter needle should be used when withdrawing the contents of an ampule. These products have a 5 micron filter incorporated in them to remove any particulate matter which may fall into the ampule when opened. The filter needle should be removed and replaced with a regular needle before injecting the drug into the solution.

Vials are made of glass or plastic and have a rubber stopper through which a needle is inserted to withdraw or add to the contents. When withdrawing solution from a vial, an equal volume of air is usually drawn up in the syringe and injected into the vial before withdrawing the contents. Some medications are packaged under pressure or may produce gas (and therefore pressure) upon reconstitution. In these situations, air should *not* be injected into the vial before withdrawing the drug. Vials may be labeled for single use or multiple dose use. Multidose products contain a preservative to inhibit microbial contamination after the vial has been opened, and may be withdrawn from more than once. Single-use vials do not contain preservatives and should be discarded after use.

Some manufacturers supply antibiotics in powder form in oversized vials or bags. These minibottle or minibag containers typically have a 100 ml capacity and the drug is reconstituted using a suitable diluent. In addition, each container is equipped with its own hanger so that it can be hung as a piggyback container. The advantage to this type of system is that the drugs are ready for use once they are reconstituted and do not have to be transferred to another container. Large-scale preparation is facilitated by manufacturers' piggyback containers.

Working with Needles and Syringes

Needles and syringes are used for virtually all parenteral product preparation. Syringes consist of a barrel and a plunger (**Figure 20–7**). They range in capacity from 0.3 ml to 60 ml.. Volumes are marked along the barrel. Needles range in size from 3/8 inch to 3 1/2 inches or longer and consist of a shaft and a hub (**Figure 20–8**). The thickness of the needle is represented by gauge size, with 29 gauge being the finest and 13 gauge the thickest. Needles of 26 to 29 gauge are most commonly used for subcutaneous and intradermal injections. Larger gauge needles (18 to 25) are used for intramuscular injections.

In preparing parenteral products, the gauge of the needle used should be the smallest practical size. If a large gauge needle is used, there is a risk of **coring** when injecting into a vial or I.V. container. Coring occurs when a needle rips a piece of the vial stopper at the injection site. This piece then falls into the container and creates a situation of particulate matter contamination.

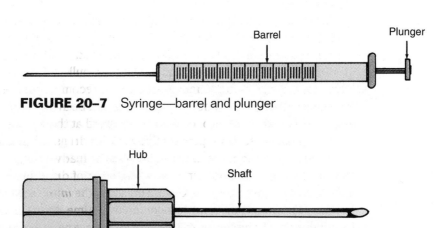

FIGURE 20–7 Syringe—barrel and plunger

FIGURE 20–8 Needle—shaft and hub

Safety Considerations

Administering drugs involves many considerations, including opening the glass ampules, various effects of the medications, and needle sticks.

Opening Glass Ampules

The process of opening a glass ampule presents risks related to broken glass. If proper technique is not used, the ampule may shatter and cut the fingers or hand. In addition, glass splinters may be thrown from the ampule when opened. These splinters could strike the eye when working in a horizontal laminar airflow hood. To reduce the risk of shattering the ampule, it is essential that it not be forced open. Most ampules have a weak spot that can be located by rotating the ampule slightly if it does not snap open with moderate pressure. It is also useful to wrap an alcohol wipe around the top of the ampule when opening to provide some protection to the fingers if the ampule shatters and to reduce the possibility of glass splinters becoming airborne.

Local and Systemic Effects of Medications

Medications may be absorbed into the body through the skin and by inhalation, thus resulting in undesirable effects when significant exposure occurs. Such effects may be localized (confined to the site of exposure, such as the skin), or systemic (within the body). An example of a local effect would be a rash or redness. An example of a systemic effect would be low blood pressure from exposure to nitroglycerin.

It is extremely important to take precautions to avoid undue exposure to medications. Anyone suffering from allergies to particular medications should wear gloves and work in a vertical laminar airflow hood when handling these products. Any medication spilled on the skin should be washed off immediately. Proper technique is vital to avoid unnecessary exposure to medications.

There is much concern about the handling of, and exposure to, cancer chemotherapy agents (also referred to as cytotoxic drugs). Some of these agents have been shown to have the potential of producing serious adverse effects. It is not clear, however, to what extent this may occur from exposure in the workplace. Therefore, it is important to follow recommended procedures for handling these substances.

In January 1986, the federal Occupational Safety and Health Administration (OSHA) released recommendations on safe handling of cytotoxic drugs by health care personnel. The American Society of Health System Pharmacists (ASHP) has subsequently released technical assistance bulletins on handling cytotoxic and hazardous drugs, which incorporate these recommendations and those of other agencies and organizations. Technicians must be aware of these recommendations and strictly follow the procedures established at their place of employment.

It is possible to be exposed to hazardous drugs in various ways. According to the ASHP, "This exposure may be through the inadvertent ingestion of the drug on foodstuffs (e.g., workers' lunches), inhalation of drug dusts or droplets, or direct skin contact." The danger is due not only to the *immediate* effects of a toxic drug, but also to how much exposure occurs over time. In other words, the effects may be cumulative. Long-term exposure *may* produce serious effects such as cancer, impaired fertility, and organ damage, although this has not been proven. Clearly, preventing unintended exposure to these substances is essential.

The ASHP has established four goals for handling hazardous drugs.

1. Protect and secure packages of hazardous drugs.
2. Inform and educate all involved personnel about hazardous drugs and train them in the safe handling procedures relevant to their responsibilities.
3. Do not let the drugs escape from containers when they are manipulated (i.e., dissolved, transferred, administered, or discarded).
4. Eliminate the possibility of inadvertent ingestion or inhalation and direct skin or eye contact with the drugs.

Proper procedures must be in place and *followed* to prevent inadvertent exposure to cytotoxic drugs. This includes the use of appropriate equipment (vertical laminar airflow hoods, gowns, gloves) and appropriate storage and disposal of these agents. While the consequences of exposure to cytotoxic drugs remain unclear, reducing the possibility of such exposure is an essential goal of all involved.

Needle Sticks

It is easy to accidentally stick oneself with a needle in an I.V. admixture area. It is, however, relatively easy to avoid such occurrences. Although the needles used within the pharmacy should normally be "clean" (i.e., not contaminated by blood from another person), needle sticks are a cause of concern. The site of injury may become infected, the resulting bleeding may contaminate other products, and there may be adverse reactions caused by exposure to any drug contained in the needle.

Needle sticks can be avoided by working carefully and not rushing when preparing parenteral products. Extra care must be taken in recapping a needle, as this procedure is often a source of needle sticks. Finally, never reach into a disposal box (sharps container) or attempt to pack down discarded syringes in these boxes. Do not fill the sharps containers more than three-fourths full.

Role of the Technician

The technician is a vital part of a parenteral admixture program. The exact role that a technician plays will vary among states due to differences in pharmacy laws. In addition, as mentioned, the degree to which parenteral admixture services are provided varies considerably among different institutions. However, technicians generally are responsible for the following:

- preparing labels and/or sorting computer-generated labels
- maintaining proper stock and supplies in the parenterals area
- assembling drugs and solutions to be used for admixtures
- reconstituting manufacturers' piggyback vials and additives
- preparing I.V. admixtures under a pharmacist's supervision
- assigning lot numbers and maintaining appropriate records for batch preparations
- preparing prefilled syringes
- preparing parenteral nutrition base solutions
- labeling completed admixtures
- delivering completed admixtures to appropriate areas
- maintaining workload statistics
- maintaining dispensing records and/or patient charges

- ensuring that all needles, syringes, and chemotherapy are properly discarded
- ensuring that no stock is outdated or deteriorated
- ensuring that medications are appropriately stored (refrigerator, freezer)
- maintaining the parenterals area in a neat and orderly manner

Summary

The parenterals technician must be a meticulous, motivated person. Due to the nature of the products prepared, any errors may have disastrous consequences to the patient. The technician must work with the pharmacist, who is responsible for checking and supervising all the technician's activities. Quality and accuracy must never be compromised. All work must be carried out in a diligent, professional manner. The technician is a key player in the functioning of a pharmacy parenterals admixture service.

ASSESSMENT

Multiple Choice Questions

1. Injectable medications account for what percentage of all drugs administered in the hospital?
   - a. 40 percent
   - b. 50 percent
   - c. 80 percent
   - d. 30 percent
   - e. 20 percent

2. Drugs are given by injection when
   - a. the patient is unable to take oral medication
   - b. the patient refuses to take oral medication
   - c. there is a need for rapid drug action
   - d. the drug may be destroyed in the gastrointestinal tract
   - e. all of the above

3. The most important characteristic of an injectable solution is
   - a. color
   - b. viscosity
   - c. dispersability
   - d. sterility
   - e. fluidity

4. A drug can be sterilized by
   - a. moist heat
   - b. gas
   - c. filtration
   - d. none of the above
   - e. all of the above

5. Pyrogenic contamination may cause the patient to have
   - a. fever
   - b. chills
   - c. infection
   - d. a and b
   - e. a and c

6. Particulate matter in an intravenous solution may
   a. cause phlebitis
   b. cause dermatitis
   c. block blood flow in small blood vessels
   d. rupture a blood vessel
   e. all of the above

7. To maintain an aseptic work environment, the technician should
   a. thoroughly wash hands
   b. wear gloves
   c. wear a clean gown
   d. wear a face mask
   e. do all of the above

8. Solution osmolality is a characteristic that results from
   a. the degree of acidity
   b. the degree of alkalinity
   c. a neutral pH
   d. the number of dissolved particles
   e. the number of undissolved particles

9. Intravenous solutions may be administered as
   a. infusions
   b. bolus
   c. piggyback
   d. saddleback
   e. a, b, and c

10. Vertical laminar airflow hoods
   a. should not be used to prepare cytotoxic drugs
   b. protect the operator from hazardous drugs
   c. do not require cleaning
   d. are not used in hospitals
   e. none of the above

True/False Questions

11. ___T___ As a general rule the more concentrated the solution, the less stable it is.

12. ___F___ There is no need to be concerned about exposure to cytotoxic drugs.

13. ___F___ Intramuscular, intravenous, and subcutaneous routes of injection are interchangeable.

14. ___F___ Visual inspection of parenteral products ensures that the drug is safe and stable.

15. ___T___ The pH of a sterile solution can affect both stability and compatibility.

Matching

16. _____ intradermal b
17. _____ subcutaneous g
18. _____ intramuscular d
19. _____ intravenous a
20. _____ intra-arterial f
21. _____ intrathecal c
22. _____ intracardiac e

a. used for large volume injection
b. injected within the skin
c. injected into the spinal fluid
d. common injection sites are the gluteus and deltoid
e. injected into a chamber of the heart
f. injected into a major artery
g. injected into the loose tissue layer below the skin

Bibliography

American Society of Health Systems Pharmacists. ASHP technical assistance bulletin on handling cytotoxic and hazardous drugs. *Practice Standards of ASHP 1995–1996.*

American Society of Health Systems Pharmacists. ASHP technical assistance bulletin on quality assurance for pharmacy-prepared sterile products. *Practice Standards of ASHP 1995–1996.*

Hunt, M.L., Jr. (1990). *Training manual for intravenous admixture personnel* (4th ed.). Chicago: Precept Press.

Turco, S., & King, R.E. (Eds.) (1987). *Sterile dosage forms.* Philadelphia: Lea & Febiger.

21 Basic Biopharmaceutics

COMPETENCIES

Upon completion and review of this chapter, the student should be able to

1. Describe the basic principles of biopharmaceutics.
2. State the objective of measuring plasma drug concentration.
3. Define bioavailability parameters of a drug.
4. Identify pharmaceutical and physiologic factors that affect the absorption of a drug.
5. Describe the process of drug absorption, distribution, and elimination.
6. Describe the basic terms in gene therapy.

Introduction

Bioavailability is a term used to evaluate how a drug product dissolves and reaches the target site after administration to a subject. It is defined in biopharmaceutics as the rate and extent of absorption of a drug product after administration. Many drug products are marketed by more than one pharmaceutical manufacturer. The method of manufacturing and the composition of the final formulation can markedly affect the bioavailability of a drug. It is important for health care personnel to understand biopharmaceutics and be able to select products that will produce equivalent therapeutic effects. In order to facilitate drug product selection, guidelines have been developed by the Food and Drug Administration (FDA) and the U.S. Pharmacopeia/National Formulary (USP-NF) for performing bioavailability and bioequivalency studies. All drug products must meet bioavailability specifications to be marketed. The rationale of a bioavailability study is to compare the systemic availability of a test product with a control (reference) in a crossover design in healthy, nonobese subjects.

Purpose of Bioavailability Studies

Bioavailability studies are performed for both new chemical entities and new formulation of an approved drug. New drugs must be clinically proven to be safe and effective prior to marketing. Generic products must demonstrate that their bioavailability is similar to a brand or reference drug product that is already on the market.

In vivo bioavailability studies are human studies performed to characterize the pharmacokinetics of a drug. Bioequivalence studies are useful in comparing the bioavailability of the same drug (same salt or ester) with various drug products. Once the drug products are demonstrated to be bioequivalent, the clinical efficacy and the safety profiles of these drug products are assumed to be similar.

Methods to Assess Bioavailability

The three methods generally used to measure the bioavailability of a drug are (1) measure the plasma drug level, (2) measure the urine drug level, and (3) measure the pharmacologic effect directly. The selection of a method depends on the objective of the study and the analytical method available. The bioavailability parameters studied generally include:

1. Plasma drug concentration data
    -   time of peak plasma (blood) concentration (t_{max})
    -   peak plasma concentration (C_{max})
    -   area under the plasma level–time curve (AUC)

2. Urinary drug excretion data
    -   cumulative amount of drug excreted in the urine
    -   rate of drug excretion in the urine
    -   time for maximum urinary excretion

3. Direct pharmacologic effect data
    -   When there is no direct method for measuring drug concentrations in plasma or urine, pharmacologic effects may be used; however, these measurements are generally more variable.

Measurement of Drug Concentration

After a drug is administered to the test subjects, plasma or urine samples are collected over a period of time. The samples are then assayed with a validated method to obtain the information necessary for calculating the bioavailability parameters.

Relative and Absolute Availability

Relative availability is the availability of a drug product when compared with an orally administered reference standard. Absolute availability is the availability of a drug product when compared with an intravenously administered standard. The relative availability of a drug product given at the same dose as the reference may be calculated using the following equation:

$$\text{Relative availability} = \frac{[AUC]_{product}}{[AUC]_{standard}}$$

$$\text{Absolute availability} = \frac{[AUC]_{PO}}{[AUC]_{IV}}$$

The area under the drug plasma concentration–time curve (AUC) is useful as a measure of the total amount of unchanged drug that reaches the systemic circulation. F is the fraction of the dose absorbed. After I.V. administration, the entire dose is placed into the systemic circulation instantaneously, and the drug is considered to be completely available and F is equal to 1. For oral drugs, F may vary from 0 (no drug absorption) to 1 (complete drug absorption).

Pharmaceutical Factors That Affect Drug Bioavailability

Disintegration

A solid drug product administered orally has to disintegrate into small particles and dissolve before the process of absorption takes place.

Dissolution

Dissolution is the process by which a chemical or drug becomes dissolved in a solvent. In biologic systems, drug dissolution in an aqueous medium is an important step prior to systemic absorption. Drugs with poor aqueous solubility dissolve slowly and will be incompletely absorbed. Thus, dissolution tests discriminate against formulation factors that may affect drug bioavailability.

Consideration of the Route of Drug Administration

Drugs may be given by oral, parenteral, enteral, inhalation, transdermal (percutaneous), intranasal, and implantation routes for systemic or local therapeutic effects. The choice of the route of drug administration depends on several factors including patient compliance, disease states, therapeutic effect, and adverse effects. Many drugs are not administered orally because of instability or potential degradation by digestive enzymes in the gastrointestinal tract. For example, insulin is administered subcutaneously (SC) or intramuscularly (IM) because it will be destroyed in the intestine. The rate of drug absorption after a subcutaneous or intramuscular injection is generally slower than that of an intravenous injection, and the onset time of the drug will be slower. Some drugs are injected to the site of action such as intrathecal injection into the spinal fluid and intra-pleural injection into the pleural (lung) cavity. The most common route of drug administration is oral.

Factors Affecting Oral Drug Absorption

The systemic absorption of a drug is dependent on (1) the physicochemical properties of the drug, (2) the nature of the drug product, and (3) the anatomy and physiologic functions at the site of drug absorption. A thorough understanding of the physiologic and pathologic factors affecting drug absorption is important in drug selection and the avoidance of potential drug-drug and drug-nutrient interactions.

Anatomic and Physiologic Considerations

The enteral system consists of the alimentary canal from the mouth to the anus. The major physiologic processes that occur in the gastrointestinal (GI) system are secretion, digestion, and absorption. *Secretion* includes the release of digestive enzymes into the lumen of the alimentary canal. Both saliva and pancreatic secretions are involved in the digestion of carbohydrates and proteins. Other secretions such as mucus protect the linings of the lumen of the GI tract. *Digestion* is the breakdown of food constituents into smaller structures in preparation for absorption. Both food and drugs are mostly absorbed in the proximal area (duodenum) of the small intestine. The process of *absorption* is the entry of constituents from the lumen of the gut into the body. Absorption of drugs may be affected by the presence of food and other substances such as antacids. Protein drugs may be digested by enzymes in the gastrointestinal tract.

Drugs administered orally pass through various parts of the enteral canal. The total transit time, including gastric emptying, small intestinal transit, and colonic transit ranges from 0.4 to 5 days. The most important site for drug absorption is the small intestine. Small intestine transit time ranges from 3 to 4 hours for most healthy subjects. If absorption is not completed by the time a drug leaves the small intestine, absorption may be erratic or incomplete. The small intestine is normally filled with digestive juices and liquids, keeping the lumen contents fluid. In contrast, the fluid in the colon is reabsorbed, and the lumenal content in the colon is either semisolid or solid, making further drug dissolution erratic and difficult. The normal physiologic processes of the alimentary canal may be affected by diet, contents of the GI tract, hormones, the visceral nervous system, disease, and drugs. Thus, drugs given by the enteral route for systemic absorption may be affected by the anatomy, physiologic functions, and contents of the alimentary tract. The absorption of drug may be altered in Crohn's and other inflammatory gastrointestinal diseases.

Oral cavity

Saliva is the main secretion of the oral cavity, and has a pH of approximately 7. Saliva contains ptyalin (salivary amylase), which digests starches. Mucin, a glycoprotein that lubricates food, is also secreted and may interact with drugs. Approximately 1500 ml of saliva are secreted per day.

Esophagus

The esophagus connects the pharynx and the cardiac orifice of the stomach. The pH of the fluids in the esophagus is between 5 and 6. The lower part of the esophagus ends with the esophageal sphincter, which prevents acid reflux from the stomach. Tablets or capsules may lodge in this area, causing local irritation. Very little drug dissolution occurs in the esophagus.

Stomach

Acid secretion and gastric emptying in the stomach are dependent on the presence of food. The fasting pH of the stomach is about 2 to 6. In the presence of food, hydrochloric acid is secreted by parietal cells and the stomach pH decreases to between 1 and 2. Some drugs will dissolve in the acid environment while other drugs may precipitate out because of lower pH. Thus, food may enhance or delay the absorption of drug due to its influence on stomach emptying and acid secretion.

Food and liquid are emptied by opening the pyloric sphincter into the duodenum. Stomach emptying is influenced by the food content and osmolality. Fatty acids and mono- and diglycerides delay gastric emptying. High-density food generally is emptied from the stomach more slowly.

Duodenum

The pH of the duodenum is about 6 to 6.5 due to the presence of bicarbonate. The pH is optimum for enzymatic digestion of protein and peptide food. Pancreatic juice containing enzymes is secreted into the duodenum from the bile duct. Some insoluble drugs are solubilized by pancreatic secretions and become better absorbed. Pancreatic lipase secretion hydrolyses fats into fatty acid. The complex fluid medium in the duodenum helps to dissolve many lipophilic drugs with limited aqueous solubility. The duodenum is the principal site of drug absorption because it has a very large surface area for drug absorption. Some drugs are not absorbed beyond the small intestine.

Jejunum

The jejunum is the middle portion of the small intestine in between the duodenum and the ileum. Digestion of protein and carbohydrates continues after receiving pancreatic juice and bile in the duodenum. This portion of the small intestine generally has less contractions than the duodenum and is preferred for in vivo drug absorption studies. Drug absorption continues in this part of the intestine.

Ileum

The ileum is the terminal part of the small intestine. This site has fewer contractions than the duodenum and may be blocked off by catheters with an inflatable balloon and perfused for drug absorption study. The pH is approximately 7, with the distal part as high as 8. Due to the presence of bicarbonate secretion, acid drugs will dissolve. Bile secretion helps to dissolve fats and hydrophobic drugs. The ileocecal valve separates the small intestines from the colon.

Colon

The colon lacks microvilli and is very limited in drug absorption due to the more viscous and semisolid nature of the lumen contents. The colon is lined with mucin, which functions as lubricant and protectant. The pH in this region is 5.5 to 7. A few drugs such as theophylline and metoprolol are absorbed in this region. Drugs that are absorbed well in this region are good candidates for an oral sustained-release dosage form. The colon contains both aerobic and anaerobic microorganisms that may metabolize some drugs. For example, L-dopa and lactulose are metabolized by enteric bacteria. Crohn's disease affects the colon and thickens the bowel wall. The microflora also become more anaerobic. Absorption of clindamycin and propranolol are increased, whereas other drugs have reduced absorption with this disease.

Rectum

The rectum is approximately 15 cm long, ending at the anus. In the absence of fecal material, the rectum has a small amount of fluid (approximately 2 ml) with a pH of approximately 7. The rectum is perfused by the superior, middle, and inferior hemorrhoidal veins. The inferior hemorrhoidal vein (closest to the anal sphincter) and the middle hemorrhoidal vein feed into the vena cava and back to the heart. The superior hemorrhoidal vein joins the mesenteric circulation which feeds into the hepatic portal vein and then to the liver. Drug absorption by rectal administration may be variable depending on the placement of the suppository or drug solution within the rectum. A portion of the drug dose may be absorbed via the lower hemorrhoidal veins from which the drug feeds directly into the systemic circulation; some drug dose may be absorbed via the superior hemorrhoidal vein which feeds into the mesenteric veins to the hepatic portal vein to the liver, and metabolized prior to systemic absorption.

Drug Disposition and Elimination

Once a drug is absorbed, it is carried to various tissues and organs in the body by the blood. The drug is delivered simultaneously to all tissues and organs. Elimination is the irreversible loss of a drug from the site of measurement. Drug elimination occurs mostly by metabolism in the liver or excretion in the kidney. Metabolism is the conversion of one chemical form to another, whereas excretion is the irreversible loss of the chemically unchanged drug.

Distribution of a drug to various body tissues occurs at various rates depending on blood supply. Drug distribution is also affected by protein binding within the plasma and tissue organs. In general, the barrier to drug diffusion is the biological membranes. Lipophilic drugs tend to diffuse across biological membranes easily. Polar drugs diffuse more slowly across biological membranes and tend to be distributed within the extracellular fluid.

The elimination half-life is defined as the time it takes for the drug plasma concentration or amount to decrease by one-half in the body. Most drugs are metabolized by the liver or eliminated by the kidney. Some are eliminated through the gall bladder by biliary secretion. Later, the same drug may be reabsorbed in the intestine. This process is known as enterohepatic cycling.

Some drugs may be rapidly metabolized in the liver after oral administration and the bioavailability becomes very small, a process generally known as first pass effect. Drug elimination may also occur by active secretion in the renal tubules. Drug filtration may occur by glomerular filtration.

Gene Therapy

Many diseases occur as a result of genetic defects or errors in the gene involved in producing essential enzymes or proteins in the body. Genetic information is now known to reside in chromosomes housing helical strands known as deoxyribonucleic acid (DNA) within the nucleus. The Human Genome Initiative was created several years ago to study all human genes. This national effort is now yielding information on many serious diseases involving congenital defects, cancer, AIDS, infection, and disorders involving the immune system. Strategies are now available to alter or block the transcriptional process in the DNA to moderate many disease processes. By altering the DNA sequence so that the complementary strand is transcribed instead of the normal "sense" gene, the DNA would not be able to make a copy of normal RNA which participates in protein synthesis. The aberrant copies of RNA may "pair up" (hybridize) with other RNAs that complement it and block protein synthesis. The medication used in targeting DNA or RNA using this technique is an antisense drug. Many oligonucleotides have been designed to target viral disease and cancer cells in the body. Antisense drugs against HIV and other viruses are now in early phases of clinical trial.

When a gene's nucleotide base sequence that controls a specific body function is known, the antisense DNA strand can be synthesized. Such strands can then be introduced into cells where they attach themselves to the complementary sense DNA strands, thereby depressing transcription of these genes. This procedure has been done successfully in cell culture for the cancer-causing gene that produces human larynx squamous carcinoma.

The first example of human gene therapy started in 1990 with FDA-approved PEG-ADA (made by Annexion Inc., Piscataway, NJ) for adenosine deaminase (ADA) deficiency, a serious rare genetic disorder weakening the immune system and resulting in easy infection. Two girls were reinfused with genetically altered white blood cells withdrawn from their bodies with the gene corrected. The altered cells live and function normally for an extended period. Gaucher's disease, a rare genetic disease involving a defective metabolic enzyme glucocerebrosidase, is another disease that is being considered for gene therapy. Gene therapy is experimental and the long-term impact of therapy is not known.

Summary

Biopharmaceutics considers the interrelationship of the physicochemical properties of the drug, the dosage form, and the routes of administration on the systemic absorption of drugs.

Drug absorption in the gastrointestinal tract is dependent upon the rate of drug dissolution, stomach emptying, pH at the site of absorption, and the presence of a passive or carrier-mediated transport system.

Distribution of a drug to various tissues depends on the blood perfusion, diffusion, transport, and protein binding of the drug. The extent of distribution is measured by the apparent volume of distribution of the drug. The rate of drug elimination is measured by the elimination half-life. The factors affecting bioavailability are (1) pharmaceutical factors, (2) physiologic factors, (3) route of administration, and (4) elimination pathways. The two major factors limiting drug bioavailability are dissolution and first pass effect. Both drug plasma and urine data are used to determine the bioavailability of a drug. Bioavailability information is helpful in selecting drug products.

ASSESSMENT

Multiple Choice Questions

1. Which of the following parameters measures the extent of bioavailability?
   a. AUC (area under the curve)
   b. plasma drug concentration
   c. rate of absorption
   d. volume of distribution

2. After an I.V. bolus administration, what percent does the plasma drug concentration decrease after one half-life?
   a. 50
   b. 0.5
   c. 5
   d. 10

3. Substituting metoprolol in place of nadolol (with the consent of the physician) is considered a
   a. pharmaceutic substitution
   b. biological equivalent
   c. therapeutic alternative
   d. generic substitution

4. Which of the following pharmaceutic factors most affects the systemic absorption for an oral drug product?
   a. shelf life of the drug
   b. the size of the tablet
   c. disintegration
   d. dissolution

5. What is the pH of the stomach in the presence of food?
   a. 1–2
   b. 3–7
   c. 6–8
   d. 9–12

6. What is the principal site of drug absorption?
   a. stomach
   b. colon
   c. rectum
   d. duodenum

7. Where is the most important site for a drug to be metabolized?
   a. rectum
   b. liver
   c. kidney
   d. muscle

Bibliography

Banker, G.S., & Rhodes, C.T. (Eds.). (1990). *Modern pharmaceutics* (2nd ed.). New York: Marcel Dekker, Inc.

Benet, L., Levy, G., & Ferraiolo, B. (1984). *Pharmacokinetics—A modern view*. New York: Plenum Publishing Corp.

Evans, W.E., Schentag, J.J., & Jusko, W.J. (1992). *Applied pharmacokinetics: Principle of therapeutic drug monitoring, Applied therapeutics* (3rd ed.). Vancouver, WA.

Gibaldi, M. (1984). *Biopharmaceutics and clinical pharmacokinetics* (3rd ed.). Philadelphia: La and Febiger.

Shargel, L., & Yu, A. (1993). *Applied pharmaceutics and pharmacokinetics* (3rd ed.). Norwalk, CT: Appleton & Lange.

Taylor, W., & Diers Caviness, M.H. (Eds.). (1986). *A textbook for the clinical application of therapeutic drug monitoring, Abbott Laboratories*.

Welling, P. (1986). *Pharmacokinetics: Process and mathematics*. American Chemical Society.

Yu, A.B.C., & Fong, G.W. (1996). Biotechnologic products. In L. Shargel et al. (Eds.), *Comprehensive pharmacy review* (3rd ed.). Baltimore, MD: Williams and Wilkins.

The Actions and Uses of Drugs

COMPETENCIES

After completion and review of this chapter, the student should be able to

1. List various dosage forms and routes of administration of drugs.
2. Detail certain food-drug interactions.
3. Cite some major effects of drug-drug interactions.
4. Describe factors affecting drug activity.
5. Explain certain disease states and how drug therapy affects them.
6. List the clinical applications of various drug categories described in this chapter.
7. Match the generic name and the common trade name of drugs used in pharmaceutical therapy.

Introduction

A drug is a substance that affects a biological system in a potentially useful way. The goal of rational drug therapy is to prevent, modify, or cure particular disease states. There are literally thousands of clinically useful drugs and hundreds of facts about each drug. To gain a basic understanding about drug therapy it is not necessary to memorize all the minute facts about each drug. The essential element in this quest for drug knowledge is to understand the basic principles of pharmacology and try to apply these principles to alter the course of the disease or alleviate the symptoms. The pharmacy technician plays the essential role of assisting the pharmacist in preparing and dispensing medication. This chapter is designed to provide technicians with the necessary tools to understand how and why a drug is prescribed.

This chapter is divided into two sections. The first section deals with factors that modify drug actions and patient response. The second section includes the major classification of drugs (generic and common trade names) and the role of these medications in the treatment of some common medical conditions.

Factors That Modify Drug Action

Route of Administration

Drugs are introduced into the body in a variety of ways. The most common methods involve swallowing or injecting. The method of administration chosen by the clinician depends on various factors (e.g., speed of onset of drug action that is required, relative side effects of the drug, the setting in which the drug will be used). The two major routes of administration are enteral and parenteral.

Enteral Administration

Oral administration

Drugs placed in the mouth and swallowed are referred to as oral medications. They are prescribed p.o., which is the Latin abbreviation for *per os,* "by mouth." This method of administration is usually the least expensive and most user friendly. It is ideal for the outpatient setting and for patients with a busy lifestyle. Oral administration is associated with a low risk of infection. The disadvantage of this method is that it cannot be used in an emergency situation because the onset of action is slow.

For an oral drug to be absorbed it must first pass through the walls of the gastrointestinal tract and the blood vessels before entering the blood stream. Blood from the gastrointestinal tract passes through the liver where the drug is metabolized into an inactive or active derivative. This process is called the **first pass effect.** The inactivation of some drugs is so great that they may be useless when administered orally. This first pass effect also accounts for the fact that the oral dose of some drugs is much larger than the intravenous dose (I.V. drugs bypass the gastrointestinal tract and directly enter the bloodstream).

Oral medications cannot be administered to an unconscious patient or to a patient who is vomiting. The oral route of administration also presents a problem for drugs that are destroyed by an acid environment (pH of the stomach is approximately 2).

Sublingual administration

Drugs placed in the mouth and held under the tongue are said to be administered sublingually (prescribed s.l.). The underside of the tongue is rich in capillary beds and provides a large area for absorption of drugs. Drugs are quickly absorbed from this route so the onset of action is quite fast. A good example is nitroglycerin sublingual administration. This drug is administered for rapid relief of anginal chest pain, because the onset of action is within minutes.

Sublingual administration bypasses the liver so the first pass effect does not present a problem. The sublingual route also bypasses the stomach so destruction of the medication by the acidic nature of the stomach need not be considered.

Buccal

Buccal administration of a drug is similar to sublingual except that the medication is placed between the cheek and the gum (*bucca* is Latin for "cheek"). This method also has similar advantages to sublingual administration (rapid absorption, bypasses liver, etc.). One disadvantage of both methods is that the patient has to be adequately instructed to self-administer the medications. Many patients start out correctly placing the medication under the tongue (s.l.) or between cheek and gum (buccal), but eventually swallow the medication. This negates the advantage of sublingual or buccal drug administration.

Parenteral Administration

Parenteral ("around the GI tract") administration involves puncturing the skin. The most common methods of parenteral administration of drugs are intravenous (I.V.), intramuscular (I.M.), and subcutaneous (S.C.).

Intravenous

Drugs are injected directly into the bloodstream when using intravenous administration. This method provides a rapid onset of action because the drug is immediately absorbed. Immediate onset of action is a definite advantage in emergency situations and for patients who are unconscious. The disadvantage is that extreme care must be exercised for dosing and administration. Once a medication is administered by this route there is no turning back. In many instances the therapeutic level of drugs may be close to the toxic level so careful monitoring is necessary. The rate of administration must be carefully controlled to minimize adverse effects. The I.V. method of drug administration presents an increased risk of infection because the injection may introduce bacteria through contamination. Intravenous administration has also been associated with pain and local irritation at the site of the injection.

Intramuscular

Intramuscular administration involves drugs that are injected directly into the muscle which is rich in blood vessels. The drugs then pass through the capillary walls and enter the bloodstream. Intramuscular administration of a drug will decrease the rate of absorption and thus minimize shock to the system. The rate of absorption depends on the formulation of the drug (e.g., oil-based substances are absorbed more slowly, water-based substances more rapidly). Long-acting preparations can also be administered by I.M. injection. Disadvantages include variable rates of absorption, pain, and local irritation.

Subcutaneous

Subcutaneous administration involves drugs that are injected beneath the skin which permeate the capillary walls to enter the bloodstream. The rate of absorption is proportional to the blood flow in the area of the injection. A disadvantage is that it is limited to only those medications that are highly soluble, low volume, and nonirritating.

Other Methods of Administration

Inhalation

Inhalation administration involves drugs that are rapidly absorbed across the large surface area of the mucous membrane of the respiratory tract. This method requires that the drugs be nebulized or aerosolized. The inhalation method is particularly useful for patients who have respiratory complaints (asthma). The drugs are administered via metered dose inhalers and are delivered directly to the site of action—the respiratory tract—with minimal systemic side effects. Metered dose inhalers are easy to use and are suitable for self-administration. The inhalation route of administration is also utilized for volatile anesthetics used during surgery.

Topical

Topical administration is useful for local administration of a drug when systemic action is not necessary or desirable. Topical application is most often associated with dermatological preparations (skin cream, ointment, lotion) and ophthalmic preparations used for glaucoma, cataracts, eye infections, etc.

Transdermal

Transdermal administration involves drugs that are formulated to be included in a patch, which is applied to the skin, whereby the medication seeps out of the patch and is absorbed through the skin. This method is used for a wide variety of conditions (pain, motion sickness, etc.).

Vaginal

Vaginal medication, in the form of a cream, gel, ointment, or suppository, is inserted into the vagina. This method is convenient and economical and is used to treat various vaginal disorders (yeast infections, local irritation, vaginal dryness). Many vaginal preparations are available without a prescription.

Rectal administration

Rectal drug administration involves the absorption of the drug (usually formulated as a suppository or enema) through the rectal mucosa. This method is ideal for unconscious or vomiting patients (e.g., compazine suppositories). It is also used for infants and children (e.g., Tylenol™ suppositories). Rectal administration is also ideal for bowel cleansing (e.g., Fleets™ enema). A disadvantage of rectal administration is that the rate and extent of absorption can be unreliable. Also, many patients tend to have a natural aversion to rectal administration. Patients must be instructed to properly self-administer suppositories and enemas. One common problem is that patients do not leave the suppositories/enema in place for the appropriate amount of time, and thus greatly decrease the absorption of the drug.

Food-Drug Interaction

For drugs administered by mouth the rate of absorption is influenced by the **pH** of the stomach and intestines, gastric emptying time and the presence or absence of food in the stomach. The possibility of **food-drug interactions** is a major source of concern for health professionals and patients alike. Patient education concerning the proper time to take certain medications in relation to meals can greatly diminish the potential for the occurrence of a serious food-drug interaction. The manufacturer's prescribing information usually addresses the appropriate time to take medication with regard to meals, fluid, and other drugs. **Table 22–1** lists the effects of food on the absorption of some selected medications.

Drug-Drug Interactions

Drugs may interact with other drugs according to several mechanisms.

Altered drug metabolism

Most drugs are biotransformed or metabolized by the body. **Metabolism** refers to the process of making a drug more polar or more water soluble. This process often results in drug inactivation and excretion. Metabolism can also result in an inactive drug (called a "prodrug") transformation into an active drug. The major organ of metabolism is the liver. Certain enzymes in the liver are responsible for major metabolic reactions. This enzyme system is called the **cytochrome P450 system.** Many drugs are metabolized by this system. The rate of inactivation and excretion of these drugs is dependent on the activity of this group of liver enzymes. The cytochrome P450 system can be induced (increased in activity) by certain drugs. This increase in activity will speed the metabolism of other drugs metabolized by the cytochrome P450 system (and speed the metabolism of the inducing agent). Increasing the metabolism of certain drugs may lead to an increase in excretion of the drug resulting in lower blood levels for these drugs. Lower drug blood levels may result in a subtherapeutic level, which is a common scenario for drug-drug interaction (e.g., one drug inducing the metabolism of another drug). An example of this type of interaction is phenobarbital increasing the metabolism of oral contraceptives thereby causing failure of conception control. Examples of other potent inducing substances include phenytoin, carbamazepine, rifampin, griseofulvin, and primidone.

TABLE 22–1 **Food Effects on Absorption of Drugs from the GI Tract**

Decreased by Food	Increased by Food
Atenolol	Chlorothiazide
Ceclor, Cephalexin	Diazepam
Erythromycin stearate (film-coated tabs)	Dicoumarol
Ketoconazole	Erythromycin estolate
Rifampin	Erythromycin ethylsuccinate
Sotalol	Griseofulvin
Alcohol	Hydralazine
Ampicillin, Amoxicillin	Labetalol
Ibuprofen	Metoprolol
Diclofenac	Nitrofurantoin
Piroxicam	Phenytoin
Cimetidine	Propranolol
Hydrocortisone	Spironolactone
Levodopa	
Metronidazole	
Methyldopa	
Digoxin	
Aspirin	
Nafcillin	
Penicillin G, V	
Sulfonamides	
Tetracycline, Doxycycline	

Other drugs and chemicals can be potent inhibitors of the cytochrome P450 system and thereby prolong the action of other drugs metabolized by this system. An example of this type of interaction is cimetidine decreasing the metabolism of theophylline, which may result in a potentially toxic increase in theophylline blood level. Potent inhibitors of the cytochrome P450 system include disulfuram, chloramphenicol, isoniazid, and erythromycin.

Altered drug absorption

Certain drugs may inhibit the absorption of other drugs leading to decreased blood levels of the affected drug. The rate of absorption of certain drugs can be slowed by drugs that decrease gastric motility. Because the small intestine is a major site of drug absorption, any drug that decreases the speed in which orally administered drugs pass from the stomach to the small intestine (site of absorption) will decrease the absorption rate (e.g., morphine, codeine). Conversely, drugs that increase gastric motility will increase the rate of absorption (metoclopramide, cisapride).

Decreased absorption of drugs can also occur by the formulation of an insoluble complex between agents such as calcium, aluminum, or magnesium (which can be present in certain vitamins and antacid preparations) and drugs such as tetracycline, doxycycline, ofloxacin, and ciprofloxacin.

Alteration of gastrointestinal pH can also affect the absorption of drugs. Drugs are absorbed at a specific pH. For example, aspirin (an acid) is absorbed best in the acid environment of the stomach. If a patient takes an antacid which changes the pH of the stomach and then takes aspirin, much less aspirin will be absorbed.

Absorption of drugs can be affected by the binding of drugs in the gastrointestinal tract. An example of this type of interaction occurs with the drug sucralfate, which is commonly used for the treatment of ulcers. If sucralfate is administered with certain drugs (e.g., digoxin, phenytoin, tetracycline, theophylline), then sucralfate will significantly reduce the absorption of these drugs.

Altered drug distribution

Once drugs are absorbed they are distributed throughout the blood as both free drug molecules and bound drug molecules. The bound drugs are bound to a protein in the plasma called albumin. It is the free drug molecules that produce the drug action; the bound drug molecules are inert. Certain drugs can displace other drugs from their binding sites to albumin, thus creating more "free" drug in circulation. This increase in free drug may greatly increase the drug's action. A serious drug interaction between phenylbutazone and warfarin occurs by this mechanism. Phenylbutazone will displace warfarin from binding to albumin (creating more free warfarin in circulation) and cause an increase in the pharmacological effect of warfarin. This increase in warfarin's action can result in bleeding or even hemorrhage.

Altered drug elimination

Most drug interactions involving elimination or excretion occur in the kidney. Certain drugs may increase or decrease the elimination of another drug thereby increasing or decreasing the blood levels of the affected drug. An example of this type of interaction occurs between probenecid and sulfonamides. Probenecid decreases the excretion of sulfonamides and can lead to sulfonamide toxicity.

Addition, synergism, antagonism

A drug interaction can occur when certain drugs have an additive effect if given together (addition). Sometimes when two drugs are given together the response elicited is greater than the combined response of the individual drugs (synergism). Another type of drug interaction can occur when one drug inhibits the actions of another drug (antagonism).

Patient-Associated Factors Altering Drug Action

Age

Drug metabolizing enzymes may not fully develop in infants or may be depressed in elderly and debilitated patients. Drug dosages which may be suitable for the average adult patient may actually be toxic in these patient populations. Elderly patients may have concomitant illnesses which predispose them to problems with drug excretion and metabolism (hypertension, diabetes, hepatic and renal disease). Dose reductions may be appropriate in these patients.

Smoking and alcohol use

Smoking and prolonged alcohol use have been shown to induce hepatic enzymes leading to an increase in the rate of metabolism for certain drugs. The dose of certain drugs which are therapeutic for the general population may actually be subtherapeutic in these patients. Similarly, if these patients stop smoking and drinking alcohol, their maintenance doses of certain drugs may now actually be toxic.

Body weight

Many drugs are dosed according to body weight (mg of drug/kg of body weight). When patients lose or gain a great deal of weight, dose adjustments may have to be made for certain drugs to ensure adequate drug response.

Pregnancy status

Before a drug is prescribed for a woman of childbearing years it is essential to know if she may be pregnant. Many drugs have been determined to have harmful effects on the developing fetus (teratogens) and should not be prescribed during pregnancy. A small number of drugs can be prescribed if the benefits outweigh the risks. The "pregnancy category" of each drug is part of the manufacturer's prescribing information and should be checked before prescribing drugs to women who are or may be pregnant. These categories detail the relative risk of prescribing these drugs (categories A through X, where A is the most benign and X is absolutely contraindicated).

Classification of Drugs

This section includes the major classification of drugs with representative drugs in each class. Over-the-counter (OTC) preparations (drugs not requiring a prescription) will be asterisked (*). Some of these drugs may be OTC in lower strengths, but may require a prescription in higher strengths.

Analgesics and Antipyretics

Analgesics are drugs that are used to relieve pain. Antipyretics are drugs used to reduce fever. Many drugs are both analgesic and antipyretic. The ideal way to treat pain is to eliminate the underlying cause; however, since that is not always possible, symptomatic relief is usually indicated. The type of analgesic chosen to relieve pain is dependent on the type of pain experienced by the patient, the side effect profile of the agent chosen, and concomitant conditions exhibited by the patient. The analgesic chosen should be given an adequate therapeutic trial and will often require a dose adjustment based on the individual pain relief requirements for each patient. Pain control should be initiated with the weakest effective agent having the least side effects. For mild to moderate pain, peripherally acting agents (acetaminophen, nonsteroidal anti-inflammatory agents [NSAIDS], or aspirin) are preferred over centrally acting agents (opioids). More severe pain may require narcotic analgesics. Many clinicians consider morphine the first line agent when treating moderate to severe pain. The best judge of pain intensity is the patient. Pain involves both a physical and a psychological component, and both aspects need to be considered when choosing a medication. Pain can also be acute or chronic. Under normal circumstances acute pain quickly subsides as the healing process occurs, thus decreasing the painful sensations.

When acute pain persists for a longer period, perhaps months, it is classified as chronic pain. Patients with chronic pain may require long-term analgesic use. The side effects and adverse effects associated with the medication become all the more important for the patient experiencing chronic pain. Pain medication should be administered on a regular basis "by the clock," so that the next dose is administered before the effect of the previous one wears off.

Generally, clinicians use the World Health Organization Analgesic Ladder for pain control when treating chronic pain.

Step 1. *Mild to moderate pain:* Treat with nonopioid analgesics.

Step 2. *Moderate pain:* Patients failing step 1 should be treated with an oral opioid analgesic indicated for moderate pain combined with a nonopioid analgesic if necessary and adjuvant (additional) medication (if necessary).

Step 3. *Severe pain:* Patients failing step 2 should be treated with an opioid intended for severe pain (I.V. or p.o.), and a nonopioid analgesic (if necessary) and an adjuvant medication (if necessary).

Nonopioid Analgesics

Generic Name	Common Trade Name
Acetaminophen (*)	Tylenol
Acetylsalicylic acid (*)	Aspirin
Choline/magnesium trisalicylate	Trilisate
Diflunisal	Dolobid
Etodolac	Lodine
Fenoprofen	Nalfon
Ibuprofen (*)	Advil, Motrin
Ketoprofen (*)	Orudis
Ketorolac	Toradol
Meclofenamate	Meclomen
Mefenamic acid	Ponstel
Naproxen (*)	Naprosyn
Naproxen sodium	Anaprox

Opioids Commonly Used for Moderate to Severe Pain

Generic Name	Common Trade Name
Codeine	Various generic
Hydrocodone combinations	Vicodin, Lortab, Lorcet
Meperidine	Demerol
Oxycodone combinations	Percodan, Percocet, Tylox
Pentazocine	Talwin
Propoxyphene	Darvon

Opioids Used for Severe Pain

Generic Name	Trade Name
Butorphanol	Stadol
Fentanyl	Duragesic
Hydromorphone	Dilaudid

Generic Name	Trade Name
Levorphanol	Levo-Dromoran
Methadone	Dolophine
Morphine	Roxanol, MS Contin
Nalbuphine	Nubain
Oxymorphone	Numorphan

Adjuvant Medications

Antihistamines, Corticosteroids, Psychostimulants, Tricyclic antidepressants, Anticonvulsants, and oral local anesthetics

Anesthetics

Anesthetic drugs relieve pain by blocking the transmission of painful impulses. These painful impulses are transmitted via nerve conduction. Some general anesthetics are administered through inhalation (called volatile anesthetics) and some are administered I.V. or I.M. General anesthetics depress the nerve pathways that carry painful signals to the brain. General anesthetics are used during surgery to produce sedation, muscle relaxation, and analgesia.

General Anesthetics

Generic Name	Trade Name
Enflurane	Ethrane
Etomidate	Amidate
Halothane	Fluothane
Isoflurane	Forane
Nitrous oxide	Various brands
Propofol	Diprivan
Thiopental	Pentothal

Local anesthetics also block pain conduction by nerves. They are used for local nerve blocks, spinal nerve blocks, and epidural nerve blocks.

Local Anesthetics

Generic Name	Trade Name
Bupivacaine	Marcaine
Dibucaine	Nupercaine
Lidocaine	Xylocaine
Mepivacaine	Carbocaine
Procaine	Novocain
Tetracaine	Pontocaine

Antacids/Acid Neutralizers

Antacids

Antacids ("against acid") are one of the cornerstones of peptic ulcer therapy. Their main mechanism of action is to neutralize stomach acidity, which is no small task, because the pH of the stomach is between 1 and 2. Antacids react with gastric acid to form a neutral component resulting in the reduction of gastric acidity. Lower gastric acidity promotes healing of ulcers. Many antacids contain either aluminum, magnesium, calcium, or sodium bicarbonate. Simethicone is often included in antacid preparations to decrease flatulence. Antacids are available without a prescription. Caution should be advised when taking antacids with certain drugs. The absorption of some drugs can be greatly diminished when administered with antacids (e.g., tetracycline, ofloxacin, doxycycline).

Antacids

Main Ingredient	Common Trade Name
Aluminum hydroxide (*)	AlternaGEL
Calcium carbonate (*)	Tums, Rolaids
Magnesium/aluminum (*)	Maalox, Mylanta, Gaviscon
Simethicone (*)	Flatulex, Mylicon, Mylanta Gas
Sodium bicarbonate (*)	Alka Seltzer

H2 Antagonists

The secretion of gastric acid is initiated by the actions of a chemical messenger called histamine. Gastric histamine blocking drugs, called H2 antagonists, interfere with the action of histamine in the stomach and inhibit the formation of gastric acid. Many H2 blockers are now available without a prescription.

H2 Antagonists

Generic Name	Common Trade Name
Cimetidine (*)	Tagamet
Famotidine (*)	Pepcid
Nizatidine (*)	Axid
Ranitidine (*)	Zantac

Proton pump inhibitors

One primary mechanism for the synthesis of stomach acid (hydrochloric acid, -HCL) requires that a proton H+ is readily available. This proton needs to be "pumped" into special cells in the stomach (parietal cells). If this pump is inhibited, the production of gastric acid will also be inhibited. This pump can be inhibited by a group of drugs called proton pump inhibitors.

Proton Pump Inhibitors

Generic Name	Common Trade Name
Lansoprazole	Prevacid
Omeprazole	Prilosec

Gastro-protective agents

Gastro-protective agents also protect the gastric mucosa and aid in the treatment of stomach ulcers.

Gastro-Protective Agents

Generic Name	Common Trade Name
Misoprostol	Cytotec
Sulcralfate	Carafate

Anthelmintics

Anthelmintics are agents that specifically target gastrointestinal infestation of worms. The most common type of worms include pinworm, ascarids, whipworm, and hookworm. Worm infestation can occur due to ingesting food or beverages that contain these parasites. The most prevalent types of foods known to be contaminated with these parasites include fresh fruit, raw vegetables, milk, fresh water fish, and raw meat. It is important for a physician to correctly identify the parasite, because drug therapy is directed at specific parasites.

Anthelmintic Drugs

Generic Name	Common Trade Name
Mebendazole	Vermox
Niclosamide	Niclocide
Piperazine citrate	Various generic
Pyrantel pamoate	Antiminth
Thiabendazole	Mintezol

Antidiarrheals

Diarrhea, characterized by loose watery stools, usually results from an increase in activity of the gastrointestinal tract caused by infection, toxins, or drugs. As a result of this increase in activity, fecal matter spends less time in the GI tract, resulting in inadequate stool formation. Less fluid is absorbed from the GI tract. Therapy is usually aimed at decreasing GI activity (antimotility agents) and increasing the absorption of fluid (adsorbents). Diarrhea may also be due to irritable bowel syndrome. Drugs that inhibit GI spasms (anticholinergic/antispasmodics) are useful in treating diarrhea spasms associated with this disorder.

Adsorbents

Generic Name	Common Trade Name
Bismuth Subsalicylate (*)	Pepto Bismol
Cholestyramine	Questran
Kaolin/Pectin (*)	Kaopectate

Antimotility Agents

Generic Name	Common Trade Name
Diphenoxylate	Lomotil
Loperamide (*)	Imodium

Antispasmodics

Generic Name	Common Trade Name
Belladonna alkaloids	Donnatal, Levsin
Clidinium (plus chlordiazepoxide)	Librax
Dicyclomine	Bentyl
Glycopyrrolate	Robinul
Propantheline	Pro-Banthine

Antianginal Agents

Angina is a condition that manifests as chest pain which may be sudden in onset, pressing in nature. The pain may also radiate down the left arm. The recognized cause of angina is coronary blood flow which is insufficient to meet the oxygen demand of the body. There are many potential causes of angina. The imbalance in oxygen delivery relative to the demands of the body may be due to some obstruction in coronary blood flow possibly due to deposits of cholesterol along the lumen of blood vessels. Another possible cause of anginal pain may be due to spasms of vascular smooth muscle. The goal of therapy is to increase the coronary blood flow and decrease the resistance to this blood flow by using drugs known as vasodilators (e.g., nitrates). Nitrates relax coronary arteries, decrease coronary vasoconstriction, and increase myocardial perfusion. Another class of drugs which will bring about vasodilatation is calcium channel blockers. Calcium channel blockers decrease calcium entry into cardiac and smooth muscle cells. They cause a decrease in smooth muscle tone and decrease vascular resistance, and thus increase the supply of blood to major organs of the body. Another goal of therapy would be to decrease the oxygen demands of the heart, which can be accomplished by depressing the "work of the heart," thus decreasing cardiac output and heart rate. Drugs called beta adrenergic blockers decrease the oxygen demand of the heart and decrease chest pain.

Nitrates

Generic Name	Common Trade Name
Isosorbide dinitrate	Sorbitrate, Isordil
Isosorbide mononitrate	ISMO, Imdur
Nitroglycerin	Nitrostat, Nitropaste, Nitro-Dur, Nitrodisc Deponit, Transderm-Nitro

Calcium Channel Blockers

Generic Name	Common Trade Name
Amlodipine	Norvasc
Bepridil	Vascor
Diltiazem	Cardizem
Felodipine	Plendil
Isradipine	DynaCirc
Nifedipine	Procardia
Verapamil	Isoptin, Calan, Verelan

Beta Blockers

Generic Name	Common Trade Name
Acebutolol[+]	Sectral
Esmolol	Brevibloc
Metoprolol	Lopressor
Nadolol	Corgard
Pindolol[+]	Visken
Propranolol	Inderal

[+] Not recommended for angina

Antiarryhthmic Drugs

An **arrhythmia** is a dysfunction in the heart's beating or rhythm which is a result of an abnormal electrical conduction in the myocardium. The primary pacemaker of the heart (the S.A. node) sets the rate and keeps the other cells in the system from firing spontaneously. If the rhythm of the pacemaker is "out of sync" with spontaneously firing cells in the bundle of His or Purkinje fibers (or in the atria), an abnormal rhythm may develop. An arrhythmia can occur for various reasons. Basically, arrhythmias occur because certain regions of the heart are: (1) beating too slowly (sinus bradycardia), (2) beating too fast (sinus or ventricular tachycardia, atrial flutter, or premature ventricular tachycardia, atrial or ventricular premature depolarization), (3) beating automatically without regulation from the electrical impulses which originate from the natural pacemaker cells in the S.A. node (multifocal atrial tachycardia, atrial fibrillation, ventricular fibrillation), and (4) allowing impulses to travel along an **alternate pathway** of electrical conductance to areas of the heart leading to electrical disturbances (AV reentry, Wolf Parkinson White syndrome). Antiarrhythmic drugs are divided into classes (1 through 4) based on their mechanism of action.

Antiarrhythmic Drugs

Generic Name	Common Trade Name
Class 1A	
Disopyramide	Norpace
Procainamide	Pronestyl
Quinidine	Quinidex, Quinaglute
Class 1B	
Lidocaine	Xylocaine
Mexiletine	Mexitil
Phenytoin	Dilantin
Tocainide	Tonocard
Class 1C	
Flecainide	Tambocor
Class 2	
Esmolol	Brevibloc
Propranolol	Inderal
Class 3	
Amiodarone	Cordarone
Bretylium	Bretylol
Class 4	
Verapamil	Calan, Isoptin

Other Agents Used for Arrhythmia

Generic Name	Common Trade Name
Adenosine	Adenocard
Digoxin	Lanoxin
Moricizine	Ethmozine
Sotalol	Betapace

Anticoagulants/Antithrombics/Thrombolytics

Drugs known as **anticoagulants** inhibit the ability of the blood to form clots. Platelets (components of blood) can stick to vessel walls and initiate the formation of a **thrombus,** which is defined as a clot that is formed in a blood vessel or a heart chamber. A thrombus can stop or slow blood flow, which may result in tissue ischemia, stroke, and heart attack. **Antithrombotic** agents prevent platelet aggregation. **Thrombolytic** agents are drugs that degrade clots already formed.

Anticoagulants

Generic Name	Common Trade Name
Heparin	Liquaemin
Warfarin	Coumadin

Antithrombic Agents

Generic Name	Common Trade Name
Aspirin (*)	Aspirin
Dipyridamole	Persantine
Ticlopidine	Ticlid
Ibuprofen (*)	Motrin

Thrombolytic Agents

Generic Name	Common Trade Name
Streptokinase	Streptase
Tissue plasminogen activator	TPA
Urokinase	Abbokinase

Anticonvulsants

Anticonvulsants or antiepileptic drugs are agents used to control seizures. A seizure is defined as a sudden, excessive, and disorderly discharge of brain nerve cells (neurons). Seizures may be due to various causes: structural abnormalities, scars, tumors, inflammation, alteration in blood gasses, pH, electrolytes, or glucose availability. Types of seizures include generalized or grand mal, absence or petit mal, partial (simple and complex), and status epilepticus. It is important to determine the specific type of seizure exhibited by the patient because the choice of anticonvulsant therapy depends on seizure type.

Anticonvulsants

Generic Name	Common Trade Name
Carbamazepine	Tegretol
Clonazepam	Klonopin
Clorazepate	Tranxene
Diazepam	Valium
Ethosuximide	Zarontin
Fosphenytoin	Cerebyx

Generic Name	Common Trade Name
Gabapentin	Neurontin
Lamotrigine	Lamictal
Phenobarbital	Luminal
Phenytoin	Dilantin
Primidone	Mysoline
Valproic acid	Depakote

Antiemetics

Agents used to relieve symptoms of nausea and vomiting are called **antiemetics.** Vomiting (emesis) is triggered by activation of certain chemoreceptor trigger zones in the brain. Nausea and vomiting can be caused by a variety of conditions (e.g., pregnancy, motion sickness, general gastrointestinal distress, hepatitis). It may also be drug induced. Chemotherapy agents are especially notorious for causing nausea and vomiting. Drug-induced nausea and vomiting can be especially problematic when they lead to dehydration, electrolyte depletion, and metabolic imbalance. Drugs used to treat emesis span a wide variety of therapeutic classes.

Antiemetics

Generic Name	Common Trade Name
Dexamethasone	Decadron
Droperidol	Inapsine
Granisetron	Kytril
Metoclopramide	Reglan
Ondansetron	Zofran
Prochlorperazine	Compazine

Antihistamines and Decongestants

Histamine is a chemical messenger which controls a wide range of physiological responses associated with various medical conditions (inflammation, allergic reactions, hay fever, common colds, and motion sickness). Some histamine-like reactions include itching, rash, reddening, and inflammation of the skin. Antihistamines are divided into first generation and second generation classifications. The first generation antihistamines are more likely associated with sedating side effects. The second generation antihistamines are less sedating and usually longer acting.

Decongestants are agents commonly employed in cold remedies. They are vasoconstrictors, because they cause shrinkage of mucous membranes and improve air passage through the nose.

First Generation Antihistamines

Generic Name	Common Trade Name
Brompheniramine (*)	Dimetapp
Chlorpheniramine (*)	Chlor-Trimeton
Cyproheptadine	Periactin
Diphenhydramine (*)	Benadryl
Hydroxyzine	Atarax, Vistaril
Meclizine (*)	Antivert, Bonine
Promethazine	Phenergan
Pyrilamine	Rynatan (pyrilamine + other ingredients)
Tripelennamine	PBZ

Second Generation Antihistamines

Generic Name	Common Trade Name
Astemizole	Hismanal
Cetirizine	Zyrtec
Loratadine	Claritin

Decongestants

Generic Name	Common Trade Name
Ephedrine (*)	Bronkotabs (plus other ingredients)
Phenylepherine (*)	Neosynephrine
Phenylpropanolamine (*)	Comtrex (plus other ingredients)
Pseudoephedrine (*)	Sudafed

Antihypertensives

Hypertension is defined as sustained elevated diastolic pressure greater than 90 mm Hg, accompanied by elevated systolic blood pressure greater than 140 mm Hg. Elevated blood pressure can result from increased peripheral vascular smooth muscle tone and increased arterial resistance, which can result in vascular damage, thus compromising functions of the heart, brain, and kidneys. Hypertension can lead to congestive heart failure, myocardial infarction, renal damage, and stroke. The goal of drug therapy is to reduce blood pressure by reducing vascular volume using diuretics, by relaxing blood vessels using vasodilators, by inhibiting the sympathetic nervous system using blocking agents (beta blockers and nerve ending blockers), and by inhibiting the renal mechanism involved with the development of hypertension by using angiotensin converting enzyme inhibitors (ace inhibitors and angiotensin 2 receptor antagonists).

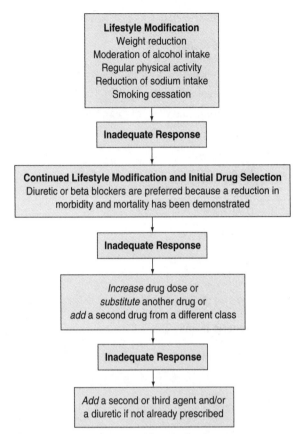

FIGURE 22–1 Stepwise approach to therapy for hypertension

Drug therapy of hypertension is usually individualized. A stepwise approach to patient care is initiated (**Figure 22–1**). Lifestyle modification (nondrug therapy) should be initiated before beginning drug therapy.

Diuretics

Generic Name	Common Trade Name
Bumetanide	Bumex
Furosemide	Lasix
Hydrochlorothiazide	Hydrodiuril, Esidrix
Spironolactone	Aldactone
Triamterene/Hydrochlorothiazide	Dyazide

Sympathetic Blocking Agents (B Blockers)

Generic Name	Common Trade Name
Atenolol	Tenormin
Labetalol	Trandate
Metoprolol	Lopressor

Generic Name	Common Trade Name
Nadolol	Corgard
Propranolol	Inderal
Timolol	Blocadren

Ace Inhibitors

Generic Name	Common Trade Name
Benazepril	Lotensin
Captopril	Capoten
Enalapril	Vasotec
Fosinopril	Monopril
Lisinopril	Prinivil, Zestril
Quinapril	Accupril

Angiotensin 2 Antagonists

Generic Name	Common Trade Name
Losartan	Cozaar

Calcium Channel Blockers

Generic Name	Common Trade Name
Amlodipine	Norvasc
Diltiazem	Cardizem
Felodipine	Plendil
Isradipine	DynaCirc
Nicardipine	Cardene
Nifedipine	Procardia
Nimodipine	Nimotop
Verapamil	Calan, Isoptin

Nerve Ending Blockers (Alpha Blockers)

Generic Name	Common Trade Name
Doxazosin	Cardura
Prazosin	Minipress
Terazosin	Hytrin

Direct Vasodilators

Generic Name	Common Trade Name
Diazoxide	Hyperstat
Hydralazine	Apresoline
Minoxidil	Loniten
Nitroprusside sodium	Nitropress

Other

Generic Name	Common Trade Name
Clonidine	Catapres
Methyldopa	Aldomet

Anti-Infectives/Antivirals/Antibiotics

Anti-infective and antibiotic drugs have the ability to destroy or inhibit the growth of microorganisms without destroying the host cells. They are selective in their toxicity. This selective toxicity does not mean that they are without side effects. Drug concentrations must be carefully controlled to maximize effectiveness and minimize side effects. Choice of anti-infective therapy depends on the following:

1. The *nature* of the infective microorganism and its *sensitivity* to various anti-infectives.
2. The *site of the infection*—the anti-infective agent must be able to reach the site of the infection in sufficient concentration to be effective. Many drugs are not able to cross into the brain and therefore are not effective for infections involving the central nervous system.
3. The *safety* of the anti-infective agent—some agents have more side effects and toxicity to organs than other agents. This difference in toxicity profile must be carefully considered when choosing an agent.
4. *Patient variable factors*—choice of agents always depends in part on the present physiological condition of the patient. Some antibiotics are not recommended for pediatrics (e.g., fluoroquinolones). Many agents require dose adjustments based on renal status or liver function.
5. *Economic factors*—the cost of an anti-infective agent is important. If the chosen antibiotic is too expensive, the patient may not purchase it or may purchase an insufficient quantity, thus leading to patient noncompliance.

Anti-infective agents are usually effective against certain types of microorganisms. Some agents are more selective than other agents. The identity and drug sensitivity of the microorganism must be determined as soon as possible so that the correct therapy will be chosen. Microbiological cultures of these organisms are obtained from the laboratory and drug sensitivities are determined to aid the clinician in determining the correct agent. Anti-infective agents are usually grouped based on their mechanism of action and structure. They can be either bacteriocidal (meaning they destroy the microorganisms) or bacteriostatic (inhibit the growth of microorganisms) in their mode of action.

Inhibitors of cell wall synthesis (penicillins, cephalosporins)

Penicillins and cephalosporins are perhaps the most widely used group of antibiotics. They are used for many different types of infections including respiratory, ear, urinary tract, central nervous system, and venereal infections. A major adverse reaction associated with penicillin is the hypersensitivity reaction, an allergic reaction which can prove to be fatal in some cases. If a patient is allergic to penicillin there may be a cross-sensitivity allergic reaction to cephalosporins. Caution should be exercised before prescribing a cephalosporin-type antibiotic to a penicillin-allergic patient.

Penicillins

Generic Name	Common Trade Name
Amoxicillin	Amoxil
Amoxicillin/Clavulanate	Augmentin
Ampicillin	Polycillin, Principen, Omnipen
Ampicillin/Sulbactam	Unasyn
Benzathine penicillin G	Various brands
Dicloxacillin	Dynapen
Methicillin	Various brands
Mezlocillin	Mezlin
Nafcillin	Unipen
Penicillin G	Various brands
Penicillin V	Various brands
Piperacillin	Pipracil
Piperacillin/Tazobactam	Zosyn
Procaine penicillin G	Various brands
Ticarcillin	Ticar
Ticarcillin/Clavulanate	Timentin
Related Agents	
Aztreonam	Azactam
Imipenem/Cilastatin	Primaxin

Cephalosporins

Generic Name	Common Trade Name
Cefaclor	Ceclor
Cefadroxil	Duricef
Cefamandole	Mandol
Cefazolin	Kefzol
Cefixime	Suprax
Cefoperazone	Cefobid
Cefotaxime	Claforan
Cefotetan	Cefotan
Cefoxitin	Mefoxin
Cefpodoxime	Vantin

Generic Name	Common Trade Name
Cefprozil	Cefzil
Ceftazidime	Fortaz
Ceftizoxime	Cefizox
Ceftriaxone	Rocephin
Cefuroxime	Zinacef, Ceftin
Cephalexin	Keflex
Cephalothin	Keflin
Cephradine	Velosef
Loracarbef	Lorabid

Folic acid antagonists

Folic acid is a necessary requirement for the production of bacterial DNA. Without folic acid, bacteria cannot grow and divide. Folic acid antagonists are drugs that specifically inhibit the production of folic acid in bacteria, preventing the multiplication of these bacteria. Folic acid antagonists are used in many different types of infections (e.g., urinary tract, skin, gastrointestinal, and respiratory infections).

Folate Antagonists

Generic Name	Common Trade Name
Silver sulfadiazine	Silvadene
Sulfacetamide	Bleph 10, Sulamyd
Sulfamethoxazole/Trimethoprim	Bactrim, Septra, Co-trimoxazole
Sulfasalazine	Azulfidine
Sulfisoxazole	Gantrisin
Trimethoprim	Trimpex

Protein synthesis inhibitors

Bacterial growth requires the production of certain proteins which are necessary for growth and division. Protein synthesis occurs inside the bacterial cell in the ribosomes. Certain antibiotics inhibit the ribosomal production of proteins and thus retard the growth of bacteria. These antibiotics are usually "broad spectrum" in that they are effective against a wide variety of bacterial infections (e.g., chlamydia, Rocky Mountain spotted fever, Lyme disease, cholera). Protein synthesis inhibitors include tetracycline, aminoglycosides, macrolides, chloramphenicol, and clindamycin.

Tetracyclines

Generic Name	Common Trade Name
Demeclocycline	Declomycin
Doxycycline	Vibramycin
Minocycline	Minocin
Tetracycline	Achromycin

Aminoglycosides

Generic Name	Common Trade Name
Amikacin	Amikin
Gentamicin	Garamycin
Neomycin	Mycifradin
Netilmicin	Netromycin
Streptomycin	Various brands
Tobramycin	Nebcin

Macrolides

Generic Name	Common Trade Name
Azithromycin	Zithromax
Clarithromycin	Biaxin
Erythromycin	Eryc, E-Mycin, Illotycin

Miscellaneous

Generic Name	Common Trade Name
Chloramphenicol	Chloromycetin
Clindamycin	Cleocin

Urinary tract antiseptics and fluoroquinolones

Fluoroquinolone antibiotics exert their effect by inhibiting the replication of bacterial DNA. These agents have primarily been employed to treat urinary tract infections, but have also been used in respiratory and gastrointestinal infections.

Fluoroquinolones

Generic Name	Common Trade Name
Ciprofloxacin	Cipro
Enoxacin	Penetrex
Lomefloxacin	Maxaquin
Nalidixic acid	NegGram
Norfloxacin	Noroxin
Ofloxacin	Floxin

Urinary Tract Antiseptics

Generic Name	Common Trade Name
Methenamine	Urised, Hiprex
Nitrofurantoin	Macrodantin

Antimicrobial agents

Antimicrobial drugs are useful in treating tuberculosis (TB) and leprosy. In recent years there has been a resurgence of TB largely due to the emergence of resistant microorganisms. Multidrug usage has become the mainstay of therapy to increase effectiveness and decrease microbial resistance.

Drugs for TB

Generic Name	Common Trade Name
Aminosalicylic acid	Various brands
Cycloserine	Seromycin
Ethambutol	Myambutol
Isoniazid	INH
Pyrazinamide	Various brands
Rifampin	Rifadin

Drugs for Hansen's Disease (Leprosy)

Generic Name	Common Trade Name
Clofazimine	Lamprene
Dapsone	Avlosulfon

Antifungal agents

Antifungal drugs are used to treat infections caused by fungi (e.g., candida albicans, aspergillis). Fungal infections can be superficial and confined to the skin or have systemic involvement (severe infections).

Antifungal Agents

Generic Name	Common Trade Name
Amphotericin B	Fungizone, Abelcet
Fluconazole	Diflucan
Flucytosine	Ancobon
Itraconazole	Sporanox
Ketoconazole	Nizoral
Clotrimazole	Lotrimin, Mycelex
Econazole	Spectazole
Griseofulvin	Fluvicin, Grisactin
Miconazole	Monistat
Nystatin	Mycostatin

Antiprotazoal agents

Antiprotazoal agents are used to treat infections caused by parasites (e.g., amebiasis, giardia, malaria, toxoplasmosis).

Antiprotazoal Agents

Generic Name	Common Trade Name
Chloroquine	Aralen
Metronidazole	Flagyl
Pentamidine	Pentam 300
Primaquine	Various brands
Pyrimethamine	Daraprim

Antiviral agents

Antiviral agents are useful in treating infections caused by a virus (human immunodeficiency virus [HIV], cytomegalovirus, herpes).

Antiviral Drugs

Generic Name	Common Trade Name
Acyclovir	Zovirax
Amantadine	Symmetrel
Didanosine	Videx
Famciclovir	Famvir
Foscarnet	Foscavir
Ganciclovir	Cytovene
Ribavirin	Virazole
Rimantadine	Flumadine
Stavudine	Zerit
Trifluridine	Viroptic
Vidarabine	Vira-A
Zalcitabine	Hivid
Zidovudine	Retrovir

Antineoplastics

Antineoplastic drugs are "cell toxins" used to treat cancer. Cancerous tumors are derived from normal cells which have undergone abnormal growth. Antineoplastic agents affect both normal cells and cancerous cells because they are difficult to selectively distinguish. Antineoplastic agents usually work by affecting some portion of the "cell growth cycle," which is accomplished primarily by damaging cellular DNA and/or affecting DNA repair of cells. Some antineoplastic agents may also work by inhibiting hormones responsible for tumor activation or by blocking specific binding sites (receptors) on cell surfaces and thus preventing the activation of tumor-promoting agents. Antineoplastic drugs are extremely toxic and can cause many adverse effects (e.g., hair loss, nausea, vomiting, bone marrow depression, anemia, mouth sores).

Antineoplastics

Generic Name	Common Trade Name
5-Fluorouracil	5-FU
Asparaginase	Elspar
Bleomycin	Blenoxane
Busulfan	Myleran
Carboplatin	Paraplatin
Carmustine	BiCNU
Chlorambucil	Leukeran
Cisplatin	Platinol
Cladribine	Leustatin
Cyclophosphamide	Cytoxan
Cytarabine	Cytosar-U
Dacarbazine	DTIC-Dome
Dactinomycin	Actinomycin D
Doxorubicin	Adriamycin
Estramustine	Emcyt
Etoposide	VePesid
Fludarabine	Fludara
Flutamide	Eulexin
Goserelin	Zoladex
Hydroxyurea	Hydrea
Idarubicin	Idamycin
Ifosfamide	Ifex
Interferon	Betaseron, Actimmune, Intron-A
Leuprolide	Lupron
Levamisole	Ergamisol
Lomustine	CeeNu
Mercaptopurine	Purinethol
Methotrexate	Rheumatrex
Mitomycin	Mutamycin
Mitoxantrone	Novantrone
Paclitaxel	Taxol
Procarbazine	Matulane
Tamoxifen	Nolvadex
Teniposide	Vumon
Thiotepa	Thioplex
Vinblastine	Velban
Vincristine	Oncovin
Vinorelbine	Navelbine

Antitussives

The cough reflex is an important protective reflex. It can help clear the secretions or dislodge foreign matter from the respiratory tract. If cough becomes severe and impinges on the performance of daily functions (work, sleep) it becomes necessary to inhibit this reflex. Coughs can be induced by irritations to the throat or by common cold symptoms produced by a release of histamine (postnasal drip). In these instances, a cough syrup containing an antihistamine may be effective to dry the nasal secretions. Many cough-control products are in combination with guaifenesin, an expectorant.

Other coughs involve irritation of the cough control center in the brain. These types of coughs may require narcotics (e.g., codeine, hydrocodone, or hydromorphone), which decrease the sensitivity of the central cough center to peripheral stimulation and decrease mucosal secretions. These agents can cause central nervous system depression and constipation. Dextromethorphan, a synthetic derivative of codeine, suppresses the response of the central cough center. It does not cause the CNS depression or constipating effects of the codeine derivatives.

Antitussives

Generic Name	Common Trade Name
Codeine plus expectorants	Tussi-Organidin NR
Guaifenesin plus codeine	Robitussin A-C
Guaifenesin (*)	Robitussin
Guaifenesin plus antihistamine or decongestants, or cough suppressant (*)	Robitussin CF, Robitussin DM
Hydrocodone plus decongestant or antihistamines	Hycomine, Tussionex

Bronchodilators

Bronchodilators relax the bronchial smooth muscle and reverse bronchoconstriction, which is the hallmark of chronic obstructive lung disease (COPD) and asthma. Other factors associated with chronic lung disease include loss of lung elasticity and chronic inflammation. Chronic inflammation can result from constant exposure to irritants (e.g., cigarette smoke, environmental pollutants), constricted bronchial passages, or increased secretions. Bronchodilators cause the relaxation of bronchial muscle and induce bronchodilation.

Bronchodilators

Generic Name	Common Trade Name
Albuterol	Ventolin, Proventil
Bitolterol	Tornalate
Epinephrine	Primatene
Ipratropium	Atrovent
Isoetharine	Bronkosol
Isoproterenol	Isuprel
Metaproterenol	Alupent

Generic Name	Common Trade Name
Pirbuterol	Maxair
Salmeterol	Serevent
Terbutaline	Brethaire, Brethine
Theophylline	Theo-Dur

Other drugs used in bronchial disorders include agents that decrease the inflammatory response (e.g., steroids and inflammatory cell stabilizers).

Steroids

Generic Name	Common Trade Name
Beclomethasone	Beclovent
Dexamethasone	Decadron
Flunisolide	AeroBid
Triamcinolone	Azmacort

Inflammatory Cell Stabilizers

Generic Name	Common Trade Name
Cromolyn	Intal
Nedocromil	Tilade

Cardiac Stimulants and Drugs Used in Heart Failure

Cardiac stimulants are used in emergency situations to stimulate the heart in conditions such as cardiac arrest. They can increase the contractility of the heart and allow for an increase in cardiac output. Many cardiac stimulants are also used to treat shock.

Heart failure occurs when the heart can no longer pump enough blood to meet the metabolic demands of the body. It can often result from prolonged and severe hypertension. Drug therapy for congestive heart failure (CHF) involves improving myocardial contractility (improving the pumping action of the heart).

Cardiac Stimulants

Generic Name	Common Trade Name
Dobutamine	Dobutrex
Dopamine	Intropin
Epinepherine	Various brands
Isoproterenol	Isuprel
Norepinepherine	Levophed

Heart Failure Drugs

Generic Name	Common Trade Name
Amrinone	Inocor
Digoxin	Lanoxin
Dobutrex	Dobutamine
Milrinone	Primacor

Drugs Affecting the Central Nervous System

Hypnotics, Anxiolytics, Sedatives, Tranquilizers, Antiparkinson Agents

Hypnotics and sedatives are drugs intended to produce sleep. These agents are usually not intended for long-term use. Many of the agents in this group are also anxiolytic agents. Anxiety is an unpleasant state of tension, apprehension, or uneasiness that may arise from a known or unknown source. Anxiolytic agents are intended to reduce anxiety and restlessness, and produce a feeling of "calm." Tranquilizers are drugs intended to produce a sense of detached calmness without mental depression. These agents are used in the treatment of mental and emotional disorders.

Anxiolytic Agents and Hypnotics

Generic Name	Common Trade Name
Alprazolam	Xanax
Buspirone	BuSpar
Chlordiazepoxide	Librium
Clonazepam	Klonopin
Diazepam	Valium
Flurazepam	Dalmane
Hydroxyzine	Vistaril, Atarax
Lorazepam	Ativan
Midazolam	Versed
Temazepam	Restoril
Triazolam	Halcion
Zolpidem	Ambien

Barbiturates

Generic Name	Common Trade Name
Amobarbital	Amytal
Pentobarbital	Nembutal
Phenobarbital	Luminal
Secobarbital	Seconal
Thiopental	Pentothal

Nonbarbiturate Sedatives

Generic Name	Common Trade Name
Chloral hydrate	Noctec

Tranquilizers/Antipsychotics

Generic Name	Common Trade Name
Chlorpromazine	Thorazine
Fluphenazine	Prolixin
Haloperidol	Haldol
Loxapine	Loxitane
Thioridazine	Mellaril
Thiothixene	Navane
Trifluoperazine	Stelazine

Antiparkinson's Agents

Parkinsonism is a progressive neurological disorder of muscle movement. This disease is characterized by tremors, muscle rigidity, and bradykinesia (slowness in initiating and carrying out voluntary movements). The cause of Parkinsonism has been linked to a deficiency in a substance called dopamine, an important chemical messenger in the brain. The primary goal of drug therapy is to restore dopamine levels in the brain.

Currently available drugs used to treat Parkinsonism will only offer temporary relief. They will not alter or reverse the disease process.

Generic Name	Common Trade Name
Amantadine	Symmetrel
Bromocriptine	Parlodel
Levodopa	Larodopa
Levodopa/Carbidopa	Sinemet
Selegiline	Eldepryl

Hormones

Hormones are chemical messengers produced by the body to regulate various metabolic functions. In certain disease states the supply of these natural chemical messengers is diminished or absent. Some examples of hormones and their functions are as follows:

- Growth hormone regulates growth.
- Thyroid hormone regulates the activity of many metabolic functions.
- Corticotropin regulates corticosteroid release from the adrenal gland which regulates blood pressure and the ability of the body to withstand stress.

- Oxytocin induces uterine contraction during labor.
- Estrogen and progesterone regulate ovarian function.
- Testosterone regulates male sexual response.
- Insulin from the pancreas regulates blood glucose, etc.

The preceding examples are only a few of the important hormones that play a role in normal metabolic function. The deficiency of these hormones can lead to such conditions as hypertension, diabetes, and sexual dysfunction. Hormones can be supplemented in the form of drugs.

Hormone Replacement Agents

Generic Name	Common Trade Name
Steroid replacement	
Dexamethasone	Decadron
Fludrocortisone	Florinef
Hydrocortisone	Hydrocort
Prednisone	Deltasone
Thyroid replacement	
Levothyroxine	Synthroid
Liothyronine	Cytomel
Liotrix	Thyrolar

Insulin and oral hypoglycemic drugs

Insulin, a hormone secreted by the pancreas, plays a major role in the regulation of blood glucose. An absolute or relative lack of insulin can cause diabetes mellitus, a disorder characterized by an elevation in blood glucose. Diabetes can be life threatening without proper treatment.

Diabetes can be divided into two groups, insulin-dependent diabetes mellitus (IDDM or Type I) and noninsulin-dependent diabetes mellitus (NIDDM or Type II). Insulin-dependent diabetes most commonly afflicts children, but can occur in adults. The disease is characterized by an absolute deficiency of insulin. Type I diabetic patients require treatment with insulin injections to avoid hyperglycemia (high blood glucose).

In Type II diabetes or noninsulin-dependent diabetes, the pancreas still retains some function and can secrete variable levels of insulin. The goal in treating Type II diabetes is to maintain blood glucose concentrations within normal limits and prevent the development of long-term complications of the disease. Weight reduction, exercise, and diet modifications are necessary; however, pharmacological intervention with oral hypoglycemic agents may also be necessary.

Insulin Preparations

Generic Name	Common Trade Name
Human insulin	Humulin
Insulin zinc insulin, Isophane insulin,	Iletin
Protamine zinc insulin, Semilente insulin,	
Ultralente insulin, Zinc insulin	

Oral Hypoglycemic Agents

Generic Name	Common Trade Name
Acarbose	Precose
Acetohexamide	Dymelor
Chlorpropamide	Diabinese
Glipizide	Glucotrol
Glyburide	Micronase, DiaBeta
Metformin	Glucophage
Tolazamide	Tolinase
Tolbutamide	Orinase
Troglitazone	Rezulin

Laxatives

Constipation can be caused by various factors (e.g., low fiber diets, certain drugs, prolonged immobilization). Laxatives are used to speed the transit of food through the gastrointestinal tract and reverse constipation. Some of these agents are termed mild laxatives, and include **bulk forming** agents used for constipation of short duration. Other types of laxatives are stronger or **stimulant type** laxatives used for more prolonged constipation. Other agents used in constipation are called **stool softeners.** These agents interact with the feces and produce softer stools and easier passage of feces through the colon.

Bulk Forming Laxatives

Generic Name	Common Trade Name
Calcium polycarbophil	Mitrolan
Methylcellulose	Cologel
Psyllium	Metamucil

Stimulant Laxatives

Generic Name	Common Trade Name
Bisacodyl	Dulcolax
Senna	Senokot

Stool Softners/Other

Generic Name	Common Trade Name
Docusate	Colace
Glycerin	Various brands
Lactulose	Chronulac
Mineral oil	Various brands
Saline solutions	Milk of Magnesia, Citrate of Magnesia

Pharmaceuticals Developed through Biotechnology

Biotechnology methods are used in the development and production of many new drugs. This technology involves the use of recombinant DNA technology. The first DNA recombination experiments involved inserting a mammalian gene (a segment of DNA) coding for a specific protein into a bacterial host. The bacteria replicated this gene and produced the desired protein. Recombinant DNA technology provides a mechanism to "copy" naturally occurring proteins in large quantities. The first proteins to be made by recombinant DNA technology were human insulin and human growth hormone.

Each year many new agents are produced by recombinant DNA technology. These agents are useful in the treatment of a wide variety of medical disorders (e.g., cancer, anemia, hepatitis).

Summary

The information in this chapter will serve to provide the pharmacy technician with the basic knowledge necessary to assist the pharmacist in the task of preparing and dispensing medication. Many new drugs are marketed each year. Technicians must continually update their drug knowledge to keep informed of the new drugs and new dosage forms.

ASSESSMENT

Multiple Choice Questions

1. Which route of administration allows a drug to bypass the first pass liver destruction?
    a. p.o.
    b. s.l.
    c. neither a nor b

2. The method of drug administration most often used in emergency situations when immediate onset of action is required is
    a. I.M.
    b. I.V.
    c. p.o.
    d. none of the above

3. The presence of food in the stomach can influence the absorption of certain drugs
    a. True
    b. False

4. Drug-drug interactions can occur due to competition for liver metabolism sites
    a. True
    b. False

5. Which drug is considered a "strong narcotic" reserved for severe pain?
   a. Naproxen
   b. Acetaminophen
   c. Propoxyphene
   d. Morphine

6. An agent classified as a general anesthetic is
   a. Amikacin
   b. Halothane
   c. Warfarin
   d. Phenytoin

7. Cimetidine, Ranitidine, and Famotidine are classified as
   a. diuretics
   b. H2 blockers
   c. psychotropics
   d. anti-inflamatory agents

8. Which of the following drugs is used in congestive heart failure?
   a. Diphenhydramine
   b. Amitriptyline
   c. Acyclovir
   d. Digoxin

9. Each of these drugs is a diuretic except
   a. Furosemide
   b. Triamterene
   c. Spironolactone
   d. Vinblastine

10. Each of these drugs is a beta lactam antibiotic drug except
    a. Amoxicillin
    b. Erythromycin
    c. Dicloxacillin
    d. Piperacillin

11. Diazepam and Lorazepam are considered useful agents in treating
    a. congestive heart failure
    b. infections
    c. anxiety
    d. angina

12. Which agent is useful in treating TB?
    a. Doxycycline
    b. Penicillin
    c. Furosemide
    d. Isoniazid

13. Which agent is considered an antiviral drug?
    a. Phenobarbital
    b. Meclizine
    c. Acyclovir
    d. Cisplatin

14. Which drug can be used as part of a cancer chemotherapy regime?
    a. Meprobamate
    b. Vinblastine
    c. Bumetanide
    d. Hydralazine

15. Which drug can be used in treating asthma?
    a. Albuterol
    b. 5 Fluorouracil
    c. Chlorpromazine
    d. Captopril

Matching

Generic Name		Trade Name	
16. __f__	Propranolol	a.	Dalmane
17. __e__	Digoxin	b.	Hydrodiuril
18. __d__	Zidovudine	c.	Thorazine
19. __g__	Acetaminophen	d.	Retrovir
20. __h__	Warfarin	e.	Lanoxin
21. __i__	Meperidine	f.	Inderal

22. ___j___   Theophylline   g.   Tylenol
23. ___c___   Chlorpromazine   h.   Coumadin
24. ___b___   Hydrochlorothiazide   i.   Demerol
25. ___a___   Flurazepam   j.   Theodur

Bibliography

Goodman, L.S., & Gillman, A. (eds.) (1996). *The pharmacological basis of therapeutics* (9th ed.). New York: McGraw Hill.

Harvey, R., & Champe, P. (eds.). (1997). *Lippincott's illustrated reviews pharmacology* (2nd ed.). New York: Lippincott Raven Publishers.

Rakel, R. (1998). *Conn's current therapy.* Philadelphia: W.B. Saunders Publishers.

Woods, A.L. (1994). *The nurse's drug handbook* (7th ed.). New York: Delmar Publishers.

Administration of Medications

COMPETENCIES

Upon completion and review of this chapter, the student should be able to

1. Specify the drug information that should be reviewed by the health care practitioner prior to administering a drug to a patient.

2. Describe the clinical and/or technical concerns required for administering medications by the following routes: oral, topical, rectal, vaginal, intraocular, intranasal, into the ear.

3. Identify five methods in which the person administering medications can reduce medication errors.

4. Discuss the characteristics and professional concerns of a drug administrator/drug technician.

5. Differentiate the directions that should be given to a patient receiving a buccal tablet and a gelatin capsule.

6. Differentiate labeling requirements between internal and external drug preparations.

7. List five situations in which a drug is discontinued or drug administration is interrupted.

8. Describe the procedure to be followed if a patient states "I cannot swallow that large tablet."

9. Discuss some causes of medication errors. Explain the universal policy to be observed if a medication error is detected.

10. List the requirements for each health care practitioner who accepts the responsibility for the administration of medications.

Introduction

This chapter focuses on the clinical, professional, and technical aspects of medication **administration.** While policies and procedures vary from institution to institution (and the institution's policy takes precedence over what is written here), the person who administers medications must always respect the dignity, privacy, safety, and autonomy of the patient. Patient cooperation is essential to the administration of most forms of medications. Even those patients who appear comatose, confused, or otherwise compromised should have the proposed procedure explained to them. Each health care practitioner who accepts the responsibility for the administration of medications must become familiar with the patient population, with the institution's policies concerning medications, with the approved methods of medication administration, with the formulary and other resources that are available for reference and information, and with the institution's expectations of the person who administers medications. All are most serious responsibilities.

Medication Orders

Drug administration is initiated with the physician's (prescriber's) order. No drug is given to a patient without physician authorization. There are a number of different kinds of medication orders. Orders written in the chart at the time of admission, which may be subsequently increased, decreased, or deleted, are the most common type of medication orders. Other types of drug orders include verbal orders that may be given by the physician to a nurse or pharmacist, usually via the phone, when unusual circumstances arise. Prior to initiation, verbal orders should be repeated to the prescriber. Verbal orders are always reduced to writing in the patient's chart, signed by the order taker, and co-signed by the physician on the next visit to the hospital. Verbal orders should be co-signed by the physician within 24 hours or as specified by hospital policy.

Stat orders are orders for drugs that should be immediately administered. The immediacy relates to the patient's condition such as pain relief, clinical distress, drug or allergic reaction. The person administering drugs always gives top priority to making sure the patient receives a "stat" drug in timely fashion. *PRN* orders are written by the physician to be given to the patient only if required by the patient's condition. Standing orders sometimes accompany a patient on admission to the hospital or are the printed drug regimens prescribed by the physician or a physician group to treat particular conditions (e.g., women who are admitted to the obstetrical unit preceding childbirth). These orders may be prewritten and signed by the physician or stamped on the chart with the physician's signature.

Hospital policy may permit drug orders to be written by persons other than medical physicians including **physician assistants,** clinical nurse practitioners, dentists, **podiatrists,** and pharmacists. These policies must be known and observed.

Information Needed on Drug Order

To properly administer a drug, the following information is needed for each drug order:

- patient's full name, room number, and bed number
- name of drug (clearly written), dosage strength (e.g., 10 mg), dosage schedule (e.g., q.d., stat, t.i.d.)
- route of administration (e.g., sublingual, subcutaneous, instill in left eye)
- length of time drug is to be given (e.g., for 24 hours, 1 week, length of hospital stay, as needed)
- prescriber's signature

The drug order is entered into the patient's medication order forms and transmitted to the pharmacy to be filled. The person who administers the drug verifies the label on the drug by comparing it with the order on the patient's medication record.

The Medication Administrator or Medication Technician

The person who will administer drugs to the patient should be in good health, free of communicable infections (a head cold, a sore throat, an open lesion). This is of importance for both the patient and the drug administrator. Patients are susceptible to **nosocomial** infections. Often the patient is weak, has had surgery or radiation therapy, and the immune system may be compromised for these or other reasons (e.g., aging process, malnutrition). The drug administrator who is at a low physical ebb due to exhaustion or poor health is more likely to make a drug administration error than a person who is well, alert, and fully attentive. In addition, a drug administrator (e.g., nurse, pharmacist, technician) who is in poor health is more apt to pick up an infection from a patient. So it is important for any person who gives direct patient care to assure and maintain good health through proper nutrition, exercise, and healthy living habits. In case of an upper respiratory infection or other indisposition the drug administrator should inform the supervisor for a change of assignment away from direct patient care for the duration of the illness. If the patient is in isolation due to an infectious, transmittable disease, the drug administrator should follow hospital policy regarding use of gloves and masks when giving direct patient care. In all events the person who is about to administer drugs should thoroughly wash his or her hands before handling any drugs and rewash the hands between patients when hospital policy or aseptic technique requires it.

The **medication technician** or **medication administrator** should appreciate the responsibility inherent in the role. This person should be knowledgeable about the responsibilities of the other members of the health team regarding drug administration and be able to communicate with them. The medication technician should always give priority to patient care, treating each patient with dignity and professional concern regardless of physical or mental impairment, lifestyle orientation/religious beliefs, or cultural background. It is necessary that the medication technician be totally familiar with the policies and procedures that prevail in a particular hospital and always know the physician, nurse, or pharmacist to whom he or she directly reports. Any unusual physical or emotional change noted by the technician during medication rounds should be immediately reported to the charge nurse. Professional confidentiality regarding any patient in the technician's care is of prime importance. Patients at all times have a right to have personal matters respected and held in confidence. Technicians should report to work dressed in professional attire, with name identification badge, in keeping with the dignity of the position and the respect they should expect from others.

Administration of the Drug

Patient Rights

Nearly every patient in the hospital will receive drugs during the stay. Each patient is entitled to the "five rights" for safe, appropriate drug administration. Drug rights of the patient include the right drug, right dose, right dosage form or right dosage route, right time, and administered to the right patient. These rights should be memorized and checked prior to each drug administration.

Right Patient

The first right requirement is to verify that the right patient is the one to receive the drug. The patient should be addressed by his or her name and then the patient identification arm band should be checked. Just addressing the person by name is not sufficient. Persons may respond positively, even if they have not clearly heard their name due to distractions, deafness, or language barriers. Beds are often shifted to different positions in the room, so identifying a person as the patient in room 120 bed 3 is insufficient information and may be misleading.

The Right Drug

The right drug is verified by checking the physician's (prescriber's) order sheet and the nurse's (or pharmacist's) drug administration form or drug cardex or drug summary on computer profile. Thousands of drugs are available and many sound alike, are spelled alike, and look alike. One or two letters in a name can mean an entirely different drug. The prescriber must be contacted if there are any questions or doubts concerning the order. Most drugs used in hospitals today are in unit-dose packages. The name is clearly visible on each drug dosage form. Labels should be checked three times before the drug is administered.

The Right Dose

Accurate **dosage strength** is critical to beneficial drug administration. Giving the wrong strength, particularly to children or infants, can be and has been fatal. The right dose is further checked with special care given to decimal points. A zero before the decimal (e.g., 0.1 mg) should be noted; care should be given if there is a zero after the decimal, which can be misleading (e.g., 1.0 is one not ten). Drug firms have addressed this problem and now label their drugs accordingly.

Proper dosage strength should never be presumed by anyone in the prescribing, dispensing, and administering process. Physicians must clearly indicate the desired strength on the medication order; pharmacists are expected to further verify dosage to be sure it is within appropriate therapeutic limits; nurses are expected to further check that the dosage strength ordered by the physician was accurately dispensed by the pharmacist or pharmacy technician. After the drug and dosage strength have gone through these three checkpoints, the last checkpoint resides with the person who administers the drug to the patient. If any dosage changes have been made along the way, the change should be clearly indicated on the patient's chart and other medication records.

Right Dosage Form

In addition to assurance that the right drug in the right strength has been selected, it is important to check and be sure that the drug is in the right dosage form. Drugs come in many different dosage forms. Liquids come as solutions, tinctures, suspensions, syrups, and elixirs. Oral solid dosage forms come as **tablets,** gelatin **capsules, caplets, enteric-coated tablets, extended-release capsules,** sublingual tablets, and buccal tablets. External preparations include creams, ointments, and lotions. Some medications in ointment form contain potent active ingredients. The length of the ointment strip must be carefully measured by the drug administrator. Injectable medications must be carefully checked to be sure whether the injection should be administered by intramuscular, intravenous, subcutaneous, or other route of administration. Drop-type drugs must be checked and used only as indicated for the eye, ear, or nose. There are many suppository dosage forms, such as rectal, vaginal, urethral. Dosage forms are NOT interchangeable, so it is important that it is the right drug, administered in the right dosage form. It is also important to note when a drug dosage form has been changed by the prescriber [e.g., an injectable drug (I.M.) is changed to an oral dosage (p.o.)]. Every drug order should include the route of administration. If a question arises, proper dosage form should be confirmed before the drug is administered.

Right Time

Time of drug administration (i.e., **dosage schedule** or frequency) is an important factor in pharmacotherapy. Drugs should be given at the time ordered—with an ordinary deviation of a half hour, unless timing is critical. Diabetics should always receive their **hypoglycemic** drugs a half hour before meals, unless otherwise specified. Patients on therapeutic drug monitoring are involved in pharmacokinetic laboratory studies. Dosage time is related to drug half-life and the time the phlebotomist will draw the blood for the serum analysis. Time of drug administration can be a critical factor in pharmacokinetic laboratory results. Time of a drug can be of great concern to the patient who is waiting. A patient who has been ordered an analgesic for the relief of pain to be given every 4 hours for the first 24 hours after the operation should receive this drug on time. Delays for this patient increase the pain and anxiety and slow the recovery process.

Review

Prior to drug administration the medication technician should become familiar with the following information regarding the drug:

- general and special uses or indications
- usual dose or dosage range
- special precautions (e.g., do not give with food; observe patient for rash)
- side effects that may occur
- foods or drugs that should not be given with the drug
- time when onset of action is expected

By reviewing this information before administering the drug, mistakes and errors can be avoided and the patient's well-being better ensured. Hospital policy will indicate how involved the medication technician becomes in providing this information to the patient. Generally the registered nurse or the pharmacist has the responsibility to answer drug information questions and to counsel the patient on proper drug use.

Oral Drug Administration

After the patient has been properly identified, the patient is either given the medication to swallow, to place under the tongue (sublingual), or to place between the cheek and the gum (buccal tablets) or the medication is appropriately injected, inserted, instilled, or inhaled in case of respiratory drug therapy. If the patient is to self-administer an oral tablet, the nurse, pharmacist, or technician should remain with the patient until the drug has been swallowed. Drugs are never left at the patient's bedside without a doctor's order. Drugs left at the bedside may be forgotten, may be discarded, or may be hoarded for future use. The patient should be instructed to place a sublingual tablet (e.g., nitroglycerine) under the tongue and leave it there until it dissolves. A patient ordered a buccal tablet should be told to place the tablet between the gum and the cheek and also allow it to dissolve. Throat and/or mouth troches or lozenges should not be swallowed or chewed but allowed to remain in the oral cavity until dissolved. In the case of a medicated mouthwash used for oral and throat infections, the patient should be told to swish the liquid around in the mouth and then either swallow or expectorate according to the nature of the substance and the dosage directions.

Usually the patient should be given an adequate amount of water (at least 4 ounces) to allow for easy swallowing, dissolution of the tablet or capsule, and prevention of esophageal erosion. Esophageal erosion can occur when an oral medication lodges and remains in the esophagus and does not move into the stomach. Particular care must be given to tablets with a corrosive potential, such as a compressed potassium chloride tablet.

The exceptions to the rule for administering sufficient water with an oral dosage form are in the cases of cough syrups intended to soothe and work in the throat area, medicated mouthwashes intended to be swallowed or expectorated, and after administering either a buccal or sublingual tablet. There are times when a liquid other than water may be indicated. If there is no contraindication, the patient may prefer to follow the drug with milk or a fruit juice. However, there are some definite contraindications. The person administering the drug should know the liquids that should not be administered with particular medications (e.g., fruit juices and sodas, such as cola beverages, should never be given with penicillin tablets; milk or milk products should not be given with the mycin-type antibiotics or certain laxatives, such as Dulcolax™).

Before leaving the patient, the person administering the drug should make sure the patient has taken the drug and has had no difficulty in swallowing the medication or following other instructions. If the patient asks questions about the drugs, an adequate answer should be given. If the person administering the drug is limited either on time or knowledge when the question was asked, a follow-up visit should be made. But such answers as "that is what the doctor orders" or "this is given to you to make you feel better" are not adequate answers. They are in fact dismissing the patient's questions and need for information. The patient is entitled to information regarding the drugs he or she is ordered. In most cases the technician will refer these questions to the nurse or pharmacist responsible for the care of the patient who will further discuss the question.

Topical Drug Administration

A topical drug is one applied to the skin. The person applying an ointment should wear disposable gloves. The area should be cleaned and any remaining ointment removed. Ointments should be applied in thin layers using cotton swabs or a tongue depressor. Liquid medications such as lotions and suspensions should first be shaken well and then applied as directed with quick sprays. Both the patient and the drug administrator should be careful not to inhale the aerosol spray. In some cases directions may require that the area be covered with sterile gauze after application. Special care should be given to burn-injured patients, because they are most susceptible to infections.

Eyedrop and Eye Ointment Application

Always aseptically clean hands by a good scrub or wear disposable gloves before instilling eyedrops. To preserve the cleanliness of the delivery orifice, do not touch the tip of the dropper or container to the patient's eye or an external surface.

Position the patient with head back. The lower lid can gently be pulled forward to create a well into which the drop or drops can be inserted. Accurately apply the drop or number of drops as directed. Many eyedrops have systemic effects; therefore, additional drops should not be given. Before the drops are administered, check the label for name and strength and directions for use, including which eye;

or if directed, both eyes should be treated. Check labels for expiration date. Never use any expired drug. If an ointment is used, apply a thin line of ointment to the slightly retracted lower lid without allowing the tip of the tube to touch the eye. After instillation of either eyedrops or ointment, instruct the patient to close the eye for a few minutes to permit the dispersion of the drug through the eye. If a tear appears, wipe it away with sterile gauze. If there is any noticeable change in the eye (increased redness, discharge, or signs of irritation), report it right away to the supervising nurse or pharmacist.

Administration of Ear and Nose Preparation

To instill eardrops, the patient should be sitting with the unaffected ear on the shoulder, or lying down with the affected ear facing up. For an adult the ear should be gently pulled up and back, and for a child the ear gently pulled down and back, to make the ear canal more accessible. Drops are inserted directly into the canal without touching the tip of the dropper or nozzle to the ear. The patient should remain positioned for a few minutes to keep the drops from running out of the ear. If a cotton plug is ordered, it should be sterile and gently placed just at the opening of the canal. Administer only the prescribed number of drops after carefully reading the label.

Nose drops should be applied with the head resting on the back of the neck. The patient should be instructed to breathe through the mouth. Instill the required number of drops and instruct the patient to keep his or her head back a few minutes and not to blow the nose for a few minutes. Nose sprays are used with the patient's head in an upright position. The spray is applied by squeezing the applicator bottle quickly and firmly while it is placed in the tip of the nostril. Repeat the process with other nostril. Use only as directed, because active ingredients in the spray enter directly into the circulatory system and may have untoward systemic effects. Other drugs in nebulizer form come with specific instructions in the package insert. These should be carefully followed to properly administer the drugs.

Application of Transdermal Drugs

Transdermal drugs, often called drug patches, consist of an active drug ingredient inside a patch held in place by small adhesive tapes. The drug is applied externally for internal or **systemic action.** A drug such as nitroglycerine (for chest pain) is placed in a transdermal patch on the skin where it is picked up by the bloodstream for action over a sustained period of time. The area where the patch is applied should be clearly dry and free of hair (e.g., upper arm or inside forearm). The patch should not be applied to any area that is irritated, calloused, or scarred. The location of the patch should be rotated when a new patch is applied. Do not place the patch below the knee or elbow. Care should be taken that the patch does not come off at night or during bathing. If the patch does fall off, check with the supervisor.

Insertion of Suppositories

Prepare a treatment by checking the label on the box. Make sure the suppository feels firm. The cocoa butter base may begin to soften or melt at warm temperature. If this occurs, briefly place the suppository, with foil wrapper intact, in cold water to increase firmness. Have a tube of lubricating ointment and a pair of disposable gloves on hand. Inform the patient concerning the drug administration procedure and position the patient as instructed. Drape the patient and provide for privacy. For rectal insertion, patient should be on one side with under leg extended and other leg flexed at knee. For vaginal insertion, patient should be on her back with knees flexed and legs spread apart. Drug administrator should put on gloves and remove suppository foil wrapper. A rectal suppository should be inserted into the rectal opening beyond the anal sphincter. Instruct the patient not to strain, which would expel the suppository. Rectal ointment and vaginal suppositories and ointments are inserted using an applicator that accompanies the suppository or cream. Further directions for use are found in the package insert.

Injectable Drug Administration

There are many techniques and various routes for the use of injectable medications. Injectable drugs can be given directly into a blood vessel (intravascular), into a vein (intravenous), into an artery (intra-arterial), into select muscles (intramuscular), under the skin (hypodermic or subcutaneous), into the skin (intradermal), into the spinal cord (intrathecal), into the heart (intrapericardiac).

Many of these injection techniques require special manipulative skill. They are considered invasive procedures, frequently using very potent drugs. Information and competency development is beyond the scope of this manual.

Discontinuance of Drug Administration

Persons involved in drug administration need to be very alert to the times when drug discontinuance, interruption of dosage schedules, or modification of scheduled dosage patterns are prescribed or indicated.

Drug administration should be withheld if the patient gives evidence of experiencing an adverse drug reaction (e.g., hives; a rash occurring on the body, face, neck, arms or legs; difficulty in breathing; double vision or seeing various colors that are not objectively present). If the drug administrator observes any of these conditions or the patient speaks about them, the supervising nurse should be contacted before the next dose is given. In other clinical situations there may be hospital policy or physician orders that direct stoppage of drug due to certain indicators. For example, do not give digoxin if apical pulse rate falls below sixty beats per minute.

Surgeons and/or anesthesiologists usually discontinue all standing medication orders prior to the patient going to surgery. At that time drugs needed prior to, during, and immediately after surgery are reordered. A drug administrator must carefully scrutinize the preoperative and postoperative drug orders for the surgical patient. Mistakes in this area could jeopardize the surgical outcome.

The patient may be scheduled for physical therapy, X ray, or other activities that take the person off the floor during the times of medication administrations. If this occurs, the supervising nurse should be contacted as to the appropriate action to take regarding giving the medication when the patient returns.

Other interruptions of drug administration can occur when the patient's orders read "nothing by mouth" and the patient is on oral drug therapy. In some situations, for various reasons, the patient may refuse to take the drug. In each case the supervising nurse, the pharmacist, or the prescribing physician must be contacted to clarify what is the appropriate action to be taken regarding drug administration.

If a patient is in a program for therapeutic drug monitoring (TDM), the drug dosage schedule and/or laboratory phlebotomy schedule may have to be modified according to the halflife of the drug to obtain the accurate drug blood serum levels that are required for optimum drug therapy dosing. These patients may require an individualized drug dosage administration schedule to be planned by the physician, pharmacist, and medical technologist. Information regarding interrupted drug administration, refusal of the patient to take one drug, and modified drug schedules should always be charted in the medication records and reported to the supervising nurse.

Unit-Dose Drug Administration

A unit-dose drug comes individually packaged and labeled and requires no further packaging or labeling. This system cuts down on the problem of medication errors and preserves the integrity and safety of the product. In a unit-dose drug delivery system, a pharmacist checks every drug order prior to the administration of the drug. The unit-dose system provides each patient with a storage bin, usually in a medication cart, in which no more than a 24-hour supply of drugs is available for the individual patient. The package is opened at the patient's bedside and the name, label, strength, and patient are once again checked against the medication cardex.

Crushing Medications

Crushing medications to assist patients who have difficulty swallowing pills or capsules is recommended only after serious consideration and consultation between the physician and the pharmacist. Medications are designed in tablet or capsule form to ensure their absorption in the correct area of the gastrointestinal tract and to eliminate or minimize digestive problems. Crushing may seriously interfere with these safety measures. Crushing cannot be used for enteric-coated or sustained-action (e.g., Pronestyl-SR) medications. Notify the pharmacy about the need to crush specific medications and follow the pharmacist's advice regarding the safety of this action.

If crushing is necessary and approved by institution policy, each medication must be crushed individually, mixed with a palatable fruit (apple sauce, jello, etc.), and given to the patient separately. Attempt to give the patient as much of the drug in the first spoonful so very little is wasted if the patient refuses the remainder. *Never mix all the patient's medications in one cup.*

Internal and External Medications

Any caregiver who has been in practice for an extended period of time can cite examples of inaccuracies that they read about, heard about, or were involved in. One that comes to mind was the elderly monk, admitted to the hospital for a severe scalp burn when someone attempting to dry up a wet lesion dropped a sunlamp on his head. The burn became infected and he was admitted to the hospital. His first morning in the hospital, his caregiver poured out and left at the bedside 2 ounces of mouthwash in a small waxed paper cup, the same as the one the patient had been given with a liquid medication the previous evening. When the caregiver returned to assist him with oral hygiene, she asked what happened to the mouthwash. She got the simple answer, "I swallowed it." The aide reported it, the patient was carefully monitored, and outside of severe **diuresis** was fortunately discharged with no other apparent side effects.

This story illustrates the fact that one cannot be too careful in providing medications for hospitalized persons.

Internal medications (to be swallowed/ingested/injected) and external medications (to be applied to the outside of the body or an adjoining orifice) should always be kept separate. These drugs are labeled differently. External preparations require a red, external use label. Black or another color is used for internal medications. Drugs labeled for topical use are also external preparations.

Ancillary labels should be carefully read and followed (e.g., "Shake well before using," "Refrigerate," "Do not refrigerate," "For external use only").

Medication Teaching

The provision of medication information to patients and their families takes some preparation and planning. Information on the patient's readiness to learn, education level, best learning method (verbal, written, demonstration), and time available for teaching (e.g., expected discharge date) is needed to prepare to teach.

Readiness to Learn

With today's shorter lengths of stay, the best time for patient teaching may be a narrow window. Signs of readiness to learn include stable physical condition, pain control, patient alertness and the ability to concentrate for at least short periods of time, and patient interest in learning about medication. Much of this information may be found in the patient's record and from other members of the health care team. When the time frame available for teaching is particularly short, the teaching plan may include instruction done by others along the patient's "continuum of care," including long-term care facility staff, home care/visiting nurse, outpatient pharmacy, and family.

Education Level

Years of schooling alone may not be the only guide to how to deliver information, but it does provide a starting point. When the patient's education has been of a basic level, it is best to address the teaching to an eighth-grade level. Avoid the use of scientific or medical terminology and give examples to support and reinforce learning. Take clues from the patient; this is ultimately the best guide on patient understanding, application, and retention. Age and developmental level should also be considered in planning teaching. Examples of teaching approach based on developmental stages are as follows:

- ask adolescents if they want parents present during teaching session
- provide the elderly patient with memory aids such as medication calendars or pillboxes
- let preschoolers handle/play with equipment before a procedure

Learning Method

How a person learns is a complex and individual process, but learning is facilitated when a number of methods and senses are involved. Methods of instruction may include a combination of the following: written materials, verbal instruction, demonstration, providing examples, video/audio tapes, and question and answer. Information is best absorbed when given over a period of time (e.g., give written material to the patient to read in the morning and return later in the day to discuss the information and answer questions). Taking time for a follow-up telephone call to the patient or providing a number for the patient to call with questions after discharge is another way to reinforce valuable information given to the patient under the stressful circumstances of illness, hospital discharge, or transfer to another facility.

Teaching Plan

Learning will best be accomplished if it is guided by a plan. Formation of a teaching plan will focus on the needs of the patient and the information to be taught. Learning objectives should be developed prior to initiating teaching. Objectives should be stated as outcome objectives (i.e., what the patient will learn by the completion of instruction). Objectives should be practical, achievable, and measurable. Include the patient's objectives in the plan when possible. Examples of teaching/learning objectives are as follows:

- the patient will be able to list three signs of digitalis toxicity that require physician notification
- the patient describes rotation of sites for insulin injection
- the patient's son demonstrates correct insulin injection technique

Objectives provide a basis for evaluating the effectiveness for teaching. The ultimate objective is that the patient has the information and skill necessary for safe medication administration.

Teaching Process

Select the most suitable and comfortable location to provide instruction. A comfortable location with limited distractions will allow the patient to concentrate on the information and ask questions. Prior to initiating teaching, the teaching plan and the objectives should be reviewed. At least two methods of instruction are recommended to improve understanding and retention. When possible provide the patient with written material from a patient teaching text, from a computerized program, or from the instructor. When a preprinted text is used it needs to be reviewed for content, education level, size of type, and so forth prior to giving it to the patient. When time permits, teaching of complex information should be given in more than one session. The definition of "complex" information will vary according to the patient, but learning that requires cognitive and psychomotor capabilities is considered "complex." Examples of complex learning include: self-injection, taking radial pulse prior to cardiac medication, and taking a child's temperature. In each of the situations the patient or family members need to have information on the reason for the procedure, the skill or procedure, and what action they are to take based on the results, such as a radial pulse of 45 per minute or a temperature of 102°F. When teaching complex information, a second or third teaching session should be scheduled to provide the patient an opportunity to absorb the information, formulate questions, and give a return demonstration as indicated. To provide the most comprehensive information in a timely manner, the teaching plan should involve and be communicated to other members of the health care team, including the physician, nurse, dietitian, case manager, and visiting nurse.

Reinforcement

Provide patients with praise and encouragement during their learning process. Describe their progress in terms of readiness for discharge, self-independence, accomplishment of a skill, or being knowledgeable about their medication.

Evaluation of Learning

Since the ultimate goal of the teaching process is to affect learning and change behavior, the evaluation of learning is the final stage of the teaching/learning process. According to the nature of the information, the evaluation method may include a short written test, requesting the patient verbally state the information and give a return demonstration (e.g., taking a pulse).

Professional Responsibility for Drug Administration

Drug administration is the shared privilege and responsibility of different health disciplines—each one with carefully delineated functional activities. Physicians or physician delegates, such as physician assistants and nurse practitioners, have the responsibility to prescribe rational and selective drug therapy, dependent upon the patient's medical profile and the drug's therapeutic characteristics.

The pharmacists are responsible to screen these orders for rationality and appropriateness in particular, individualized cases. In some instances the pharmacist is invited to participate in the multidisciplinary planning of a particular patient's drug regimen. The pharmacist evaluates the choice of drug for a particular pathology, and if doubt arises, the physician is contacted. Further consideration is given to the drug dose, the time intervals between cases, the patient's past drug history regarding allergies, drug sensitivities, and past untoward drug reactions. The pharmacist further considers the drug benefit/risk ratio regarding the possibility of a drug-drug interaction, a drug-food interaction or a drug-laboratory test interaction. If there is apparent serious drug risk involvement, the pharmacist further consults with the physician regarding appropriate drug administration. If the pharmacist evaluates the regimen to be within the bounds of sound therapy, the drug is dispensed, for an inpatient, through the nursing service in most situations. If the pharmacy completely controls the drug-usage process, a medication technician may then assume the final responsibility for proper drug administration.

However, in most institutions, the nursing department in collaboration with the pharmacy department is responsible for the final step in the drug-usage process (i.e., administration of the drug and observation of the patient regarding the therapeutic outcome of the drug action. According to hospital policy the task of actually giving the medication to a patient may be delegated to a technical assistant or trained medication technician. Yet, the responsibility of the drug's outcome remains with the licensed health professionals involved.

Basically, the right drug, for the right reason, must be given to the right patient at the right time, in the right dosage strength and in the right drug dosage form. This is the core responsibility of the drug administration process. Responsibility for the outcome is shared by the professionals of medicine, nursing, and pharmacy.

Legal Responsibilities in Drug Administration

Many states and many health care institutions have very specific policies and procedures that must be carried out exactly as written. Presently many states require a registered nurse to administer all medications. At the same time other states and health institutions, due to fiscal, technical, personnel, and patient loads, are changing and/or modifying existing regulations. Basic requirements do not change, even if the assigned or designated personnel change.

Every hospital is required to have a policy and procedural manual to ensure patient safety and patient care. It is necessary that these policies and procedures be known and observed by the persons involved in drug administration activities.

When medication errors are made, they are usually related to the patient's "five rights." To prove negligence, it must be established that drug administration policy was not followed, careless shortcuts were taken, and/or the medication order and administration procedure were not adequately checked by the responsible licensed professional. Adequate patient drug-use control, drug-use evaluation, and drug-use surveillance must be top priorities to ensure patient safety. Detected errors must be reported immediately to the licensed supervisor.

All medication errors should be reviewed using a performance improvement process in which the policy, procedure, actions of the individuals involved, and environmental factors are reviewed and considered. The goal of the performance improvement process is to identify individual and system problems which, if corrected, will help to avoid future errors.

New Trends in Drug Administration

Drug administration methods are frequently called drug delivery systems. Drug firms have made large investments in researching and developing new methods to target drug administration dosage forms to maximize effectiveness and to limit unwanted systemic effects. The future may see pharmacy technicians specializing in the maintenance, utilization, and monitoring of these new and often unique devices and drug administration delivery systems.

If contemporary trends, particularly the working definition for pharmaceutical care, continue to prevail, pharmacy technicians of the future may require the knowledge, judgment, techniques, and skills to participate in the health care team as competent pharmacy medication technicians.

Summary

The administration of medication is a serious responsibility, requiring the possession of clinical information and skills. It includes not only information about the drugs being given, but also the proper procedures for safe administration and documentation. Skills in administration ensure that the patient receives medication in the safest and most therapeutic manner with the least chance of mistakes, untoward reactions, or spread of infection.

ASSESSMENT

Multiple Choice Questions

1. The drug administration process begins with
   a. the physician's prescription
   b. the pharmacist dispensing the drug
   c. the nurse evaluating the patient
   d. the technician's assignment
   e. the request for a drug

2. Medication orders include
   a. drugs ordered by the physician after medical rounds
   b. telephone drug orders in emergencies
   c. standing drug orders for particular patient categories
   d. "stat" orders to be immediately administered
   e. all of the above

3. A PRN drug is administered
   a. routinely
   b. at night before sleep
   c. before meals
   d. when the patient's condition requires it
   e. immediately

4. Patient rights include
   a. right drug
   b. right time
   c. right dosage strength
   d. right dosage form
   e. all of the above

5. Prior to administering a drug, the medication technician should
   a. know the patient's age, sex, and weight
   b. know the usual dose or dosage range of the drug
   c. check with the supervising nurse or pharmacist before each drug is administered
   d. warn the patient of any possible side effects
   e. all of the above

6. A drug may be left at the patient's bedside if
   a. the patient requests that the drug be left
   b. the patient is asleep
   c. the patient is in X ray
   d. the patient wants to discuss the drug with the pharmacist
   e. none of the above

7. At least 4 ounces of water should be given following the drug administration of
   a. a buccal tablet
   b. a medicated mouthwash
   c. an aspirin tablet
   d. cough syrup
   e. a sublingual tablet

8. Sufficient water given after administration of a solid oral dosage form
   a. assists the patient in swallowing
   b. prevents esophageal irritation
   c. aids drug solubility
   d. all of the above
   e. none of the above

9. After administration of eyedrops the patient should be advised to
   a. not move his or her head
   b. not to sneeze
   c. close the eye(s) for a few minutes
   d. immediately wipe away any tears
   e. stay in a darkened room

10. Transdermal drug patches are placed
    a. on the upper arm or inside forearm
    b. below the knee
    c. directly above the wrists
    d. on the most accessible spot
    e. where directed by patient

11. Outcomes of the performance improvement process for medication errors include
    a. identifying problems in the medication administration process
    b. determining the need for staff education
    c. reducing the possibility of future errors
    d. all of the above

12. When administering an enteric-coated medication to a child or geriatric patient, the administrator may take the following action(s):
    a. give crushed in applesauce
    b. dissolve in water
    c. give with sufficient juice
    d. give sublingually

True/False Questions

13. __T__ Drug administration requires a physician's or other authorized prescriber's drug order.

14. __F__ If a person appears to be in serious distress, the medication technician selects a drug to bring relief.

15. __T__ Any unusual or newly occurring physical or mental change observed by the medication technician should be reported promptly to the supervising nurse.

16. __T__ Patient confidentiality regarding drugs, disease, and other personal and clinical matters is a responsibility of the medication technician.

17. __F__ If a drug is not available as ordered as a capsule, the medication technician may substitute a tablet with the same active ingredient or strength.

18. __T__ All drug discrepancies and errors must be immediately reported to the supervising nurse and/or pharmacist.

Matching

19. __b__ ointment   a. internal drug

20. __b__ topical preparation   b. external drug

21. __a__ tablet

22. __a__ elixir

23. __a__ intramuscular injection

Bibliography

Gourley, D.R., Wedemweyer, H.F., & Norvell, M. (1986). Administration of medications. In T. R. Brown & M. C. Smith (Eds.), *Handbook of institutional pharmacy practice* (p. 352). Baltimore: Williams & Wilkins.

24 Drug Distribution Systems

COMPETENCIES

Upon completion and review of this chapter, the student should be able to

1. Outline the responsibility of the pharmacist and the role of the pharmacy technician in the drug distribution functions.

2. Differentiate among the four major drug distribution systems.

3. Describe the purpose, functions, and advantages of the unit-dose drug distribution system.

4. Distinguish the main differences between a decentralized and a centralized drug distribution system.

5. Explain why the pharmacist must review a physician's direct medication order.

6. List the information that is included on a medication order.

7. Briefly explain the four methods in which physicians' original orders are directly transmitted to the pharmacy.

8. List the drug distribution activities that can be generated through computerization.

9. Describe various ways in which the pharmacy technician is directly involved in the computerization process.

10. List the check points required by the pharmacist and by the pharmacy technicians when a physician's medication order is received in the pharmacy.

Introduction

Drug control is one of the pharmacist's most important contributions to health care. With the advent of new regulations and the constantly changing health care system, methods of distributing and controlling drugs must undergo continuous reevaluation and review. Only then can efficient systems that meet changing requirements be ensured. Advancing technology will permit the pharmacist to move from traditional product-focused dispensing to that of a patient advocate and provider of clinical services. The pharmacist will assume a larger role in improved therapeutic outcomes in disease management. Greater efficiency and economy in disease therapy will be ensured.

The role of the technician in the area of dispensing and drug distribution is to assist the pharmacist. Technicians are an integral and important component of the health care team, in which they primarily assist the pharmacist. The legal responsibility for dispensing remains with the pharmacist.

After reviewing this chapter, the student should have a good understanding of drug distribution systems. The technician should be able to classify the different types of distribution systems and actively participate in system planning and development. They should be able to clearly define the role of the technician in a distribution system.

Drug Distribution Systems

The Pharmacy and Therapeutics Committee is responsible for the development of broad policies and procedures that provide for the proper distribution of medications and pharmaceutical aids to patients. The drug distribution systems in use today are variations of four concepts: floor stock, patient prescription, combined floor stock and patient prescription, and unit dose. Additional components of the drug distribution system are covered in other chapters of this manual and include intravenous admixtures, controlled drug distribution, and interdepartmental requisitions.

Complete Floor Stock System

In the complete floor stock system of distribution, all medications are stocked on the nursing unit, with the possible exception of some rarely used and very expensive medications. Medications that require an expanded level of professional supervision and control, such as antineoplastic agents and antibiotics, may not be included in floor stock supplies. The nurse is totally responsible for all aspects of preparation and administration of medications. This method of dispensing is strongly discouraged because of several inherent disadvantages.

- There is increased potential for medication errors, as medication orders are not reviewed by the pharmacist. Thus, a nurse may select the wrong medication to administer from the vast array of drugs and dosage forms available.
- Economic loss may occur because of misappropriation or diversion by hospital personnel and lost medication charges. Expired, contaminated, and deteriorated drugs remaining on the unit may also mean economic loss and possible patient harm if administered from the floor stock supply.
- Increased drug inventory is necessary because of multiple inventories on each nursing unit. Thus, drug inventory control is poor.
- Storage and control problems occur because of limited storage facilities on nursing units.

Individual Prescription System

In the individual prescription system of dispensing, a multiple days' supply of each medication is dispensed for the patient on receipt of prescriptions or orders. The nurse transcribes and prepares individual prescriptions or orders from the physician's original written order and forwards the request to pharmacy for filling. Commonly, a 3- to 5-day supply is provided by pharmacy. When the original supply is exhausted, the nurse prepares another request and the whole process is repeated. A tremendous amount of time and manpower is required. Maintenance of drug containers on the nursing staff in an organized, easily accessible method is wasteful of nursing time. Pharmacy is usually responsible for charges and credits which are individually entered into the patient's account or forwarded to the business office for processing. Altogether, much time is required of all participants. Although this system is an improvement over the floor stock system, it is not an efficient or practical method of drug distribution.

Combined Floor Stock and Patient Prescription System

In the combined floor stock and patient prescription system of drug distribution, the primary method of dispensing is the individual prescription order supplemented with a limited number of floor stock items. This method possesses the benefits of both systems. The floor stock items are generally over-the-counter medications (e.g., aspirin, acetaminophen, laxatives, vitamins) and selected controlled drug medications. Although this system is far superior to the two previous systems discussed, it also exhibits the disadvantages of both systems.

Unit-Dose Drug Distribution System

Unit-dose distribution represents a significant refinement of the individual prescription order system and is considered to be the safest, most economical method of distributing drugs in health care institutions. It is considered to be a hospital system, not simply a pharmacy system, because it involves many departments and disciplines in its planning, development, and operation.

The unit-dose system has been preferred to the floor stock or individual system of drug distribution by many authorities, including the federal government. It has proved to be the most effective drug distribution system available today. Following are the advantages of this type of system over the conventional approach:

- reduction in medication errors
- improved drug control
- decrease in the overall cost of medication distribution
- more precise medication billing
- reduction of medication credits
- reduced drug inventories throughout the institution

Numerous variations of unit-dose systems have been implemented throughout the world, but all share several common features. In all systems, unit-dose packages of drugs are dispensed from pharmacy in a ready-to-administer form that requires no additional manipulation, measurement, or preparation by the nurse who administers the medication.

A large- or small-volume injection may be considered a unit dose, but it is not normally distributed in the same manner. Virtually all other medications can be dispensed as a unit-dose package, which is defined as containing the particular dose of the drug ordered for the patient. For example, a unit-dose liquid may contain from a fraction of a milliliter to 60 or more milliliters, but it is the exact amount ordered by the physician. A unit dose of tablets or capsules may contain one or more or a fraction of a commercial dosage form, but it is the amount ordered to be administered. A single-unit package contains one discrete dosage form such as one tablet, 5 ml of a liquid, or a prefilled syringe containing 25 mg in 1 ml. A single-unit package may also be a unit-dose package if it contains the dose prescribed.

Centralized Dispensing

In centralized dispensing systems, all activities required in the preparation and distribution of medications take place within the central pharmacy area.

Unit-dose medications are made available on the nursing floor one or more times daily, depending on the staff available and the logistics of moving the supplies to and from the pharmacy and nursing locations. Patients' drugs are generally dispensed in amounts needed for the next 24 hours. In some institutions, nursing units are resupplied twice or even three times daily. There may be many specific times during the day when drugs are scheduled to be administered to patients. In some cases, the pharmacy makes multiple drug deliveries each day to accommodate the need. Some drugs requiring special handling (e.g., antineoplastics, very expensive medications, and items too large to fit in pneumatic tube systems) may be hand-carried to the patient floor at the time of need.

The greatest number of technicians are usually involved in the unit-dose dispensing system. The technician assists in preparing all medication doses and fills the cabinets, carts, or cassettes. The technician utilizes the patient medication profile which has been generated by either a manual or computerized system to prepare and deliver the medication to the patient care areas.

All medications must be checked by a pharmacist before they are distributed to the patient care area. During this process, the pharmacist ensures that the correct drug and correct number of doses have been prepared. By visually inspecting the total drug supply for each patient, the pharmacist has another opportunity to confirm the absence of drug-drug interactions. The pharmacist is also able to assess the completeness of labeling, look for outdated supplies, and lastly, take full responsibility for the accuracy of the filling process.

Decentralized Dispensing

In a centralized system all doses are prepared at a central location. In a decentralized system, the doses are prepared in a **satellite pharmacy** located in or near the nursing unit. The satellite may serve several nursing units or even one or more floors. Generally, the **centralized system** allows for somewhat greater management efficiency and control; the **decentralized system** allows for closer pharmacist-physician-nurse-patient relationships. In addition, decentralization provides pharmacy services to the unit more quickly, accurately, and efficiently.

Physician's Original Order

Medications are dispensed only on the written order of a licensed physician or other licensed prescriber such as physician's assistant, nurse practitioner, or dentist. The prescriber must also be certified by the institution as qualified to have privileges in the institution.

Basic Requirements of a Complete Medication Order

A medication order should be legible, written in ink, and include the following information:

- patient's name, room number, and hospital number (The patient's age, weight, height, and gender should be included unless available in the patient's pharmacy profile.)
- name and strength of the medication (The nonproprietary or generic name is preferred, although most physicians are inclined to utilize trade names. Dosage strengths should always be written in the metric system. Topical agents such as ophthalmic solutions and nasal solutions may have their strength expressed as a percentage.)

- intravenous solution orders, both large and small volume (Both should indicate the name and strength of each additive and volume of the carrier or diluent with the flow rate or frequency, e.g., 125 ml/hr, q8h, or over 24 hours)
- route of administration (e.g., po, im, iv, pr, each eye, right ear)
- frequency of administration (e.g., b.i.d., t.i.d., qhs, qam, with meals)

It should be noted that when a prescriber verbally issues a medication order, it can only be received by a pharmacist or nurse; it cannot be received by a technician. The order is reduced to writing by the nurse or pharmacist immediately, and should be noted as a telephone order (t.o.) or verbal order (v.o.) on the medication order sheet (Physician's Order Form). The physician is responsible for countersigning this order within 48 hours. It must be emphasized that only a pharmacist or a nurse is authorized to accept telephone or verbal orders.

Transmittal of Orders to Pharmacy

A number of methods are presently in use for obtaining the physician's order. The Joint Commission on Accreditation of Healthcare Organizations (JCAHO) and most state boards of pharmacy require that the pharmacy receive the physician's original prescription—or a copy of the original prescription—when filling medication orders. A direct copy of the order is most frequently utilized. This procedure eliminates transcription errors, which are a frequent source of medication errors. It is the pharmacist's responsibility to review, interpret, and evaluate the medication order.

Traditionally the nurse was given the responsibility of transcribing the doctor's orders as written on the chart onto a pharmacy order form. However, the more people involved in reviewing, evaluating, and transcribing an order, the greater the potential for error. By receiving a direct copy of the physician's original order, the pharmacist can review, clarify, and interpret the order, which is his or her legal and ethical responsibility. This process is now almost universally accomplished by the use of no-carbon-required (NCR) physician order forms. A direct copy of the original becomes available, and can be transmitted to pharmacy for immediate processing.

Electromechanical Systems

Several electronic methods have been utilized to transmit orders from the nursing unit to pharmacy. Like any mechanical equipment, provisions must be made for backup systems in the event of mechanical failure. **Electrostatic copying machines** (photocopiers) and **facsimile transmitting equipment** (fax machines) can be used to copy or transmit orders.

Computerization

One of the most important developments which has significantly changed drug distribution systems is the utilization of computers. A medical information system (MIS) based on computer technology has developed to varying degrees based on the diverse needs of pharmacy and other departments. There are, therefore, a multitude of pharmacy computer systems available today. Different hardware systems and software programs, interfacing with other hospital departments, must be considered in the selection of a pharmacy support system.

Computerization offers the pharmacist a systematized method of order entry, patient profile development, label production, fill lists, and reports. It also provides clinical cross-checking mechanisms for allergy and sensitivity detection, dosage verification, drug interaction, and food-drug interactions.

Currently a number of programs providing comprehensive drug information can be easily accessed during order entry. These allow the pharmacist to confirm the accuracy of drug use and dosage while checking for side effects, contraindications, laboratory test interferences, and so forth. This information may be printed immediately to assist in the education of the pharmacy staff, nurses, physicians, and other professionals within the institution.

An efficient computerized order entry system can generate **patient profiles** for the pharmacist, which include all information necessary for adequately supervising appropriate drug usage within the institution. The profile includes basic patient demographic information, all scheduled and unscheduled or "prn" drugs, frequency, and cautionary statements. The complete profile is then used to generate medication administration records (MARs) for the nurse, which duplicate most of the information on the profile and tell the nurse when she is to administer drugs to each of her patients.

Other applications which can be derived from the computerized profile include dispensing orders or "fill lists" from which the technician fills patient cassettes or drug drawers for the next 24-hour period or less.

The computerized profile should also be capable of transferring charges to the patient's account by direct interface with the institution's financial program. Credits for drugs not used are also applied in the same manner.

Inventory control is managed through the computerized system by deleting items dispensed and their cost. Unused drugs returned to pharmacy are credited to the inventory and to the patient at the same time. Financial status is enhanced and pharmacy administration is provided with valuable reports which may be of importance to upper-level management.

The technician becomes directly involved in all aspects of computerization in most institutions. Order entry may be performed "conditionally" by the technician. The technician's entry is validated by the pharmacist before the order is activated. Other areas in which the technician's computer ability is utilized include floor stock entry, special patient charges and credits, labeling, report generation, and housekeeping or end-of-day functions. The areas of computerization and the technician's involvement are unlimited.

Physician's Order Entry Process

The institution's information or computer system may enable a physician to enter and transmit orders directly to various departments such as pharmacy, laboratory, and radiology. This is accomplished by utilizing the keyboard or using a **video display terminal (VDT).** With the latter system, the physician utilizes a light pen and selects the desired drug, dosage strength, frequency, and other necessary information from various menus. The physician may also be alerted immediately of possible drug interactions, overdoses, formulary status of the drug ordered, availability, and needed laboratory monitoring.

Receiving the Medication Order

The role functions of both the technician and the pharmacist are shown in Table 8–2 of Chapter 8. The responsibilities are clearly defined for each individual in the dispensing system.

The Pharmacist's Role

It is the responsibility of the pharmacist to review and interpret every medication order prior to dispensing the medication. With the use of a computerized or manual patient profile, the pharmacist is able to evaluate the patient's complete medication regimen.

The Patient's Profile

A patient profile is a complete listing of the patient's medications. For those institutions that do not utilize computers, the profile form is designed to list all medications, strengths, directions, and patient data in addition to quantities and date dispensed. Depending on the institution, some profiles contain clinical data such as laboratory results, and antimicrobial culture and sensitivity reports. Previously used but discontinued drugs are also visible.

When the unit-dose distribution system is used, a profile must be maintained so that the pharmacy may schedule, and the technician may prepare and distribute, individual medication doses according to the appropriate dosing schedule.

The drug profile system enables the pharmacist to identify potential drug interactions, dosage changes, drug duplications, overlapping therapy, and any drug that is contraindicated because of allergy or sensitivity. A complete patient profile should include but not be limited to the following information:

- patient's full name, location, age, weight, sex, hospital number, and admitting physician's name
- provisional diagnosis, secondary diagnosis, and confirmed diagnosis, if available
- allergies, sensitivities, and idiosyncrasies
- drug history from the patient interview
- name of medication dispensed, strength, dosage, directions for use, quantity dispensed, date and initials of pharmacist
- I.V. therapy, e.g., large- and small-volume intravenous solutions with or without additives, hyperalimentation fluids, chemotherapy, etc.
- laboratory data if known (e.g., electrolytes, creatinine, cultures, and sensitivities)
- diet (e.g., low-sodium, diabetic)
- selected diagnostic data related to coronary disease, diabetes, hypertension, etc.
- initials of dispensing technician and checking pharmacist

By receiving a copy of the complete physician's order, the pharmacist is able to seek information concerning laboratory test results, nursing procedures, and dietary intake which might have been ordered. The pharmacist can then monitor possible drug-laboratory interactions, food-drug interactions, and other aspects of the patient's therapeutic program.

The pharmacist is also responsible for checking the technician's work in all aspects of the dispensing procedure:

- verification of the order entry on the patient's profile to ensure that transcription or entry of the doctor's medication order is correct
- verification of drug selection, to be certain that the proper medication was set up for dispensing
- checking of the drug label and contents to make certain that the finished product is complete, accurate, and ready for use
- checking unit-dose cassettes against the profile generated fill list to verify that the drugs dispensed are correct and properly labeled. This process allows the pharmacist to conduct a final check of all unit-dose drugs to which the patient will be exposed.

Technician's Role

It is the responsibility of the technician who receives the written prescription order to prepare the medication for dispensing. When the physician's order copy is received in the pharmacy, the technician must confirm that all necessary information pertaining to the patient's identification is available in the computer or on the profile (e.g., patient name, age, room number or location, hospital identification number, patient weight, allergies and sensitivities, and the physician's name). If a nurse has received a verbal or telephone order, that name should follow the physician's name.

If all necessary information is present, the technician will enter the order onto the computerized profile or transcribe it to a hand-generated profile if that system is in use. It is the pharmacist's responsibility to review the order and the technician's order entry and validate its completeness and accuracy. The pharmacist will also take into consideration the patient's medication history, if available. (It is the policy in some hospitals to have the pharmacist interview patients on admission to obtain a drug history to assist in evaluating the patient's drug therapy.)

An important function of the technician is to answer the telephone. The technician functions in screening telephone calls and referring callers to the appropriate individuals in the department (see Table 8–2 of Chapter 8). If the question asked is beyond the technician's ability to respond accurately, the technician should be able to make an appropriate judgment and refer the caller to the person most capable of meeting the caller's needs.

Following order entry and validation, the technician prepares the drug for dispensing. The proper medication is selected from the appropriate storage site in either unit-dose form or bulk. For other than unit-dose drug distribution systems, the appropriate container must also be chosen. The technician prepares the label and counts or pours the designated quantity of the drug.

Compounding procedures

Qualified technicians may be allowed to conduct less critical compounding and manufacturing procedures under the pharmacist's direction and supervision. If two or more drugs are compounded or mixed, or prefabricated powders are reconstituted for dispensing for a single dose, it may be considered "compounding."

If more than a single dose of a compounded product is prepared for future dispensing, it is known as "manufacturing" and requires the use of a manufacturing worksheet on which all components are identified by name, manufacturer, lot number, and quantitative amounts. Compounding directions are written or printed. A new lot number is assigned from a master control record. Arbitrary expiration dates are applied and should, where possible, be based on published stability information. Packaging information is also documented. The pharmacist must check all weights, measures, and processes and the completed product for uniformity and accuracy. The names of the technician and supervising pharmacist are recorded on the worksheet. After the procedure is completed and checked, all necessary maintenance, housekeeping, and record-keeping duties are performed by the technician.

Labeling and Dispensing Medications

The technician in most cases will be responsible for labeling of medications. Labels may be computer generated, typed, or machine printed. Hand-written labels with pen, pencil, or marker are absolutely prohibited. One label should never be superimposed on another. The label should be clear, legible, and free from erasures and strikeovers. It should be firmly affixed to the container.

Patients frequently judge the efficacy of a drug by the appearance of the label attached to the container. A neat label may signify to the patient that the drug is effective and will be of benefit. A sloppily printed label will indicate lack of concern by the pharmacy and its staff. The patient (and nursing and medical staffs) may interpret this indifference as a lack of effectiveness of the drug or lack of concern for the patient's well-being. Careful attention to the label indicates that careful attention has been given to preparing the medication as well.

With the exception of unit-dose or single-use products, the label should bear the name, address, and telephone number of the institution or pharmacy. Medications should never be relabeled by nursing personnel or anyone other than personnel supervised by a pharmacist.

Other points to consider in labeling:

■ The metric system rather than the apothecary system should be utilized (e.g., 65 mg instead of 1 gr)

■ When dispensing medications, the technician should be aware of any needed accessory labels which should be attached to the container. These may include but are not limited to the following:

> "For the Eye"
> "Keep in Refrigerator"
> "Shake Well Before Use"
> "Swallow Whole: Do not Crush, Break or Chew"
> "For the Ear"
> "Poison: Not for Internal Use"
> "Take with a Full Glass of Water"

There are a multitude of accessory labels available and every pharmacy should have a representative supply on hand to assist patients and staff in understanding the appropriate use of the medication.

■ When labeling a compounded prescription for inpatient use, the name and amount or percentage of each active ingredient should be indicated on the label. Prescription labels for outpatients should indicate the name of each therapeutically active ingredient.

■ In the event the medication being labeled requires further dilution or reconstitution, the label should provide appropriate directions. (*NOTE:* Effective unit-dose systems do not require the nurse to conduct these operations; only in cases of extremely limited stability should this be allowed.)

■ Expiration dates or dates beyond which the medication should not be used should always appear on both unit-dose and prescription labels. There is little scientific information available to assist the pharmacy in determining how long the effectiveness of the medication can be ensured once it is removed from the manufacturer's original container. Many institutions will arbitrarily apply a 6-month expiration date unless the manufacturer's date arrives earlier. In no case should the expiration date exceed that of the original container. Special circumstances will require that a specific expiration date be applied. For example, many antibiotics for oral suspension when reconstituted are stable for no longer than 7 to 14 days. Packaging materials, storage conditions, light conditions, and other factors must be considered in selecting an appropriate expiration date. The primary or secondary accessory label should indicate:

■ "Expiration Date: _____ " or "Use Before _____ "

■ Parenteral medications may require special labeling in that the route of administration should be indicated (e.g., "For IM Use Only" or "Not for I.V. Use," and so forth.

■ Labels for large- and small-volume intravenous solutions should be placed on the container so as to allow for visual inspection of the solution and should be readable in the hanging position.

■ Those containers that present difficulty in labeling such as small tubes or bottles must be labeled with a minimum of the patient's name and location. If possible, the drug name and strength should also be included. The small tube or bottle should be placed in a larger container bearing a label with all necessary information.

Medication Delivery Systems

Transportation Courier

Some institutions have a centralized transportation courier system that delivers and transports medications, laboratory specimens, and supplies. In other hospitals and institutions, pharmacy technicians transport medications by providing order pickup and delivery. In a unit-dose exchange system, a technician uses a mobile cart to deliver medications in cassettes to the patient care area, exchanges full cassettes for those used during the previous 24-hour period, and returns the used cassettes to pharmacy for refilling.

Equipment

Various types of delivery equipment have been utilized to transport medications. The **pneumatic tube system** utilizes carrier cartridges that are sent from the pharmacy department directly to the terminal at the designated patient care area. All departments may be served depending on the number and location of terminals. In the event of mechanical problems, a backup system must be available to ensure rapid transfer of needed medications to the area or patient. Delays in drug delivery have been a major source of irritation for nurses and may result in medication errors when the delivery time is excessive.

Dumbwaiters or elevators are used extensively when drugs and orders are to be transferred. Unfortunately, they only move in the vertical direction. Personnel must then move materials from the elevator core area to the patient care area. Elevators and dumbwaiters are also subject to breakdown and may impose a need for technicians to utilize stairways to move medications to their destination.

Robots are utilized in some institutions. These mobile computerized mechanical devices can be programmed to follow buried guidelines in the floor to move to virtually any location in the building. They are able to detect and move around obstacles, and "speak" recorded messages. Other hospitals have found small track-mounted carts useful, which move to and from patient care areas delivering paper and supplies much like pneumatic tube systems. Their advantage is that they can handle much larger items and quantities than pneumatic tubes.

All mechanical systems are subject to failure, and provision must be made for alternate delivery methods when breakdown occurs. Drug security and control during transfer is a major concern which must always be considered in the selection and use of any transportation method. Pilferage, loss, and waste may create significant legal and financial problems.

Unit-Dose Picking Area

The area in pharmacy where unit-dose carts are filled usually consists of slanted shelves on which plastic or cardboard bins are arranged to permit easy access by the technician's hands to select the doses needed. Bins are labeled in large letters showing the drug name, both generic or nonproprietary, and trade name and strength. Circular shelves permitting one or two technicians to work with a minimum of movement are most efficient. Shelves are within easy reach and should require minimal stooping or stretching. Adequate lighting is essential. Rubber mats on the floor reduce the strain of standing too long in one place.

One or more computer terminals and printers are located within the picking area to permit the technician to generate fill lists, post charges and credits, and review patient profiles. Sufficient space should be available outside the immediate picking area for storage of transfer carts where the supervising pharmacist can also conduct the checking procedure. A telephone is essential and a small compounding and packaging area with sink and running water should be immediately adjacent to the picking area.

The number and variety of drug bins in the picking area is never static. Change is constant and it is incumbent upon the technicians to ensure that the most frequently needed drugs are most readily retrievable. Infrequently used items should be relegated to the general stock area.

Return of stock to drug bins when patients are discharged or the drug is discontinued is a major source of error. Drugs in opened containers are never reissued. Unopened expired drugs are segregated for return to the manufacturer. Unit-dose packages may be dropped into a wrong bin and, if technicians become complacent and do not read and heed labels carefully, the wrong drug or dose may be issued in another cartfill operation. The area should be kept free of clutter and trash. Maintenance of a clean picking area is absolutely necessary.

Medication Dispensing Units

Medication dispensing units or carts are available in many different configurations. They are designed to be wheeled from the nursing station to the patient's bedside, where the medication is administered directly to the patient.

Single-sided or double-sided carts may contain from a few to as many as sixty patient-identified drawers which hold those medications dispensed to each patient. The drawers may vary in length, width, and depth to accommodate the different needs of specific patient care areas.

Some newer carts also have computer terminals attached, which enable the nurse to document the administration of each drug removed from the patient's drawer. This information may then be transmitted to the pharmacy computer system or institutional mainframe for charging purposes, inventory control, and to update the patient's profile.

Individual patient bins or drawers are stored in portable cassettes. Each cassette may hold up to thirty bins. The pharmacy technician uses a mobile cart to carry filled cassettes to the nursing station, unlocks the medication cart, and removes a cassette holding the empty drawers from the previous delivery period. The technician then inserts a filled cassette for the next 24-hour period and returns to pharmacy with the empty drawers to repeat the filling process.

Proper maintenance of patient bins is an important responsibility of the technician. Each drawer or bin must be properly labeled with a computer-generated, typed, or machine-printed label showing the patient's name, room number, and physician's name. Sufficient dividers should be available to separate unit-dose packages and provide for efficient organization. In some institutions, drawer dividers serve to identify those drugs to be given at different dosing periods. For example, drugs prescribed in the early morning are located at the front of the drawer, those in the middle are to be given during the day, while those in the rear are scheduled for late evening or bedtime use. A final section might contain prn drugs. Dividers of different colors may also be used to further distinguish administration periods.

Carts and bins should be cleaned frequently. When possible, bins should be taken at regular intervals or when conditions indicate to a location where they can be thoroughly washed and sanitized.

Drug Distribution Systems of the Future

Advancing technology and decreasing cost of computerization promise to effect momentous changes in pharmacy practice. Health care will require increased utilization of the pharmacist's unique clinical knowledge. As the pharmacist becomes more involved in direct patient care, a cadre of well-educated and motivated technicians will be required to relieve the pharmacist of the labor-intensive drug distribution requirements. Those patients admitted for institutional care will require very intensive short-term care. The need for painstaking accuracy in drug therapy to ensure rapid recovery with minimal adverse effects will insert the pharmacist more firmly in the therapeutic decision-making process.

Automation will positively affect medication outcomes by influencing prescription, distribution, administration, documentation, and monitoring of every aspect of drug therapy. At the same time, automation is expected to reduce the number of pharmacists and technicians required to manage medication distribution.

A definition of automated pharmacy systems has been adopted by the National Association of Boards of Pharmacy (NABP), which states that they "include but are not limited to mechanical systems that perform operations or activities, other than compounding or administration, relative to the storage, packaging, dispensing, or distribution of medications, and which collect, control and maintain all transaction information."

Robotics

Several robotic devices are currently in use and others are being developed rapidly which will mechanize the drug distribution process. An important impetus of automation is to reduce medication errors. The tedious, repetitive tasks to which the pharmacy staff are exposed can be largely reduced by automation technology. Painstaking record keeping, repetitious movement, and physical stress inherent in existing drug distribution systems can be diminished while increasing the total output with fewer errors. It must be remembered, however, that stocking a robotic canister with the wrong drug may result in a multitude of medication errors before it is detected. Careful, serious attention with checking and cross-checking must be ensured to prevent such serious errors.

As with more traditional systems, automated dispensing may be centralized or decentralized. Decentralized devices are commonly used today, but centralized systems that require larger initial investment are under intense study in many larger institutions. Either system is interfaced with the pharmacy or institutional mainframe computer to maintain financial and inventory control. Space does not allow thorough discussion of all currently available automated dispensing systems; a few are mentioned as an introduction.

One of the simplest and earliest automated devices was the electronic tablet counter used extensively in community pharmacies, outpatient clinics, and mail-order pharmacies. Banks of counters holding the most frequently used solid oral medications are capable of increasing prescription output significantly.

A recent advance requires entering prescription information into a computer which instructs a robot to print a bar coded label. The robot then selects a container of appropriate size, labels the container, then moves to a bar coded tablet or capsule canister, counts the exact number of doses ordered, caps, and ejects the filled container onto a conveyor belt where the pharmacist then makes a final check.

"Pyxis"

A novel approach to making first-dose and frequently used medications readily available on the nursing unit is the "MedStation Rx System" produced by Pyxis Corporation. A variety of compartments are available which permit the storage of virtually any desired medication including controlled substances, intravenous solutions, and equipment. Once pharmacy has entered order changes and validated the profile, drugs on the distant patient care unit become available to the nurse.

Authorized nurses, using their passwords, have access via a touch screen computer terminal in which they are able to identify the patient's profile. Drugs ordered for prn or specific dosage periods can be selected on the screen. A drawer containing the drug opens and the nurse removes the needed dose. The profile is updated instantaneously and charges are applied. Documentation of every aspect of the process is maintained and a variety of reports can be generated. It is claimed that narcotic key searches, end-of-shift counts, and missing medications are eliminated.

ATC 212 System

Another packaging and distribution system, the ATC 212 System available from Baxter Healthcare, relieves many of the tedious picking, packaging, and cart-filling procedures required of the technician. Canisters holding a majority of the most frequently used solid oral doses can supply up to 85 percent of the drugs required for any specific nurse's station. Each dose is packaged in a film strip with the patient's name, location, and physician's name. In addition, the package provides the time at which the medication is scheduled for administration. This information is extracted from the computerized patient profile. Packaging may be organized in order of administration time. If desired, all medications due at a specific dosing period may be presented to the nurse in a single package. Even the color of each tablet or capsule can be printed on the package to assist in identification. Bar coding for drug and patient identification is also possible and may assist in eliminating some common errors. There is a substantial reduction in the time spent by technicians in picking and filling medication cassettes, and the pharmacist's checking time is also reduced significantly.

Automated Healthcare, Inc.

Currently, fifty or more hospitals throughout the United States have purchased or leased $500,000 robotic devices from Automated Healthcare, Inc., of Pittsburgh, to automate drug dispensing. This technology is based on a three-axis robot which moves horizontally and vertically along rows of bar coded prepackaged solid oral or small volume vials and ampuls. Based on the patient's computerized profile which is interfaced with the robot, the equipment selects those medications needed by the patient for the next dosing period at a very rapid rate. The collected drugs are ejected into a bin for placement in a patient identified drawer and ultimate distribution to the nurse's station. It is also capable of returning unused drugs to the appropriate peg for subsequent dispensing.

Reports indicate that the machine can process 1200 medication selections per hour and recognize 900 different medications. The error rate is reported to be one in four hundred million selections. As with other automated equipment, charges and credits are immediately passed to the patient's bill.

A caveat

None of the high-tech equipment mentioned here and none that is likely to be developed is immune to hardware failure, power failure, and software failure. Users fail as well when maintenance is delayed and the equipment is misused. There must be a backup system in place, which will depend largely on the technician and pharmacist executing a manual process to ensure that patients receive the right drug at the right time in the right dose and by the right route. The human machine will never be completely outdated.

Summary

In this chapter the technician's role has been described in relation to function in drug distribution and control. The identified functions should not be considered all-inclusive, but merely a general orientation or guideline. Only a few of the many tasks have been described. Because each pharmacy—centralized or decentralized—is an entity of its own, it would be unrealistic and undesirable to rigidly outline the exact role of the technician. After thorough orientation and in-service training, the department's policy and procedure manual should be consulted and followed carefully before starting a new position.

Because pharmacy is changing everywhere in its direction from product orientation to a patient-oriented focus, the roles of both the pharmacist and technician are undergoing dynamic changes. The technician must be willing to continue the learning process, be open to innovative services, and seriously assume some of the newer responsibilities which advancing pharmaceutical science and technology may require.

ASSESSMENT

True/False Questions

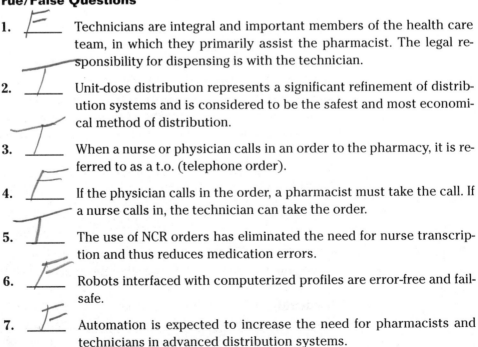

1. _F_ Technicians are integral and important members of the health care team, in which they primarily assist the pharmacist. The legal responsibility for dispensing is with the technician.

2. _T_ Unit-dose distribution represents a significant refinement of distribution systems and is considered to be the safest and most economical method of distribution.

3. _T_ When a nurse or physician calls in an order to the pharmacy, it is referred to as a t.o. (telephone order).

4. _F_ If the physician calls in the order, a pharmacist must take the call. If a nurse calls in, the technician can take the order.

5. _T_ The use of NCR orders has eliminated the need for nurse transcription and thus reduces medication errors.

6. _F_ Robots interfaced with computerized profiles are error-free and fail-safe.

7. _F_ Automation is expected to increase the need for pharmacists and technicians in advanced distribution systems.

Matching

8.	_d_	ASHP	
9.	_f_	robotics	
10.	_g_	MAR	
11.	_h_	technician order entry	
12.	_c_	pneumatic tube	
13.	_e_	JCAHO	
14.	_i_	dumbwaiter	
15.	_b_	NCR	
16.	____	scanner	
17.	_j_	facsimile equipment	

a. carrier cartridges

b. no carbon required

c. used by supermarkets and some unit-dose systems

d. national organization for health system pharmacists and pharmacy technicians

e. Joint Commission on Accreditation of Healthcare Organizations

f. computerized robot for cassette filling

g. medication administration record

h. must be validated by a pharmacist

i. elevator for transporting orders

j. fax

Completion

18. List five advantages of a unit-dose distribution system.

Bibliography

ASHP statement on unit-dose drug distribution. (1989). *American Journal of Hospital Pharmacy, 46,* 2346.

Barker, K.N., Felkey, B.G., Flynn, E.A., et al. (1998). White paper on automation in pharmacy. *Consulting Pharmacists,* 256–284.

Barker, K.N., Harris, J.A., Webster, D.B., Stringer, J.F., Pearson, R.E., Mikeal, R.L., Glotzhober, G.R., & Miller, G.J. (1984). Consultant evaluation of a hospital medication system: Synthesis of a new system. *American Journal of Hospital Pharmacy,* 41(10): 2016–2021.

Crawford, S.Y. (1990). ASHP national survey of hospital-based pharmaceutical services. *Americal Journal of Hospital Pharmacy, 47,* 2665–2695.

Freedman, G.I. (1985, February). Pharmacist-oriented drug distribution systems. *American Journal of Hospital Pharmacy, 42*(2): 383–385.

Hanan, Z.I. et al. (1975, October). Training guidelines for hospital pharmacy supportive personnel. New York State Council of Hospital Pharmacists, Commission on Supportive Personnel.

Hassan, W.E. (1986). *Hospital Pharmacy* (5th ed.). Philadelphia: Lea and Febiger.

Jeffrey, L.P., & Gallina, J.N. (1973). Pharmacy staffing patterns for unit-dose medication distribution systems. *Hospital Pharmacy, 8,* 229–231.

Mar, D.D., Hanan, Z.I., & LaFontaine, R. (1978). Improved emergency room medication distribution. *American Journal of Hospital Pharmacy, 35,* 70–73.

Posey, L.M. (1996). Drug distribution: Options for enhancing efficiency. *Consulting Pharmacists, 11,* 1219–1225.

Tribble, D.A. (1996). How automated systems can (and do) fail. *American Journal of Health-System Pharmacists, 53,* 2622–2627.

The Pharmacy and Infection Control

COMPETENCIES

Upon completion and review of this chapter, the student should be able to

1. Describe modes of transmission of pathogens.
2. Identify four aerobic pathogens responsible for nosocomial epidemics relating to infusium septicemia.
3. Utilize methods for preventing contamination of sterile products compounded in the pharmacy.
4. Describe universal (standard) precautions.

Introduction

The hospital's pharmacy plays a very important role in infection control as its products are potentially disseminated to all patients. Contamination of medications or other pharmacy products, whether caused by faulty manufacturing, handling, storage, or compounding, can have disastrous effects on many patients throughout the hospital.

The pharmacy has professional and administrative functions that are required to ensure patient safety through the proper storage and dispensing of drugs. The infection control committee should assist the pharmacy in establishing and ensuring use of aseptic procedures for all compounding and handling of drugs. Extreme caution and use of strict aseptic technique must be utilized at all times during admixture of parenteral medications, especially hyperalimentation and other intravenous fluids.

Responsibilities of the Pharmacy

Pharmacy personnel are not at high risk unless they are involved in direct patient care, such as during cardiac-arrest response. Patient morbidity and mortality can result from contaminated pharmaceuticals. The pharmacy department should participate in multidisciplinary quality assurance teams, infection control committees, and antimicrobial utilization evaluations to ensure appropriate preparation and use of pharmaceuticals. The pharmacy may participate with infection control departments in managing employee exposure to contagious patients and the selection of germicides. Responsibilities lie with strict enforcement of aseptic practices regarding sterile medication preparation and storage. It may be necessary for pharmacy personnel to participate in the identification of patients who have received specific products associated with epidemics. Other responsibilities of pharmacy departments may include managing patients' intravenous (I.V.) therapy and compounding enteral nutrition products. The pharmacy department provides oversight of the safe use of medications in other areas of the institution, for example, regular inspections for outdated multidose vials and the monitoring of storage space for refrigerated medication. Many institutions' infection control professionals provide prevalence rounds in the pharmacy department on a scheduled basis to ensure the standards of practice. The pharmacy provides information on pharmaceuticals including indications, dosage, route of administration, contraindications, adverse effects, drug interactions, and proper storage.

Work Practice Controls

Handwashing is generally considered the single most important procedure for preventing nosocomial infections and cross contamination. The purpose of handwashing for routine practices is to remove microbial contamination acquired by recent contact with infected or colonized patients or environmental sources. The purpose of antiseptic handwashing, called health care personnel handwashing by the Food and Drug Administration, is to minimize counts of both transient and resident skin flora.

Handwashing Indications

1. when hands are visibly soiled
2. before contact with particularly susceptible patients, such as the severely immunocompromised and newborns
3. after situations during which microbial contamination of hands is likely, especially those involving contact with mucous membranes, blood or body fluids, secretions, and excretions
4. after contact with inanimate sources likely to be contaminated
5. before and after drug preparation
6. before and after glove use

Antiseptics are products with antimicrobial activity that are designed for use on skin, removing both transient and resident flora, and should be used for handwashing. Examples include alcohols, chlorhexidene 2% and 4%, iodophors, parachlorometa-xylenol (PCMX), and triclosan.

Maintenance of a clean work environment assists in assuring a quality product. All work surfaces must be cleaned daily, and afterwork cleaning with a germicidal agent (usually a hospital approved germicide) is recommended.

All health care workers must use personal protective equipment (PPE) according to specific procedures. Pharmacy personnel must wear proper PPE (masks, gowns, and gloves) when preparing parenteral and hyperalimentation fluids. Always maintain the area as a sterile field with a mask, sterile gloves, and gowns.

Aseptic Technique

The basic principles underlying practices of asepsis are (1) microorganisms are capable of causing illness in humans, (2) microorganisms harmful to humans can be transmitted by direct or indirect contact, and (3) illness caused by microorganisms can be prevented by interrupting the transmission of microorganisms from reservoir to susceptible host. Asepsis is defined as the absence of pathogenic, disease-producing microorganisms. Therefore, provide a sterile field for admixture preparation.

Risks Associated with Contamination of Sterile Products

Contamination of infusates is an uncommon cause of infections, but may result in epidemics (Maki, 1992). Types of contamination are intrinsic—that which occurs during the manufacturing process—and extrinsic—that which occurs subsequent to manufacturing, during the admixture process, or while the infusate is in use (Simmons et al., 1983). Both types of infusate contamination are a less frequent cause of infection than cannula-related contamination; however, they are more likely to result in bacteremia and septic shock (Maki, 1992).

Most nosocomial epidemics of infusion-related septicemia are caused by aerobic gram-negative pathogens (Maki & Martin, 1975). The pathogens indicated include Enterobacteriaceae spp., Klebsiella, Enterobacter, Serratia marcescens, Citrobacter freundii, and Burkholderia (Pseudomonas) cepacia (Maki, 1992; Maki & Martin, 1975; Cleary, MacIntyre, & Castro, 1981). Epidemics of Candida parapsilosis fungemia have been related to the use of contaminated parenteral nutrition (PN) (Solomon et al., 1984; Plouffe et al., 1977). Intrinsic contamination of infusate has led to an epidemic of nosocomial sepsis (Felts et al., 1972). Epidemics of septicemia caused by *Staphylococcus saprophyricus* and Enterobacter cloacae have resulted from contamination of parenteral admixtures during compounding or storage (Degleux et al., 1991; Llop et al., 1993).

Clusters of postoperative infections have been associated with extrinsic contamination of propofol, an intravenous hypnotic agent; organisms isolated include *Staphylococcus aureus,* Candida albicans, Moraxella osloenis Enterobacter agglomerans, and Serratia marcescens (Centers for Disease Control and Prevention [CDCP], 1990; Bennett et al., 1995).

Surveys of in-use I.V. fluids have found contamination rates of approximately 1 to 4 percent; however, most microorganisms recovered have been skin flora that do not grow well, were not associated with infections, and are generally considered to be of low virulence (Garbea, 1984; Maki et al., 1987). Microorganisms that have the ability to proliferate in different fluids include Klebsiella, Serratia, and Enterobacter spp. Pseudomonas cepacia can multiply in 5% dextrose (Maki, 1992), C. albicans can grow slowly (Maki, 1992), whereas Staphylococcus, Proteus, Escherichia coli, Herellea, and Pseudomonas aeruginosa die slowly in dextrose (Maki & Martin, 1975). Water pathogens such as P. cepacia, P. aeruginosa, Acinetobacter, and Serratia will grow in distilled water. Ringer's solution also harbors P. aeruginosa, Enterobacter, and Serratia. Sodium chloride 0.9% can support bacterial growth. PN fluids can grow fungus very slowly, such as C. albicans and Torulopsis glabrata; proliferation can occur at 4°C after 7 days. The growth of most bacteria is inhibited in PN solutions. The addition of albumin to PN solutions increases the potential for bacterial and fungal growth.

Bacteria and fungi such as S. epidermidis, C. albicans, and E. coli survive in total nutrient admixtures (TNA), in which fat emulsion is combined with dextrose and amino acid mixtures. P. aeruginosa, S. aureus, S. epidermidis, S. faecalis, and group JK Corynebacterium displayed greater growth in TNAs as compared with PN fluids.

Contaminated pharmaceutical products have led to infections. Contaminated multidose ophthalmic solutions have resulted in Serratia marcescens keratitis and P. aeuginosa corneoscleritis; this organism was cultured from the container but not the solution (Templeton et al., 1982; Alfonso et al., 1987). According to literature, bacteria grew from 82 of 638 in-use multidose ophthalmic solutions (Hovding & Sjursen, 1982); however, when 81 opened multidose vials were tested no contamination resulted (Tammer, Sweet, & Ross, 1994).

An outbreak of sepsis resulted from an irrigation with E. cloacae–contaminated solution. Enteral nutrition preparations are associated with infections, including septicemia. Enteral nutrition preparations also support the growth of gram-negative bacteria, gram-positive bacteria, and fungi. Mineral oil used for bathing infants was contaminated with Listeria monocytogenes, which led to an outbreak of neonatal listeriosis (Schuchat et al., 1991).

Preventing Contamination of Sterile Products Prepared in the Pharmacy

The environment influences the outcome of a quality product. Its relationship to sterility and quality should be considered during any preparation. All sterile products should be prepared in a class 100 environment which can be achieved with the use of a certified vertical- or horizontal-laminar flow hood (ASHP, 1993). Laminar air-flow hoods should be operated prior to product preparation for a length of time sufficient to permit purge of room air from the work area. Check manufacturer's recommendations for each hood. Hoods should be placed in low traffic areas, preferably in a separate room, to reduce the risk of contamination. Storage within this room should be kept to a minimum and restricted to items necessary for sterile preparation only. Cardboard boxes, carpets, drapes, and other particle-generating items should not be permitted. All interior surfaces should be cleaned with an appropriate germicidal agent such as a phenolic, quaternary ammonium or alcohol. Preparation of products should be done at least 6 inches inside the hood. Certification of hoods may be required by regulatory agencies; check local standards for hood certification, such as JCAHO. The hood should be positioned to prevent room air circulation and vents from interfering with the work area airflow. Check manufacturer's recommendations for a specific agent. A suggested procedure for cleaning is to cleanse work areas before the first procedure of the day, after spills, and at least once each shift.

Housekeeping

Attention to housekeeping facilitates the proper environment for medication preparation and should be on a consistent, scheduled basis. The sterile preparation room should be maintained free of visible dust and debris. Sterile supply shelves should be maintained dust free. Routine daily cleaning of floors and horizontal surfaces should be performed with an EPA-approved germicide detergent.

Attire

Staff attire can play a role in preventing contamination. At least one professional society (ASHP, 1993) recommends wearing protective gowns, masks, and facial/head hair covers during sterile product preparation. No recommendation is given for protective garb when preparing I.V. admixtures in the Center for Disease Control and Prevention (CDC) guidelines on intravascular device–related infections (CDC, 1995).

Asepsis in Sterile Product Preparation

Use of asepsis in sterile product preparation requires that hands be thoroughly washed using an antimicrobial skin cleanser and friction for 10 to 15 seconds (Larson, 1995) prior to commencing work in the sterile preparation area. Consumption or storage of food and beverages is not permitted in the sterile preparation area as they can influence the presence of vermin. Touch contamination of sterile supplies should be avoided. Any items used for compounding of products within the hood should first be disinfected with an EPA-approved agent. Ingredients used for sterile product preparation should be checked first for package integrity and expiration dates.

Other Quality Control Issues

Additional quality control issues involve the use and maintenance of multidose vials (MDVs). Additives from MDVs which are used in the preparation of sterile products are of concern in the ultimate sterility of the end product. Persons entering MDVs must use aseptic technique, which requires the cleansing of the rubber diaphram with alcohol before insertion of a sterile needle. This procedure must be performed each time the vial is entered (CDC, 1995). Items requiring refrigeration should be maintained at temperatures according to manufacturer's recommendations. The number of entries into an MDV may affect the content's sterility (Longfield et al., 1984). There are no specific guidelines regarding the length of time an opened MDV can safely be used (CDC, 1995), and USP considers time limits on MDVs to be arbitrary (Moi & Thornton, 1991). However, the length of time an MDV remains used once opened may serve to indicate the potential for multiple entries and thus the possibility of resultant contamination. Dating vials at the time of opening may have no effect on sterility (Melnyk et al., 1993), but may be useful in preventing long-term storage and use of open vials. Some manufacturers and institutions advise a 30-day use, so consult with the infection control professional at your facility.

Upon completion of preparation, the end product should be carefully observed for the presence of particulates, leaks, cracks, or turbidity indicating contamination (Simmons, Hooton, & Mallison, 1982). *A contaminated product should be discarded.* The CDC (Simmons, Hooten, & Mallison, 1982) recommends that admixed parenterals should have a label affixed to the container stating additives and their dosage, date and time of compounding, expiration date, and identification of the person performing the compounding, Storage of pharmaceuticals should be overseen by the pharmacy for proper temperature maintenance and expiration dates. The CDC (Simmons, Hooton, & Mallison, 1982) recommends refrigeration of parenterals promptly after admixture if they are not to be administered within 6 hours of preparation. Upon commencing use, the CDC recommends parenterals be completed or discarded within 24 hours (Simmons et al., 1983).

Additional Safety Factors and Quality Control

There should be scheduled monitoring of handwashing, aseptic technique, storage of pharmaceuticals and supplies, refrigeration of medications with proper temperatures, maintenance of clean surfaces, maintenance of laminar flow hoods and work surfaces, admixture procedures, proper labeling of solutions with dates, assessment of admixture sterility, and proper use of PPE.

Infectious Disease Process—Chain of Infection

The chain of infection consists of an integrated group of six factors, which, when present, function to facilitate transmission and acquisition of infection.

1. The *causative agent* is a biologic, physical, or chemical entity capable of causing disease. Agents responsible for disease include bacteria (rickettsia, mycoplasma, and chlamydia), viruses, fungi, protozoa, helminths, and prions.

2. The *reservoir* of the agent is a place in which an infectious agent can survive, but may not multiply. A common example is the hepatitis A virus which survives in clams but does not multiply. Common reservoirs include humans, animals, the environment, and fomites. Reservoirs associated with infection are patients, health care workers, health care equipment, and the environment.

3. The *portal of exit* is the location where the agent leaves the reservoir, such as the respiratory tract, genitourinary tract, gastrointestinal tract, skin, mucous membranes, and blood. Transplacental exit permits exchange of an agent from the mother to the fetus.

4. The *modes of transmission* are the mechanisms by which agents are transferred to the susceptible host, which is accomplished by

- contact
  - direct contact—person to person
  - indirect contact—contact with a contaminated object, e.g., contaminated endoscope
  - droplet spread of large particles causing brief passage of an infectious agent in the air, usually a distance of 3 feet, e.g., talking, sneezing, or coughing
- common vehicle
  - active or direct transmission, e.g., Salmonella in food
  - passive or indirect transmission, e.g., hepatitis A virus by soiled matter
- airborne spread
  - contained within droplet nuclei, capable of traveling long distances, e.g., tuberculosis
- vector-borne spread such as insects, e.g., feet of flies, malaria, yellow fever

5. The *portal of entry* is a path by which an infectious agent enters the susceptible host. Portals of entry include the respiratory tract, genitourinary tract, gastrointestinal tract, skin and mucous membranes, and blood.

6. The *susceptible host* is a person or animal lacking effective resistance to a particular pathogenic agent. Factors that influence susceptibility include age, sex, ethnicity, socioeconomic status, marital status, disease history, lifestyle, and heredity.

Isolation Precautions

Isolation precautions include a variety of infection control measures used to prevent cross contamination and infection. Handwashing is the single most important measure to reduce the risks of transmitting organisms from one person to another. Gloves also provide a physical barrier, but can have holes either upon use or as a result of use. Therefore, it is imperative to wash hands prior to and after glove use. Gloves are used for one task only. Failure to change gloves between patient contacts is an infection control hazard.

Isolation precautions in hospitals may vary. Universal precautions with measures used for preventing contact, droplet, and airborne transmission should be a policy to ensure adequate infection control practice and to provide the standards of care mandated by state and federal guidelines. Measures used for isolating the patient include a private room, cohorting (placing patients with the same infectious agent together), and PPE. Consistent with universal standard precautions, personnel should always use PPE when involved with patient care depending on the task performed. PPE includes masks, eye protection, face shields, gowns, and protective apparel.

Universal Precautions

The Hospital Infection Control Practices Advisory Committee [HICPAC] has redesigned the categories of isolation precautions in hospitals which include universal precautions. The new system addresses universal precautions and standard precautions, and includes the use of transmission-based precautions (Garner & HICPAC, 1996). Standard precautions are used for all patient care.

Airborne precautions, used in addition to standard precautions, are for patients known or suspected to have communicable illnesses transmitted by airborne droplet nuclei. Examples include measles, varicella (including disseminated Herpes zoster), and tuberculosis.

Droplet precautions, used in addition to standard precautions, are for patients known or suspected to have serious illnesses transmitted by large-particle droplets. Examples include invasive Haemophilus influenzae type b disease, including meningitis, pneumonia, epiglottis, and sepsis; invasive Neisseria meningitidis disease, including meningitis, pneumonia, and sepsis; and other bacterial respiratory infections such as diphtheria (pharyngeal), mycoplasma pneumonia, pertussis, pneumonic plague, streptococcal pharyngitis, pneumonia, or scarlet fever in infants and young children. Certain viral infections are included: adenovirus, influenza, mumps, parvovirus B19, and rubella.

In addition to standard precautions, contact precautions are used for patients known or suspected to have serious illnesses easily transmitted by direct patient contact or by contact with items in the patient's environment. Examples include gastrointestinal, respiratory, skin, or wound infections or colonization with multidrug-resistant bacteria judged by the infection control program, based on current state, federal, regional, or national recommendations, to be of special clinical and epidemiologic significance. Enteric infections with a low infectious dose or prolonged environmental survival are included. Examples are Clostridium difficile for diapered or incontinent patients; enterohemorrhagic Escherichia coli 0157:H7; Shigella, hepatitis A, or rotavirus; and respiratory syncytial virus, parainfluenzae virus, or enteroviral infections in infants and young children. Certain skin infections that are highly contagious or that may occur on dry skin are included. Examples are cutaneous diptheria, Herpes simplex virus (neonatal or mucocutaneous), impetigo, major (noncontained) abscesses, cellulitis, or decubiti; pediculosis, scabies, Staphylococcus furunculosis in infants and young children, Herpes zoster (disseminated or in the immunocompromised host); viral/hemorrhagic conjunctivitis; and viral hemorrhagic infections (Ebola, Lassa, or Marburg).

Summary

The theory, background, and application of government and in-house regulations are described to assist the pharmacy technician in understanding and applying the methods and techniques needed to provide the utmost safety in the preparation and dispensing of sterile medications. Parenteral medications are prescribed for the most seriously ill, and therefore all means are used to provide maximum patient safety and patient care.

Infection control is an on-going attitude and so is practical application of vigilance for all members of the healthcare team. Prevention of nosocomial incidence is a serious professional responsibility for the pharmacy technician, the pharmacist, the nurse, the physician, the laboratory technician, and other caregivers. Particular consideration is given to the need for strict aseptic technique and the application of universal precautions as required in pharmacy practice.

ASSESSMENT

Multiple Choice Questions

1. Handwashing is considered
   a. the single most important procedure for preventing infections
   b. a good idea in the practice of infection control
   c. only the first step in a person's work day
   d. to be done *only* when preparing admixtures

2. Agents used for handwashing include
   a. cidex
   b. ethylene oxide
   c. sodium hypochlorite
   d. chlorhexidene or triclosan

3. Asespis is defined as
   a. an increase in pathogenic (disease producing) organisms
   b. the absence of pathogenic microorganisms
   c. a few colonies of microorganisms
   d. killing only nonpathogenic pathogens

4. *Most* nosocomial epidemics of infusion-related septicemia are caused by
   a. gram-positive pathogens
   b. fungus
   c. gram-negative pathogens
   d. protozoa

5. The causative agent for an outbreak of neonatal listerosis was
   a. safflower oil
   b. mineral oil
   c. Vaseline
   d. talcum powder

6. The mode of transmission for infectious agents is
   a. the mechanism by which an agent is transferred to the susceptible host
   b. by the direct route only
   c. by the agent responsible for airborne disease
   d. through the cutaneous tissue only

7. Personal protective equipment (PPE) must be utilized for all patient care, which includes
   a. gloves, mask, gown, and eye protection
   b. booties
   c. cloth gown
   d. hair net

8. Universal [standard] precautions must be enforced for
   a. all patients
   b. only when entering an isolation room
   c. taking care of tuberculosis patients
   d. administering drug therapy

9. Isolation precautions for use in hospitals were redesigned by
   a. JCAHO
   b. HICPAC
   c. New York State
   d. the commissioner of health

10. Failure to change gloves between patient contacts is considered
    a. the acceptable procedure
    b. an infection control hazard
    c. breech of practice
    d. not important

11. Which of the following microorganisms can multiply in solutions of 5% dextrose?
    a. Enterobacter
    b. Staphylococcus
    c. Pseudomonas
    d. Proteus

12. Which of the following disease entities may be effectively transmitted via the hands of pharmacy personnel?
    a. scabies
    b. mumps
    c. Herpetic whitlow
    d. measles

13. MDVs should be used
    a. until all contents have dried up
    b. until there are no specific guidelines for length of use
    c. until contents appear cloudy
    d. as long as sterility can be reasonably assured

14. The CDC recommends refrigeration of admixed parenterals if they are not to be administered within
    a. 24 hours of preparation
    b. 6 hours of preparation
    c. 1 hour of preparation
    d. 8 hours of preparation

Bibliography

Accreditation Manual for Hospitals 1996. (1996). Chicago: Joint Commission on Accreditation of Healthcare Organizations, 71–74.

Alfonso, E., Kenyon, K.R., Ormerod, D. et al. (1987). *Pseudomonas* corneoscleritis. *Am J Opthalmol, 103,* 90–98.

American Society of Hospital Pharmacists. (1993). ASHP technical assistance bulletin on quality assurance for pharmacy-prepared sterile products. *Am J Hosp Pharm, 50,* 2286–2398.

Bennett, S.N., McNeil, M.M., Bland, L.A. et al. (1995). Postoperative infections traced to contamination of an intravenous anesthetic, propofol. *N Engl J Med, 333,* 147–154.

Center for Disease Control and Prevention. (1995). Intravascular device related infections prevention; guideline availability; notice. *Federal Register, 60,* 49978–50005.

Center for Disease Control and Prevention. (1990). Postsurgical infections associated with an extrinsically contaminated intravenous anesthetic agent-California, Illinois, Maine and Michigan. *MMWR, 39,* 426–427, 433.

Cleary, T.J., MacIntyre, D.S., & Castro, M. (1981). *Serratia marcescens* bacteremias in an intensive care unit: Contaminated heparinized saline solution as a reservoir. *Am J Infect Control, 9,* 107–111.

Degleux, G., Le Coutour, X., Hecquard, C. et al. (1991). Septicemia caused by contaminated parenteral nutrition pouches: The refrigerator as an unusual cause. *J Parenter Enteral Nutr, 15,* 474–475.

Felts, S.K., Schaffner, W., Mely, M.A. et al. (1972). Sepsis caused by contaminated intravenous fluids. *Ann Int Med, 77,* 881–890.

Garner, J., & HICPAC. (1996). Guideline for isolation precautions in hospitals. *Infect Control and Hosp Epid, 17,* 54–80.

Gorbea, H.F., Snydman, D.R., Delaney, A. et al. (1984). Intravenous tubing with burettes can be safely changed at 48-hour intervals. *JAMA, 251,* 2112–2115.

Hovding, G., & Sjursen, H. (1982). Bacterial contamination of drops and dropper tips of in-use multidose eye drop bottles. *Acta Ophthal, 60,* 213–222.

Larson, E. (1995) APIC guideline for handwashing and hand antisepsis in health care settings. *Am J Infect Control, 23,* 251–269.

Llop, J.M., Manques, I., Perez, J.L. et al. (1993). Staphylococcus sapophyticus sepsis related to total parenteral nutrition admixtures contamination. *J Parenter Enteral Nutr, 17,* 575–577.

Longfield, R., Longfield, J., Smith, L.P. et al. (1984). Multidose medication vial sterility: An in-use study and a review of the literature. *Infect Control, 5,* 165–169.

Maki, D.G. & Martin, W.T. (1975). Nationwide epidemic of septicemia caused by contaminated infusion products: IV. Growth of microbial pathogens in fluids for intravenous infusion. *J Infect Dis, 131,* 267–272.

Maki, D.G., Botticelli, M.S., LeRoy, M.L. et al. (1987). Prospective study of replacing administration sets for intravenous therapy at 48- vs. 72-hour intervals. *JAMA, 258,* 1777–1781.

Maki, D.G.. (1992). Infections due to infusion therapy. In J.V. Bennett, P.S. Brachman, J.P. Sanford (Eds.), *Hospital infections,* (3rd ed.). Boston: Little, Brown, 849–898.

Melnyk, P.S., Shevchuck, Y.M., Conly, J.M. et al. (1993). Contamination study of multiple dose vial. *Ann Pharmacother, 27,* 274–278.

Moi, S., & Thornton, J.P. (1991). Time limit on multidose vials after initial entry. *Hosp Pharm, 26,* 805–809.

Plouffe, J.F., Brown, D.G., Silva, J. et al. (1977). Nosocomial outbreak of *Candida parapsilosis* fungemia related to intravenous infusion. *Arch Intern Med, 137,* 166–186.

Schuchat, A., Lizano, C., Broome, C.V. et al. (1991). Outbreak of neonatal listeriosis associated with mineral oil. *Pediatr Infect Dis J, 10,* 183–189.

Simmons, B.P., Hooton, T.M., Mallison, G.F. (1982). CDC guidelines for hospital environmental control: Pharmacy. *Hosp Infect Control, 2,* 28H–28I.

Simmons, B.P., Hooton, T.M., Wong, E.S. et al. (1983). CDC guidelines for the prevention and control of nosocomial infections: Guidelines for prevention of intravascular infections. *Infect Control, 5,* 183–188.

Solomon, S.L., Kabbaz, R.F., Parker, R.H. et al. (1984). An outbreak of *Candida parapsilosis* bloodstream infections in patients receiving parenteral nutrition. *J Infect Dis, 149,* 98–102.

Tamer, H.R., Sweet, B., & Ross, M.B. (1994). Use and sterility of multidose opthalmic medications. *Am J Hosp Pharm, 51,* 500–502.

Templeton, W.C. III, Eiferman, R.A., Snyder, J.W. et al. (1982). *Serratia* keratitis transmitted by contaminated eyedroppers. *Am J Opthalmol, 93,* 723–726.

26 Accreditation of Technician Training Programs

COMPETENCIES

Upon completion and review of this chapter, the student should be able to

1. State four objectives of the accreditation process for pharmacy technician training programs.

2. Articulate the primary reason for a differentiated workforce in the pharmacy profession.

3. Explain ASHP's involvement in accrediting pharmacy technician training programs rather than in evaluating competency achievement of individual pharmacy technicians.

4. List the eight areas that comprise the Accreditation Standard for Pharmacy Technician Training Programs.

5. Outline the objectives that form the basis for pharmacy technician training programs.

6. List the organizations that have endorsed the Model Curriculum for Pharmacy Technician Training.

Introduction

The objectives of the **accreditation** process for pharmacy technician **training programs** are to (1) upgrade and standardize the formal training that pharmacy technicians receive; (2) guide, assist, and recognize those health care facilities and academic institutions that wish to support the profession by operating such programs; (3) provide criteria for the prospective technician trainee in the selection of a program by identifying those institutions conducting accredited pharmacy technician training programs; and (4) provide prospective employees a basis for determining the level of competency of pharmacy technicians by identifying those technicians who have successfully completed accredited technician training programs.

The Need for Differentiated Workforce

During the past decade many of ASHP's initiatives have centered on pharmacy's movement toward becoming a full-fledged clinical profession. ASHP has long recognized that as we continue to move in this **clinical** direction, other health care professions and the public will increasingly look to pharmacy for answers to complex questions in drug therapy. With pharmacists' continuing efforts to enhance the degree to which they better utilize their knowledge and skills by providing direct patient care services, it becomes more evident that many, if not all, of the technical tasks routinely done by pharmacists must be delegated (with appropriate guidance and supervision) to nonprofessional personnel.

Development of a differentiated workforce will provide a core of well-trained pharmacy technicians who can assist the pharmacist in the delivery of pharmaceutical care by performing routine tasks that were formerly part of the traditional role of the pharmacist.

ASHP Initiatives

For over two decades ASHP, in response to an obvious void, has promulgated documents that specifically address **outcome competencies** for pharmacy technicians. However, to date these have not been uniformly recognized and accepted throughout pharmacy. While these documents are gaining a greater degree of acceptance among pharmacists, it remains clear that the job category of "technician" continues to be interpreted differently because no two technicians are necessarily measured by the same "yardstick."

ASHP has remained steadfast in its belief that an absolute prerequisite for the orderly development of pharmacy support personnel is uniform recognition and acceptance of a competency or performance standard. Moreover, it has agreed that such a standard provides the basic **objective** for supportive personnel training programs.

Early on, ASHP recognized that a competency standard alone could not suffice for development of pharmacy technician training programs. In fact, ASHP considered as part of its early deliberations about such programs whether competency-based training would be acceptable. Key to these deliberations was the realization that the structure and process of these training programs would be of secondary importance; competency outcomes would be the primary concern. Further, it was agreed that the feasibility of developing competency-based training programs, which depend largely on the ability to evaluate competency achievement, would not be difficult. Despite these considerations and due in large measure to the advice of its members, ASHP expressed uneasiness about promoting establishment of competency-based technician training programs. As a consequence, ASHP decided to follow the more traditional pattern of evaluating each training program through the process of accreditation. It is easy to understand how ASHP chose this avenue, as it already had a well-established accreditation process for postgraduate pharmacy residency training programs in place since 1963.

Accreditation is defined as the process by which an agency or organization evaluates and recognizes a program of study or an institution as meeting certain predetermined qualifications or standards. It applies only to institutions and their programs of study or their services.

Obviously, to establish an accreditation program, ASHP knew firsthand that it was necessary to develop an accreditation standard that would delineate specific facilities and process requirements in addition to competency outcome criteria. Therefore, in November 1980 the ASHP Board of Directors requested that an accreditation standard for technician training programs be developed. They also authorized implementation of an accreditation process for such programs at the earliest possible time.

An accreditation standard for pharmacy technician training programs was approved by the ASHP board in April 1982. The first program was accredited in September 1983.

Accreditation Program

As noted in the ASHP **regulations** on accreditation of pharmacy technician training programs (Appendix G), the accreditation service is conducted by authority of ASHP Board of Directors under the direction of the **Commission on Credentialing.** The commission reviews and evaluates applications and survey reports and, as delegated by the board, takes final action on all applications for accreditation in accordance with the policies and procedures set forth in the regulations.

All pharmacy technician training programs making application for accreditation by ASHP are evaluated by **site survey** against the ASHP Accreditation Standard for Pharmacy Technician Training Programs (Appendix G). Comprising eight parts, the standard outlines specific requirements for administrative responsibility for the training program, qualifications of the training site, qualification of the **pharmacy service** that is used to provide trainees with practical experience, qualifications of the pharmacy director and preceptors, qualifications and selection of the applicant, the overall structure of the pharmacy technician training program, experimentation and innovative approaches to training, and issuance of the certificate of completion.

With respect to the competency-based objectives that must be developed as a fundamental component of any ASHP-accredited technician training program, individuals are encouraged to use the Model Curriculum for Pharmacy Technician Training. Developed by pharmacy technician training program directors and ASHP staff, this document is intended to provide pharmacy technician educators with a prototype for training pharmacy technicians in all practice settings. The curriculum is divided into three components: (1) goal statements and educational objectives; (2) a curriculum map; and (3) descriptors for each of the modules of instruction. The curriculum has been endorsed by the American Association of Pharmacy Technicians, American Pharmaceutical Association, Pharmacy Technician Educators Council, and ASHP.

The ASHP accreditation standards accommodate training programs offered by hospital and health system pharmacy departments, managed care facilities, community colleges, vocational/technical institutes, proprietary agencies, and military facilities. Currently, there are over fifty-five ASHP-accredited programs that are conducted in each of these types of training facilities.

Additional information about the ASHP program for accreditation of pharmacy technician training programs can be obtained by contacting the Accreditation Services Division, American Society of Health-System Pharmacists, 7272 Wisconsin Ave., Bethesda, MD 20814, (301)657-3000, ext. 1251.

ASSESSMENT

Multiple Choice Questions

1. ASHP has accredited pharmacy technician training programs in
   a. colleges of pharmacy
   b. vocational/technical schools
   c. military schools
   d. hospital pharmacy departments
   e. all of the above
   f. none of the above

2. Continuing accreditation of a pharmacy technician training program is dependent upon
   a. a site visit
   b. adherence to accreditation standards
   c. increased number of graduates over previous years
   d. at least one graduating class every two years
   e. all of the above
   f. none of the above

3. A pharmacy technician may engage in the following activities:
   a. packaging and labeling medication doses
   b. maintaining patient records
   c. preparing intravenous admixtures
   d. inventory of drug supplies
   e. all of the above

4. A differentiated workforce is needed in pharmacy because
   a. pharmacists provide direct patient care services
   b. technicians answer complex questions in drug therapy
   c. pharmacists must perform many technical functions
   d. personnel best suited for the role perform specialized functions

Bibliography

ASHP. (1996). Model curriculum for pharmacy technician training. Bethesda, MD: *ASHP.*

ASHP accreditation standard for pharmacy technician training programs. (in press). *American Society of Health-System Pharmacists, Practice Standards of ASHP 1998–1999.*

ASHP position on long-range pharmacy manpower needs and residency training. (1980, September). American Society of Hospital Pharmacists, 37, 1220.

ASHP regulations on accreditation of pharmacy technician training programs. (in press). *American Society of Health-System Pharmacists, Practice Standards of ASHP 1998–1999.*

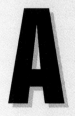

Long-Term Care

A–1: Examples of Guidelines for Automatic Stop-Order Policy in a Skilled Nursing Facility (Unless Otherwise Specified by Physician)

Drug Type

Analgesics . . . . .30 days
    Darvon, Darvocet

Antianemia drugs . . . . .30 days
    iron

* Antibiotics . . . . .7 days
    Keflex, tetracycline

* Antiemetics . . . . .4 days
    Compazine, Tigan

Anticoagulants . . . . .30 days
    Coumadin

Antihistamines . . . . .7 days
    Chlor-Trimeton, Seldane, Sudafed

Antineoplastics . . . . .30 days
    Nolvadex, Hydrea

Barbiturates . . . . .30 days
    phenobarbital

Cardiovascular . . . . .30 days
    digoxin, vasotec, quinidine

Cathartics . . . . .30 days
    Pericolace, Colace, Senokot

* Cold preparations . . . . .5 days
    Phenergan Expectorant, Robitussin

Dermatologicals . . . . .30 days
    Lidex, hydrocortisone, Synalar

Diuretics . . . . .30 days
    HCTZ, Dyazide, Aldactazide, Lasix

A–2: Medication Order Entry Flow Chart

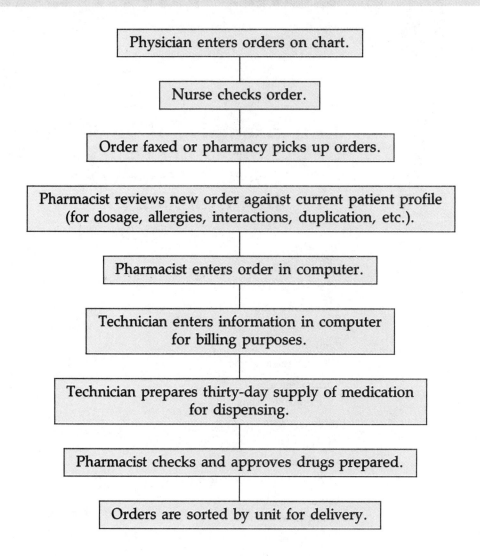

Physician enters orders on chart.

Nurse checks order.

Order faxed or pharmacy picks up orders.

Pharmacist reviews new order against current patient profile (for dosage, allergies, interactions, duplication, etc.).

Pharmacist enters order in computer.

Technician enters information in computer for billing purposes.

Technician prepares thirty-day supply of medication for dispensing.

Pharmacist checks and approves drugs prepared.

Orders are sorted by unit for delivery.

A–3: Inspection of Medication Stations

Unit: _____ Date: _____

Check (√) if in compliance. Make comments below.

		Yes	No
1.	The area is clean and well organized.	( )	( )
	Are cabinet doors and/or door to room locked?	( )	( )
	Medication carts are locked and kept in secure area.	( )	( )
2.	Are refrigerator and lighting working properly? (temperature between 36°F and 46°F)	( )	( )
3.	Is refrigerator clean and free of food and labeled "Not for the storage of flammable liquids"?	( )	( )
4.	Are external medications separated from internal medications?	( )	( )

	Yes	No
5. Medication draws are labeled with patient's name.	( )	( )
Are any medications outdated, recalled, deteriorated, broken, or contaminated?	( )	( )
6. Are thermolabile medications properly stored?	( )	( )
Are all light-sensitive medications properly stored?	( )	( )
7. Are all controlled substances stored in a double-locked cabinet?	( )	( )
8. Are records of distribution and/or administration of controlled substances maintained properly?	( )	( )
9. Are all medications properly labeled?	( )	( )
10. Are all discontinued medications returned to the pharmacy?	( )	( )
11. Multiple-dose vials are dated on first use and discarded after 30 days.	( )	( )
12. Medication brought from home is sent home or stored according to policy.	( )	( )
13. Are any of the following present?		
a. Nonapproved medications? (review floor stock list)	( )	( )
b. Samples?	( )	( )
c. Nondrug items or related items?	( )	( )
d. Flammables properly stored?	( )	( )
14. Reconstituted drugs are labeled with the date prepared and their expiration date.	( )	( )
15. Hypodermic syringes and needles are properly stored and disposed of.	( )	( )
16. Emergency trays and charts checked for adequate and proper supply of drugs; outdated drugs removed and replaced.	( )	( )
17. Medication procedure manual, formulary, and PDR are available.	( )	( )
18. Crash cart and trauma kit reviewed for outdated and missing meds.	( )	( )
19. References:		
a. Antidote chart	( )	( )
b. Approved abbreviations posted	( )	( )
c. Metric apothecary chart posted	( )	( )
d. Poison Control and Drug Information Center phone number	( )	( )
20. Are any investigational drugs present?	( )	( )
21. Previous deficiencies corrected.	( )	( )

22. Indicate follow-up required: _____

_____

_____

_____

R.Ph. _____ R.N. _____

A–4: Emergency Tray Contents

Medications

2 Aminophylline I.V. 500 mg 20 mL
12 Aromatic Ammonia Vaporoles
1 Atropine Sulfate Inj. 0.4 mg/mL, 1 mL
1 Calcium Gluconate Inj. 10% 10 mL
1 Cogentin Inj. 2 mg/2 mL Amp
1 Dexamethasone Inj. 4 mg/mL (Decadron)
1 Dextrose Inj. 50% 50 mL
1 Digoxin 0.25 mg/mL (Lanoxin) 2 mL
1 Diphenhydramine Inj. 50 mg/mL (Benadryl)
4 Epinephrine Inj. 1:100 (Adrenalin) 1 mL
10 Furosemide Inj. 10 mg/mL (Lasix) 2 mL
1 Glucagon Inj. 1 mg
1 Lidocaine 1% Inj. Topical (Xylocaine)
1 Lidocaine 2% Inj. Topical (Xylocaine)
1 Methylprednisolone Inj. 125 mg (Solu-Medrol)
1 Nitroglycerine SL Tabs 1/150 gr
1 Phenytoin Inj 100 mg/2 mL (Dilantin)
1 Sodium Bicarbonate Inj. 7.5% 50 mL
4 Cephradine 250 mg (velosef)
4 Sulfa/Trim DS (Bactrim DS)
2 Cefazolin Inj. 1 gm (kefzol, Ancef)

Supplies

1 Tubex holder
1 3 mL syringe
1 5 mL syringe
1 20 mL syringe
1 60 mL syringe
1 I.V. Cath 20 g × 1 1/4″
1 I.V. Cath 24 g × 3/4″

5 needles 25 g × 5/8″
1 needle 19 g × 1 1/2″
3 needles 20 g × 1 1/2″
2 needles 22 g × 1 1/2″
Alcohol pads
Bandages
Gauze pads
1 tourniquet (Plain)
1 tourniquet (Velcro)
Steri-Strip Skin Closures
4 Erythromycin 250 mg
4 Cipro 250 mg
2 Noroxin 400 mg

Omnibus Budget Reconciliation Act of 1990 (OBRA 90)

The Omnibus Budget Reconciliation Act of 1990 (OBRA 90) encompasses a number of laws relating to pharmacy practice.

OBRA 90 is intended to save taxpayers' money, as the full name indicates. Congress decided to reduce the government's cost for pharmaceuticals in the Medicaid program. In addition, Congress made a positive statement about the pharmacist as a health care professional who can improve the quality of a patient's drug regimen. Congress obviously believes that higher-quality patient care is more cost-effective patient care and the pharmacist has been chosen as the key player in the latest congressional effort to improve the quality of care.

OBRA 90 was not the first piece of congressional legislation to require DUR or Drug Regimen Review (DRR) by pharmacists. The Health Care Financing Administration (HCFA) promulgated regulations effective in 1990 that expand the pharmacist's functions of optimizing drug therapy in long-term care facilities.

The section of OBRA 90 that relates to the Medicaid prescription drug program is lengthy and touches upon almost every aspect of pharmacy practice.

The three main sections are:

- Manufacturer rebates to state Medicaid programs
- Mandatory drug use review (DUR), which includes patient counseling
- Government-sponsored demonstration projects relating to the provision of pharmaceutical services.

The section of OBRA 90 that recognized pharmacists as professionals whose expertise can detect potential problems with drug therapy and promote rational outcomes will be discussed.

Each individual state shall establish regulations encompassing a review of drug therapy before each prescription is filled or delivered to an individual typically at the point of sale. The review shall include screening for potential drug therapy problems due to therapeutic duplication, drug-disease contraindications, drug-drug interactions (including serious interactions with nonprescription or over-the-counter drugs), incorrect drug dosage or duration of drug treatment, drug-allergy interactions, and clinical abuse/misuse.

As part of the state's prospective drug use review program, applicable state law shall establish standards for pharmacist counseling of individuals receiving prescriptions, which includes at least the following:

1. The pharmacist must offer to discuss with each individual or caregiver of such individual (in person when practicable, or by telephone) matters which, in the exercise of the pharmacist's professional judgment he/she deems significant, including the following:
   a. The name and description of the medication.
   b. The dosage form, dosage, route of administration, and duration of drug therapy.
   c. Special directions and precautions for preparation, administration, and use by the patient.
   d. Common severe side effects or adverse affects or interactions and therapeutic contraindications that may be encountered, including their avoidance and the action required if they occur.
   e. Techniques for self-monitoring drug therapy.
   f. Proper storage.
   g. Prescription refill information.
   h. Action to be taken in the event of a missed dose.
2. A reasonable effort must be made by the pharmacist to obtain, record, and maintain at least the following information regarding individuals receiving prescriptions:
   a. Name, address, telephone number, date of birth (or age), and gender.
   b. Individual history when significant, including disease state or states, known allergies and drug reactions, and a comprehensive list of medications and relevant devices.
   c. Pharmacist comments relevant to the individual's drug therapy. Nothing in the clause shall be construed as requiring a pharmacist to provide consultation when an individual receiving benefits under this subchapter or caregiver of such individual refuses such consultation.

The Health Care Financing Administration (HCFA) has the responsibility for setting the federal guidelines for state Medicaid agencies to use in establishing pharmacist's responsibilities in counseling patients. HCFA has indicated that pharmacists could not delegate the actual counseling to ancillary personnel, but that such personnel could extend the offer to patients to receive counseling. They permit ancillary personnel to collect, record, and seek clarifications. The ultimate responsibility for ensuring that these tasks are accomplished rests with the pharmacist.

APPENDIX

B Regulatory Standards in Institutional Pharmacy Practice

B–1: ASHP Statements

Continuing Education

Pharmaceutical Care

Pharmaceutical Research in Organized Health Care Settings

Pharmacist's Role in Infection Control

Pharmacist's Role in Pharmacokinetic Monitoring

Pharmacist's Role in Substance Abuse Prevention, Education, and Assistance

Principles for Including Medications and Pharmaceutical Care in Health Care Systems

The Formulary System

The Pharmacist's Responsibility for Distribution and Control of Drug Products

The Pharmacist's Role with Respect to Drug Delivery Systems and Administration Devices

The Pharmacy and Therapeutics Committee

The Role of the Pharmacist in Patient-Focused Care

The Use of Medications for Unlabeled Uses

Unit-Dose Drug Distribution

B–2: ASHP Guidelines

Safe Use of Automated Medication Storage and Distribution Devices

Adverse Drug Reaction Monitoring and Reporting

ASHP Guidelines for Selecting Pharmaceutical Manufacturers and Suppliers

Formulary System Management

Medication-Use Evaluation

Minimum Standard for Pharmacies in Hospitals

Obtaining Authorization for Documenting Pharmaceutical Care in Patient Medical Records

Outsourcing Pharmaceutical Services

Pharmaceutical Research in Organized Health Care Settings

Pharmaceutical Services for Ambulatory Patients

Pharmaceutical Services in Correctional Facilities

Pharmacist's Role in the Development of Clinical Care Plans

Pharmacist-Conducted Patient Education and Counseling

Preventing Medication Errors in Hospitals

Providing Pediatric Pharmaceutical Services in Organized Health Care Systems

Provision of Medication Information by Pharmacists

Standardized Method for Pharmaceutical Care

The Pharmacist's Role in Home Care

B–3: ASHP Technical Assistance Bulletins

Assessing Cost Containment Strategies for Pharmacies in Organized Health Care Settings

Compounding Nonsterile Products in Pharmacies

Drug Formularies

Evaluation of Drugs for Formularies

Handling Cytotoxic and Hazardous Drugs

Hospital Drug Distribution and Control

Pharmacy-Prepared Ophthalmic Products

Quality Assurance for Pharmacy-Prepared Sterile Products

Recruitment, Selection, and Retention of Pharmacy Personnel

Repackaging Oral Solids and Liquids in Single-Unit and Unit-Dose Packages

Single-Unit and Unit-Dose Packages of Drugs

Surgery and Anesthesiology Pharmaceutical Services

The Pharmacist's Role in Immunization

Use of Controlled Substances in Organized Health Care Settings

B–4: ASHP Therapeutic Guidelines

Angiotensin-Converting Enzyme Inhibitors in Patients with Left Ventricular Dysfunction

Antimicrobial Prophylaxis in Surgery

Nonsurgical Antimicrobial Prophylaxis

B–5: ASHP Therapeutic Position Statements

Antithrombotic Therapy in Chronic Atrial Fibrillation

International Normalized Ratio System to Monitor Oral Anticoagulant Therapy

Preferential Use of Metronidazole for the Treatment of Clostridium Dificile-Associated Disease

Safe Use of Niacin in the Management of Dyslipidemias

Strategies for Identifying and Preventing Pneumococcal Resistance

Strategies for Preventing and Treating Multidrug-Resistant Tuberculosis (MDR-TB)

Strict Glycemic Control in Selected Patients with Insulin-Dependent Diabetes Mellitus

The Institutional Use of 0.9% Sodium Chloride Injection to Maintain Patency of Peripheral Indwelling Intermittent Infusion Devices

Use of Aspirin for Prophylaxis of Myocardial Infarction

Note: Copies of ASHP statements, guidelines, technical assistance bulletins, therapeutic guidelines, and therapeutic position statements may be obtained directly from the American Society of Health-System Pharmacists, 7272 Wisconsin Ave., Bethesda, MD 20814, 301-657-3000.

APPENDIX C

Materials Management of Pharmaceuticals

C–1: ASHP Technical Assistance Bulletin on the Evaluation of Drugs for Formularies

Preamble

One of the major responsibilities of a pharmacy and therapeutics (P&T) committee is to develop and maintain a drug formulary system. The formulary can be used as the basis for promoting optimal pharmacotherapy because it contains only those drugs judged by the P&T committee to be in the best interest of the patient's health needs in terms of efficacy and cost. The pharmacist is a key member of the drug evaluation team because of his or her knowledge of pharmacology, pharmacokinetics, toxicology, therapeutics, and drug purchasing.

A thorough, critical review of the pharmaceutical and medical literature is necessary for evaluating drugs proposed for admission to a formulary. Comparative data associated with a drug's efficacy, adverse effects, and cost and the determination of its potential therapeutic advantages and deficiencies require critical evaluation by the pharmacist. Drugs may be added to or deleted from a formulary based on evaluation by the P&T committee. Alternative actions might include either conditional approval for a specific time period (with subsequent reevaluation) or temporary limitation of a drug's use to an individual medical service specialty with future reassessment.

Evaluation Report Considerations

A standardized evaluation report should be developed by the pharmacy for use in the evaluation process. It is recommended that each report include the following information:

1. Generic name.
   - List the officially approved name of all chemical entities in the drug product.
2. Trade name(s).
   - List the most common trade name(s) of the drug product.
3. Source(s) of supply.
   - Identify the pharmaceutical vendors from which the drug product can be procured.
   - For a generic drug product, identify the actual manufacturer; if applicable, identify the vendors distributing the product.
4. *American Hospital Formulary Service Drug Information* classification number.
   - List the number for quick access and retrieval of information.
5. Pharmacologic classification.
   - State the pharmacologic class to which the drug belongs and any similar properties it possesses compared with existing drugs.
   - State the mechanism of action; if the mechanism of action is unknown, state this. If applicable, the mechanism of action may be compared with that of another drug or class of drugs.
6. Therapeutic indications.
   - State the uses of the drug as approved by the Food and Drug Administration; indicate whether the use is prophylactic, therapeutic, palliative, curative, adjunctive, or supportive.
   - Evaluate uses of the drug in comparison with other established forms of therapy, using, if possible, human studies for compari-

son. Comparisons should emphasize therapeutics (efficacy, incidence of treatment success, remission, sensitivity, ease of monitoring, and treatment periods required) and include a critical analysis of clinical studies in such areas as patient population, methodology, statistics, and conclusions.

- Identify non-FDA-labeled uses for the drug and those uses that show promise in investigational studies.

7. Dosage forms.
   - List all dosage forms available as approved by FDA; list unit cost.
8. Bioavailability and pharmacokinetics.
   - List bioavailability data for the most common route of administration and dosage of the drug. Other bioavailability data should be available on request by the P&T committee.
   - List pharmacokinetic data for absorption, distribution, metabolism, and excretion of the drug. For absorption, include information on the extent and rate of absorption of the drug by the usual routes of administration; the factors that might affect the rate or extent of absorption; the therapeutic, toxic, and lethal blood levels; the period of time required for onset, peak, and duration of therapeutic effect; and the half-life and factors affecting it. For distribution, include information on the usual distribution of the drug in body tissues and fluids, the drug's propensity to cross the blood-brain barrier or placenta or to appear in human milk, the drug's propensity for protein binding, and the drug's volume of distribution. For metabolism, include information on sites of metabolism, extent of biotransformation, and metabolic products and their activity. For excretion, include information on routes of elimination from the body, factors affecting elimination, and the form in which the drug is eliminated.
9. Dosage range.
   - List the dosage range for different routes of administration of the drug.
   - List initial, maintenance, maximal, geriatric, and pediatric doses for the drug.
10. Known adverse effects and toxicities.
    - Discuss adverse effects of the drug and their frequency of occurrence from research data of human studies.
    - Discuss means or methods of preventing or treating adverse effects and toxicities. Benefits of disease treatment and risks of adverse effects should be emphasized.
11. Special precautions.
    - List precautions and contraindications for certain disease states or other conditions.
    - Compare all of the preceding data with existing similar agents, where applicable.
    - List potential drug interactions if deemed clinically important.
12. Comparisons.
    - List therapeutic comparisons with other drugs or treatment regimens.
    - List cost comparison data of a standard treatment regimen with the new drug versus currently used drugs.
    - List unusual monitoring or drug administration requirements for the drug.
13. Recommendations.
    - Formulate recommendations from analysis of all of the preceding data and consideration of other factors such as medical staff preference, distribution problems, and availability of the drug. Recommend action to be taken with regard to the drug's formulary status, as follows:

    Uncontrolled: To be available for use by all medical staff.

    Monitored: To be available for use by all medical staff, but its use is to be monitored.

    Restricted: To be available for use by the medical staff of a specific service or department.

    Conditional: To be available for use by all medical staff for a specific time period.

    Deletion: To be deleted from the current formulary.

Recommended Reference Materials

This list of recommended references includes those sources that commonly provide useful information in drug evaluation; however, review of additional specialty journals or other sources may be required.

- Texts.
  1. *American Hospital Formulary Service Drug Information.*
  2. *Drug Topics Redbook Annual Pharmacists' Reference.*

3. *Facts and Comparisons.*
4. *Martindale—The Extra Pharmacopoeia.*
5. *Physicians' Desk Reference.*
6. *The Pharmacological Basis of Therapeutics.*

■ Periodicals and abstracting systems.
1. *American Journal of Hospital Pharmacy.*
2. *Annals of Internal Medicine.*
3. *Archives of Internal Medicine.*
4. *Antimicrobial Agents and Chemotherapy.*
5. *Clinical Pharmacology and Therapeutics.*
6. *Clinical Pharmacy.*
7. *Drug Therapy.*
8. Drugdex.
9. Drugs.
10. *Drug Intelligence and Clinical Pharmacy.*
11. *Hospital Formulary.*
12. *Hospital Therapy.*

13. Iowa Drug Information System.
14. *International Pharmaceutical Abstracts.*
15. *Journal of the American Medical Association.*
16. *The Lancet.*
17. *Medical Letter on Drugs and Therapeutics.*
18. *New England Journal of Medicine.*
19. Paul de Haen Information Systems.
20. *Pharmacotherapy.*

This technical assistance bulletin is supplementary to the "ASHP Statement on the Pharmacy and Therapeutics Committee,"[1] "ASHP Statement on the Formulary System,"[2] and "ASHP Technical Assistance Bulletin on Hospital Formularies,"[3] which should be consulted for further information on the formulary system.

References

1. American Society of Hospital Pharmacists. (1984). ASHP statement on the pharmacy and therapeutics committee. *Am J Hosp Pharm, 41,* 1621.
2. American Society of Hospital Pharmacists. (1983). ASHP statement on the formulary system. *Am J Hosp Pharm, 40,* 1384–1385.
3. American Society of Hospital Pharmacists. (1985). ASHP technical assistance bulletin on hospital formularies. *Am J Hosp Pharm, 42,* 375–377.

Developed by the ASHP Council on Professional Affairs. Approved by the ASHP Board of Directors, November 19, 1987. Supersedes an earlier version approved by the Board of Directors, April 30, 1981. Copyright © 1988, American Society of Hospital Pharmacists, Inc. All rights reserved.

The bibliographic citation for this document is as follows: American Society of Hospital Pharmacists. (1988). ASHP technical assistance bulletin on the evaluation of drugs for formularies. *Am J Hosp Pharm, 45,* 386–387.

C–2: ASHP Guidelines for Selecting Pharmaceutical Manufacturers and Suppliers[a]

Pharmacists are responsible for selecting, from hundreds of manufacturers and suppliers of drugs, those that will enable them to fulfill an important obligation: ensuring that patients receive pharmaceuticals and related supplies of the highest quality and at the lowest cost. These guidelines are offered as an aid to the pharmacist in achieving this goal.

Obligations of the Supplier

Pharmacists may purchase with confidence the products of those suppliers meeting the criteria presented here. Other factors such as credit policies, delivery times, and the breadth of a supplier's product line also must be considered when selecting a supplier.

Technical Considerations

1. On request of the pharmacist (an instrument such as the ASHP Drug Product Information Request Form is useful in this regard), the supplier should furnish
   a. Analytical control data.
   b. Sterility testing data.
   c. Bioavailability data.

d. Bioequivalency data.

e. Descriptions of testing procedures for raw materials and finished products.

f. Any other information that may be indicative of the quality of a given finished drug product.

Testing data developed by independent laboratories should be identified by the supplier. All information should be supplied at no charge.

2. There should be no history of recurring product recalls indicative of deficient quality control procedures.

3. The supplier should permit visits (during normal business hours) by the pharmacist to inspect its manufacturing and control procedures.

4. All drug products should conform to the requirements of the *United States Pharmacopeia—The National Formulary (USP—NF)* (the most recent edition) unless otherwise specified by the pharmacist. Items not recognized by USP—NF should meet the specifications set forth by the pharmacist.

5. To the extent possible, all products should be available in single-unit or unit-dose packages. These packages should conform to the "ASHP Technical Assistance Bulletin on Single-Unit and Unit-Dose Packages of Drugs."[1]

6. The name and address of the manufacturer of the final dosage form and the packager or distributor should be present on the product labeling.

7. Expiration dates should be clearly indicated on the package label and, unless stability properties warrant otherwise, should occur in January or July.

8. Therapeutic, biopharmaceutic, and toxicologic information should be available to the pharmacist on request. Toxicity information should be available around the clock.

9. Patient/staff educational materials that are important for proper use of the product should be routinely available.

10. On request, the supplier should furnish proof of any claims made with respect to the efficacy, safety, and superiority of its products.

11. On request, the supplier should furnish, at no charge, a reasonable quantity of its products to enable the pharmacist to evaluate the products' physical traits, including pharmaceutical elegance (appearance and absence of physical deterioration or flaws), packaging, and labeling.

Distribution Policies

1. Whenever possible, delivery of a drug product should be confined to a single lot number.

2. Unless otherwise specified or required by stability considerations, not less than a 12-month interval between a product's time of delivery and its expiration date should be present.

3. The supplier should accept for full credit (based on purchase price), without prior authorization, any unopened packages of goods returned within 12 months of the expiration date. Credits should be in cash or applied to the institution's account.

4. The supplier should ship all goods in a timely manner, freight prepaid, and enclose a packing list with each shipment. All items "out of stock" should be noted, and the anticipated availability of the item should be clearly indicated. There should be no extensive recurrence of back orders.

5. The supplier should warrant title to commodities supplied, warrant them to be free from defects and imperfections and fit for any rational use of the product, and indemnify and hold the purchaser harmless against any and all suits, claims, and expenses, including attorneys' fees, damages, and injuries or any claims by third parties relating to the products.

Marketing and Sales Policies

1. The supplier should not, without written consent, use the pharmacist's or his or her organization's name in any advertising or other promotional materials or activities.

2. The supplier should honor formulary decisions made by the organization's pharmacy and therapeutics committee, and the supplier's sales representatives should comply with the organization's regulations governing their activities.

3. The supplier should not offer cash, equipment, or merchandise to the organization or its staff as an inducement to purchase its products.

4. Discounts should be in cash or cash credit, not merchandise, and should be clearly indicated on invoices and bills rather than consisting of end-of-year rebates or similar discount practices.

5. In entering into a contract to supply goods, the supplier should guarantee to furnish, at the

price specified, any minimum amount of products so stated. If the supplier is unable to meet the supply commitment, the supplier should reimburse the organization for any excess costs incurred in obtaining the product from other sources. If, during the life of the contract, a price reduction occurs, the lower price should prevail.

6. All parties to the bidding process should respect the integrity of the process and the contracts awarded thereby.

Responsibilities of the Purchaser

It may be desirable to purchase drugs or other commodities on a competitive bid basis. The pharmacist should ensure that competitive bidding procedures conform to the guidelines below:

1. Invitations to bid should be mailed to the suppliers' home offices with copies to their local representatives (if any), unless suppliers specify otherwise.

2. Potential bidders should be given no less than 3 weeks to submit a bid.

3. The opening date for bids should be specified and honored by the purchaser.

4. The language of the invitation to bid should be clear and should indicate the person (and organization address and telephone number) the bidder should contact in the event of questions or problems. Specifications should be complete with respect to products, packagings, and quantities desired.

5. If bidding forms are used, they should contain adequate space for the bidder to enter the information requested.

6. The winning bidder should be notified in writing. Unsuccessful bidders may be informed of who won the award at what price, if they so request.

7. The quantities specified in the invitation to bid should be a reasonable estimate of requirements.

8. If the invitation to bid is offered on behalf of a group of purchasers, the individual members of the group should not engage in bidding procedures of their own and should purchase the goods in question from the winning bidder.

Reference

1. American Society of Hospital Pharmacists. (1985). ASHP technical assistance bulletin on single-unit and unit-dose packages of drugs. *Am J Hosp Pharm, 42,* 378–379.

ª Available from ASHP, 7272 Wisconsin Avenue, Bethesda, MD 20814.
Approved by the ASHP Board of Directors, November 14, 1990. Revised by the ASHP Council on Professional Affairs. Supersedes previous versions approved November 17–18, 1983, and September 22, 1989. The bibliographic citation for this document is as follows: American Society of Hospital Pharmacists. (1991). ASHP guidelines for selecting pharmaceutical manufacturers and suppliers. *Am J Hosp Pharm, 48,* 523–524. Copyright © 1991, American Society of Hospital Pharmacists, Inc. All rights reserved.

APPENDIX
D The Hospital Formulary System

D–1: The Pharmacy and Therapeutics Committee

The Pharmacy and Therapeutics Committee is a standing committee of the medical staff and is responsible to the Quality Improvement Committee. This committee shall be so selected as to represent different medical departments or divisions. A chief medical resident, a member of the nursing staff, and the director of Drug Information Services or his/her pharmacist designee, shall serve as members. A representative of the administration who has administrative responsibility for the department of pharmacy services shall also serve as a member.

The committee's duty shall be to review periodically the therapeutic agents and devices used in the hospital and clinics to ensure that their quality meets specifications of the *United States Pharmacopeia (U.S.P.), Good Manufacturing Practices,* other pertinent publications, and applicable hospital committees. This will in part be accomplished through a continually revised hospital formulary.

The committee shall function in both an advisory and an educational capacity.

1. It shall deal with contemporary problems in therapeutics.
2. It shall select for routine use within the institution and its ambulatory services and clinics, therapeutic agents that represent the best available for the prophylaxis or management of disease.
3. It shall recommend the deletion of drugs from the formulary that no longer meet the needs of the hospital patients.

The department of pharmacy services shall recommend to the committee quality control specifications, methods of distribution and control, and drug-utilization reviews.

Function

1. To serve as an advisory group to the medical staff, to the hospital administration, and to the department of pharmacy services on matters pertaining to drug utilization, drug-use control, and standards of practice concerning the use of drugs.
2. To recommend the adoption group to the medical staff, to the hospital administration, and to the department of pharmacy services on matters pertaining to drug, utilization, drug-use control, and standards of practice concerning the use of drugs.
3. To assist in the formulation and implementation of programs designed to meet the needs of the professional staff of physicians, nurses, pharmacists, and others for complete and current knowledge on matters related to drug practice.
4. To serve in an advisory capacity to the medical staff in the selection or choice of drugs that meet the most effective therapeutic quality standards and to evaluate objectively clinical and scientific data regarding new drugs or agents proposed for use in the hospital.
5. To differentiate between similar therapeutic agents and to recommend the best agent for use in the hospital.
6. To develop a formulary of accepted drugs for use in the hospital and to provide for its constant revision. This formulary shall reflect the modern teachings of pharmacotherapeutics and will present a listing of selected therapeutically effective drugs that should be the optimum in drug therapy.
7. To recommend policies regarding the surveillance of investigational drugs.
8. To study problems relating to the administration of medications and make recommendations where applicable.
9. To serve as a focal point for collecting data obtained from drug utilization reviews throughout the hospital.
10. To review and, if necessary, take action on observations made.

D–2: Definitions and Categories of Drugs to be Stocked in the Pharmacy

Formulary Drug

A formulary drug is a therapeutic agent whose place in therapy is well established. It is selected by the Pharmacy and Therapeutics Committee as essential for the best patient care. Such a drug shall be listed in the formulary and stocked in the pharmacy.

Clinical Evaluation Drug

A clinical evaluation drug is a commercially available, nonformulary agent that is temporarily made available to a particular physician or physicians for the purpose of evaluation for formulary inclusion. Any attending physician, with the approval of the chief of service, may request to evaluate a nonformulary drug. It is the responsibility of the Pharmacy and Therapeutics Committee to review these requests. If approved by the chief of service, the requesting physician shall complete a Clinical Evaluation Drug Request Form and submit it to the secretary of the Pharmacy and Therapeutics Committee. The request for the evaluation may be approved by the chair of the Pharmacy and Therapeutics Committee.

The request form will seek the following information:

- objectives of the clinical evaluation
- criteria for selection of patients who will receive the drug
- parameters to be assessed
- estimated number of patients to be studied
- duration of study

The requesting physician shall submit the results of the evaluation after an interim period of time (usually 6 months) to the Pharmacy and Therapeutics Committee.

The final report shall contain conclusions of the requesting physician and a recommendation to the Pharmacy and Therapeutics Committee concerning the drug's role relative to formulary alternatives. If admitted to the formulary, the investigating physician will be expected to assist the Drug Information Service in developing criteria for the appropriate use of the agent.

During the evaluation, the investigating physician(s) need not complete a Nonformulary Drug Request Form for each patient. The department of pharmacy services will be responsible for monitoring the usage of the evaluation drug.

Restricted Drug

A restricted drug is a therapeutic agent, admitted to the formulary, the use of which is authorized by a specific group of physicians designated by the committee (see Administrative Guidelines). The following procedures will apply:

- Drugs in the category will be dispensed only if prescribed by a full-time faculty member of the designated group of physicians.
- Other members of the medical staff may prescribe the drug for an individual patient if they have the drug order authorized by one of the designated physicians.

Investigational Drug

An investigational drug is a therapeutic agent undergoing clinical investigation. It is not approved for general use by the Food and Drug Administration. Or it has been approved by the FDA only for a cause different from that being investigated.

The medical executive committee, through the Pharmacy and Therapeutics Committee, has charged the department of pharmacy services with the administrative control of experimental therapeutic agents. This administrative control includes storage, disposition, and record keeping. In addition the pharmacy is charged with the responsibility for providing drug information relative to these agents.

In order to implement the change, physicians are asked to comply with the following procedures:

- Obtain approval for any study of investigational agents from the Institutional Review Board.
- Complete the Investigational Drug Data Form and return it to the pharmacy.
- Provide the pharmacy with a copy of the signed consent form.
- Instruct the manufacturer to supply the pharmacy with all available pharmacologic and stability data.
- Make arrangements for transfer of the drug to the pharmacy if it is to be received directly by the chief investigator.
- Arrange with the pharmacy for a minimum inventory level and indicate if the pharmacy is to reorder.

Nonformulary Drug

A nonformulary drug is any drug other than one classified as a formulary drug, evaluation drug, restricted drug, or investigational drug. Nonformulary medications may only be prescribed by chiefs of service or attending physicians. These medications will not be dispensed without the prior submission of a Nonformulary Drug Request Form.

Upon receipt of a medication order, the pharmacist will notify the prescriber if the prescribed medication is nonformulary. The pharmacist will suggest to the prescriber alternative medications in the same therapeutic class. If the prescriber still wishes to use the nonformulary medication, a Nonformulary Drug Request Form shall be submitted for each individual patient. The pharmacist will inform the prescriber that there might be a delay in obtaining the requested medication due to possible problems.

D–3: Additions to the Formulary

Requests for the addition of drugs to the formulary may be initiated by an attending physician of the medical staff. A Request for Formulary Addition Form must be completed and signed by the requesting physician, cosigned by the chief of service, and submitted to the secretary of the Pharmacy and Therapeutics Committee. Incomplete forms will be returned to the requesting physician for completion.

The Drug Information Service shall be responsible for preparing all drug evaluation reports. These reports will review the pertinent literature concerning the requested drug and will make recommendations to the committee on the appropriate formulary status of the drug.

The recommendations of the Drug Information Service will be discussed with the requesting physician. The requesters may address the committee when the drug is discussed.

The committee may admit a drug monograph to the formulary without restriction or may restrict the drug's use to the following categories:

1. Restricted to previously established criteria for use. The use of drugs in this category is regularly audited by the drug-use evaluation program of the department of pharmacy services. The audit criteria are based on the established explicit criteria.
2. Restricted to use by full-time faculty within designated departments, divisions, or services.
3. Restricted to prior approval by full-time faculty within designated departments, divisions, or services.

The formulary status of a particular drug may be reviewed and evaluated by the committee after a specific period of time, usually 6 months.

A drug that is reviewed by the committee for formulary addition becomes official on the first day of the month following the meeting upon publication in the formulary update.

D–4: Deletions from the Formulary

Drugs may be deleted from the formulary as a result of the addition of more efficacious or safer agents, or at the request of a committee member of the Drug Information Service. Drugs may also be deleted upon review of the annual Low Volume of Use report.

Proposed deletions from the formulary will be published in the formulary update so that the medical staff may comment before final action is taken. If no objections to the deletion are heard, the drug will be removed from the formulary.

E
Basic Biopharmaceutics

E-1: Core References

1. AMA drug evaluations—objective evaluations of drugs and their usage in various disease states; also contain information on the usage of drugs outside the indication in the package insert.
2. *American Druggist Blue Book and Drug Topics Book*—alphabetical listing of products, giving manufacturer, dosage forms, package sizes, and costs; also includes product identification guide and manufacturers' addresses and phone numbers.
3. *American Hospital Formulary Service*—contains extensive monographs on drugs and drug classes; excellent source for the following categories: adverse drug reactions, drug interactions, pharmacokinetics, therapeutics, and pharmacology.
4. *American Drug Index*—alphabetical listing of products giving manufacturer, chemical name, dosage forms, strengths, category of use; cross-indexed by generic and trade names; also includes manufacturers' addresses.
5. *Clinical Toxicology of Commercial Products*—provides information covering the toxicity of commercially available products and recommends appropriate emergency and supportive treatment when poisoning occurs.
6. *Drugs of Choice*—describes drugs of choice for various disease states and therapeutic problems.
7. *Facts and Comparisons*—provides product monographs, comparative information on similar products, and cost index; includes a section on investigational drugs.
8. *Handbook on Nonprescription Drugs*—contains monographs on various classes of nonprescription drugs; compares contents of products in similar classes.

9. *Handbook of Clinical Drug Data*—contains useful clinical information and numerous drug tables. The second half of the handbook is drug review monographs.
10. *Handbook of Poisoning* (Dreisbach)—provides a concise summary of the diagnosis and treatment of clinically important poisons
11. *Hanstens Drug Interactions*—comprehensive listing of drug-drug interactions and drug laboratory test interferences.
12. *Manual of Medical Therapeutics*—a reference manual ("how to") concerning disease states and drug therapy encountered by the hospital staff physician.
13. *Martindale: The Extra Pharmacopoeia*—contains extensive referenced monographs on drugs and drug classes with international coverage. Excellent source for the following categories: adverse reactions, drug interactions, foreign drugs, pharmacokinetics, therapeutics, and pharmacology.
14. *Merck Index*—a concise description of single-entity compounds, listing the general properties and other chemical information.
15. *Merck Manual*—contains a comprehensive listing of disease states and their treatment; a good, quick reference source.
16. *Meyler's Side Effects of Drugs*—comprehensive listing of drugs' side effects and adverse reactions reported worldwide.
17. *Pharm Index*—contains brief descriptions of new products, changed products, discontinued items, investigational products, and costs; also contains a review article in each update.
18. *The Pharmacological Basis of Therapeutics*—an extensive pharmacology textbook; excellent source for the following categories: ad-

verse drug reactions, pharmacokinetics, therapeutics, and pharmacology.

19. *Physicians' Desk Reference*—product package inserts arranged by manufacturer; also includes product identification guide and manufacturers' addresses and phone numbers.

20. *Problems in Pediatric Drug Therapy*—This pocket-sized handbook provides a concise, referenced compilation of clinical and pharmacological data concerning the use and effectiveness of drugs on the fetus, infant, and child.

21. *Remington's Pharmaceutical Sciences*—Excellent pharmacy textbook, including chapters on drug classes with individual drug monographs and several other chapters useful in providing drug information; excellent source for the following categories: drug interactions, pharmaceutical calculations, pharmaceutical compatibility and stability, therapeutics, and pharmacology.

Properly using the various references must be learned through experience. You must read the instructions and preface to understand the content and advantages of each reference source.

E–2: Textbooks

- *Applied Pharmacokinetics* (Evans et al.)
- *Clinical Pharmacy and Therapeutics*
- *Clinical Use of Drugs* (Young and Koda-Kimble)
- *Compendium of Pharmaceuticals and Specialties*
- *Current Therapy* (Conn)
- *Dictionario de Especialidades*
- *Drug Interaction Facts*
- *Evaluations of Drug Interactions*
- *Handbook of Antimicrobial Therapy* (The Medical Letter)
- *Handbook of Injectable Drugs* (Tissel)
- *Harriet Lane Handbook* (pediatrics)
- *Harrison's Principles of Internal Medicine*
- *Imprex: Index of Imprints Used on Tablets and Capsules*
- *Index Nominum*
- *National Drug Code Directory*
- *Organic and Chemical Drugs and Their Synonyms*
- *PDR Drug Interactions and Side Effects Index*
- *PDR for Nonprescription Drugs*
- *PDR for Ophthalmology*
- *PDR Indications Index*
- *Pediatric Dosage Handbook* (APhA)
- *Pharmacological and Chemical Synonyms*
- *Pharmacy Law Digest*

E–3: Journals

- *American Druggist*
- *American Journal of Health-System Pharmacists*
- *American Journal of Medicine*
- *American Pharmacy*
- *Annals of Internal Medicine*
- *Archives of Internal Medicine*
- *British Medical Journal*
- *Clinical Pharmacokinetics*
- *Clinical Pharmacology and Therapeutics*
- *Clinical Pharmacy*
- *Current Therapeutic Research*
- *Drug Intelligence and Clinical Pharmacy*
- *Drugs n. Drug Therapy*
- *Drug Topics*
- *Hospital Formulary*
- *Hospital Pharmacy*
- *Hospital Practice*
- *International Pharmaceutical Abstracts*
- *Journal of the American Medical Association*
- *Lancet*
- *Modern Medicine*
- *New England Journal of Medicine*
- *P & T Pharmacy Practice News*
- *Pharmacy Times*
- *Postgraduate Medicine*

E–4: Newsletters

- Clin-Alert
- Current Contents
- Drug and Therapeutics Bulletin
- Facts and Comparisons Newsletter
- FDA Drug Bulletin
- FDC Reports—The Green Sheet
- FDC Reports—The Pink Sheet
- INPHARMA
- Medical Letter on Drugs and Therapeutics
- Pharmascope
- Reactions
- SCRIP

E–5: Noncomputerized Drug Information Resources

- Adverse Reaction Titles (Excerpta Medica) (adverse drug reaction abstracts)
- deHaen Information Systems (comprehensive drug literature abstracting service)
- Drugdex (up-to-date, unbiased, referenced drug information system)
- Drug Literature Index (Excerpta Medica) (index to the drug literature worldwide)
- Guide to Parenteral Admixtures (information on the compatibility and stability of parenteral drugs)
- Identidex (tablet and capsule identification)
- Index Medicus (comprehensive index to the medical literature)
- International Pharmaceutical Abstracts (abstracts on all aspects of pharmacy and pharmacy practice)
- Iowa Drug Information System (drug and therapeutic literature abstracting system)
- Poisindex (identification and management of poisons)

E–6: Computerized Drug Information Resources

- ASHP Drug Information Source (includes ASHF Drug Information, Handbook of Injectable Drugs, and International Pharmaceutical Abstracts)
- Drug Information Fulltext (comprehensive, objective, authoritative source of evaluating drug information)
- Drugdex (up-to-date, unbiased, referenced drug information system)
- Emergindex (disease and trauma information)
- F-D-C Reports (information on food, drugs, and cosmetics)
- Identidex (tablet and capsule information)
- IDIS Drug File (information on drugs worldwide)
- Martindale (British Pharmacopoeia)
- Merck Index (compendium of information on chemicals, biologicals, and drugs)
- Physician's Desk Reference (product overviews of commonly prescribed drugs)
- PDR Drug Interactions and Side Effects Diskettes (side effects and adverse drug reactions)
- Poisindex (identification and management of poisons)
- Reprorisk (reproductive risk information)
- Side Effects of Drugs (side effects and adverse drug reactions)
- Tomes (*Toxicity, Occupational Medicine, and Environmental Series*)

E–7: Electronic Bulletin Boards

- ClinNet, (800) 882-2488 or (412) 648-7893, American College of Clinical Pharmacy (ACCP members only)
- F.I.X., (800) 262-8664 (The Formulary)

- PharmLine, (800) 247-4276, American Association of Colleges of Pharmacy (AACP members only)
- PharmNet, (800) 848-8980 (call for local number), American Society of Health-System Pharmacists (ASHP members only)

E–8: Biological Databases

- Biosis (biological abstracts and biosearch index)
- Cancerlit (cancer research information)
- Medline (premier source for biomedical literature)
- Excerpta Medica (English language abstracts of medical papers)
- Excerpta Medica-Drug File (abstracts of drug usage worldwide)

- International Pharmaceutical Abstracts (IPA) (abstracts on all aspects of pharmacy and pharmacy practice)
- Iowa Drug Information System (IDIS) (drug and therapeutic literature abstracting system)
- Pharmaceutical News Index (index to all aspects of the pharmaceutical industry)
- Toxline (comprehensive toxicology abstracting service)

F Drug Distribution Systems

F–1: ASHP Statement on Unit-Dose Drug Distribution

The unit-dose system of medication distribution is a pharmacy-coordinated method of dispensing and controlling medications in organized health care settings.

The unit-dose system may differ in form, depending on the specific needs of the organization. However, the following distinctive elements are basic to all unit-dose systems: medications are contained in single unit packages; they are dispensed in as ready-to-administer form as possible; and for most medications, not more than a 24-hour supply[a] of doses is delivered to or available at the patient care area at any time.[1,2]

Numerous studies concerning unit-dose drug distribution systems have been published over the past several decades. These studies indicate categorically that unit-dose systems, with respect to other drug distribution methods, are (1) safer for the patient, (2) more efficient and economical for the organization, and (3) a more effective method of utilizing professional resources.

More specifically, the inherent advantages of unit-dose systems over alternative distribution procedures are

1. A reduction in the incidence of medication errors.
2. A decrease in the total cost of medication-related activities.
3. A more efficient usage of pharmacy and nursing personnel, allowing for more direct patient care involvement by pharmacists and nurses.
4. Improved overall drug control and drug-use monitoring.
5. More accurate patient billings for drugs.
6. The elimination or minimization of drug credits.
7. Greater control by the pharmacist over pharmacy workload patterns and staff scheduling.
8. A reduction in the size of drug inventories located in patient care areas.
9. Greater adaptability to computerized and automated procedures.

In view of these demonstrated benefits, the American Society of Hospital Pharmacists considers the unit-dose system to be an essential part of drug distribution and control in organized health care settings in which drug therapy is an integral component of health care delivery.

References

1. Summerfield, M.R. (1983). *Unit-dose primer*. Bethesda, MD: American Society of Hospital Pharmacists.
2. American Society of Hospital Pharmacists. (1980). ASHP technical assistance bulletin on hospital drug distribution and control. *Am J Hosp Pharm, 37,* 1097–1103.

[a]In long-term care facilities, a larger supply of medication (e.g., 48 or 72 hours) may be acceptable.

Approved by the ASHP Board of Directors, November 16, 1988, and by the ASHP House of Delegates, June 5, 1989. Supersedes previous versions approved by the House of Delegates on June 8, 1981, and by the Board of Directors on April 19, 1975, and November 13–14, 1980. Copyright © 1989, American Society of Hospital Pharmacists, Inc. All rights reserved. The bibliographic citation for this document is as follows: American Society of Hospital Pharmacists. (1989). ASHP statement on unit-dose drug distribution. *Am J Hosp Pharm, 46,* 2346.

APPENDIX

G Accreditation of Technician Training Programs

G-1: ASHP Regulations on Accreditation of Hospital Pharmacy Technician Training Programs

Preamble

Pharmacists have long recognized the need for a corps of technically trained support personnel in the field of pharmacy. This need arises from the fact that the practice of pharmacy encompasses a complex set of tasks in a wide array of environments, some of which require the knowledge and judgment of a pharmacist but many others of which do not. Without the benefit of a technically trained adjunctive work force, pharmacists would be compelled to devote much of their own time and energies to the performance of technical tasks rather than to those patient care pursuits for which they have been trained.

ASHP supports the effective use of qualified technicians in all pharmacy settings; further, the Society recognizes an obligation to promulgate standards for the training of such personnel. To ensure a continuing supply of well-qualified technicians for pharmacy practice, an accreditation program is conducted by the Society.

Objectives

The objectives of the accreditation program are (1) to upgrade and standardize the formal training that pharmacy technicians receive; (2) to guide, assist, and recognize those health systems and academic institutions that wish to support the profession by operating such programs; (3) to provide criteria for the prospective technician trainee in the selection of a program by identifying those institutions conducting accredited pharmacy technician training programs; (4) to provide pharmacies

a basis for determining the level of competency of pharmacy technicians by identifying those technicians who have successfully completed accredited technician training programs; and (5) to assist in the advancement and professional development of the pharmacy technician.

Authority

The program for accreditation of pharmacy technician training programs is conducted by the authority of the Board of Directors of ASHP under the direction of the Commission on Credentialing. All matters of policy relating to the accreditation program considered by the Commission on Credentialing shall be submitted for approval to the Board of Directors of the Society. The Commission on Credentialing shall review and evaluate applications and survey reports submitted and shall be specifically delegated by the Board of Directors to take final action on all applications for accreditation, in accordance with the policies and procedures set forth herein. The minutes of all transactions of the Commission on Credentialing shall be submitted to the Board of Directors for its review.

Policies

The following policies apply to the technician training accreditation program:

1. **Initial Evaluation of Training Program.**
   a. The accreditation program shall be conducted as a service of ASHP to institutions voluntarily requesting evaluation of their programs.

b. Application for accreditation may be made upon the initiation of operation of the program. Completion and submission of application forms may occur prior to the time that the program is fully eligible for accreditation. An initial application fee, as established by the Board of Directors, shall be assessed to the institution.

c. To be eligible for accreditation, a program must have been in operation for one full training cycle and have at least one graduate. (If accreditation is granted, it shall be retroactive to the date on which a valid and complete application, including all requested supporting documents, is received by the Society's Director of Accreditation Services.)

d. Program evaluation shall be by site survey.

e. Programs shall be reviewed by pharmacists or pharmacy educators appointed by the Society's Director of Accreditation Services.

f. An annual accreditation fee, established by the Board of Directors, shall be assessed to the institution for purposes of initial and continued accreditation of the program.

2. *Certificate of Accreditation.*

a. A certificate of accreditation will be issued by the Society's Board of Directors to those institutions for whom accreditation is approved; however, the certificate remains the property of ASHP and shall be returned to the Society at any time accreditation is withdrawn.

b. Any reference by an institution to accreditation by the Society in certificates, catalogs, bulletins, communications, or other forms of publicity shall state only the following: "(name of institution) is accredited for pharmacy technician training by the American Society of Health System Pharmacists."

3. *Continuing Evaluation of Accredited Programs.*

a. The Society regards evaluation of accredited technician training programs as a continuous process; accordingly, the Commission on Credentialing shall request program directors of accredited programs to submit periodic written status reports to assist the commission in evaluating the continued conformance of individual programs to the accreditation standard. Written reports shall be required from program directors at least every 3 years.

b. Accredited training programs shall be reexamined by site visit at least every 6 years.

c. Any major change in the organization of a program will be considered justification for immediate reevaluation.

d. The annual accreditation fee as described in item 1.f. above shall cover the cost of reaccreditation.

4. *Withdrawal of Accreditation.*

a. Accreditation of a pharmacy technician training program may be withdrawn by the Society for any of the reasons stated below.

   (1) Accredited programs that no longer meet the requirements of the Society's Accreditation Standard for Pharmacy Technician Training Programs shall have accreditation withdrawn.

   (2) Accredited programs without a technician trainee for 2 consecutive years shall have accreditation withdrawn.

   (3) Accreditation shall be withdrawn if the program director is replaced by another individual whose qualifications do not meet the requirements of the Accreditation Standard.

b. The institution shall submit a new application and undergo reevaluation to regain accreditation.

c. Accreditation shall be withdrawn without prior notification of the institution of the specific reasons why its program does not meet the Accreditation Standard for Pharmacy Technician Training Programs. In such instances, the institution shall be granted an appropriate, specified period of time to correct deficiencies.

d. The institution shall have the right to appeal the decision of the Commission on Credentialing.

Accreditation Procedures

1. *Application for Accreditation.*

a. Application forms can be requested from the American Society of Health System Pharmacists, Director of Accreditation Services, 7272 Wisconsin Avenue, Bethesda, MD 20814. The application should be signed by the chief executive officer or applicable authority of the institution seeking accreditation and the director of the technician training program and submitted, along with the supporting documents specified in the application instructions, to the Society's Director of Accreditation Services. The duplicate copy should be retained for the applicant's files.

b. Once the application is received, the site is contacted to schedule a survey.

c. Background materials should be submitted to the Society's Director of Accreditation Services 45 days prior to the site survey.

2. *Site Visit.*

a. At a mutually convenient time, the Society will send a survey team to review the training program. Instructions for preparation for the site visit (list of documents to be made available to the team, suggested itinerary, etc.) will be sent to the program director well in advance. Normally, the site visit is conducted in one working day by a team of two people.

b. In the case of a program conducted by an academic institution, arrangements may be made by the institution for the survey team to conduct an onsite review of the practical training sites. Time constraints may not allow visitation of practical training sites.

3. *Survey Report.*

a. At the end of the survey, the survey team will complete an oral report that will be reviewed with the program director and chief executive officer (or his representative).

b. The oral report will then be sent in a formal written report to the institution within 45–60 days of the survey.

c. The institution will be given 30 days in which to respond to the survey report. The response should be in writing and sent to the Director of Accreditation Services.

d. The institution's accreditation application file, including the surveyors' report, plus any written comments received from the institution, will be reviewed by the Commission on Credentialing at its next meeting. The commission will resolve any factual issues at that time.

e. Notice of action taken by the commission will be sent to the chief executive officer of the institution and the technician program director. The report will indicate that the commission has acted either (1) to accredit or reaccredit the program for a period not to exceed 6 years or (2) to withhold or withdraw accreditation.

4. *Appeal of Commission Decision.*

a. *Notification of intent to appeal.* In the event that the commission shall fail to accredit or reaccredit fully a program, the institution's chief executive officer may appeal the decision of the commission to an appeal board on the grounds that the decision of the commission was arbitrary, prejudiced, biased, capricious, or based on incorrect application of the standards to the institution. The chief executive officer must notify the Director of Accreditation Services, in writing by registered or certified mail within 10 days after receipt of the commission's decision, of the institution's intent to appeal. The institution must state clearly on what grounds the appeal is being made. The institution shall then have an additional 30 days in which to prepare for its presentation to an appeal board.

b. *Appeal board.* On receipt of an appeal notice, the Director of Accreditation Services shall proceed to constitute an ad hoc appeal board. The appeal board shall consist of one member of the Society's Board of Directors, who shall be appointed by the President of ASHP and who shall serve as chair, and two directors of accredited pharmacy technician training programs, neither of whom is a member of the Commission on Credentialing, one to be named by the appellant and one by the chairman of the commission. The Director of Accreditation Services shall serve as secretary of the appeal board. As soon as appointments to the appeal board have been made, the Director of Accreditation Services shall immediately forward to all appeal board members copies of all written documentation considered by the commission in rendering its decision.

c. *Hearing.* The appeal board shall have convened in not less than 30 days nor more than 60 days from the date of receipt of an appeal notice by the Director of Accreditation Services. The Director of Accreditation Services shall notify appellants and appeal board members, at least 30 days in advance, of the date, time, and place of the hearing. The institution filing the appeal may be represented at the hearing by one or more appropriate officials and shall be given the opportunity at such hearing to present evidence (oral, written, or both) and information that refutes or overcomes the findings and decision of the Commission on Credentialing. The Director of Accreditation Services shall represent the commission at the hearing.

The appeal board shall advise the appellant of the Board's decision, in writing by registered or certified mail, within 10 days of the date of the hearing. The decision of the appeal board is final and binding on both the appellant and ASHP.

d. *Appeal board expenses.* The appellant shall be responsible for all expenses incurred by its own representatives at the appeal board hearing and shall pay all rea-

sonable travel, living, and incidental expenses incurred by its appointee to the appeal board. Expenses incurred by the other board members and the Director of Accreditation Services shall be borne by ASHP.

Approved by the ASHP Board of Directors, September 26, 1997. Developed by the ASHP Commission on Credentialing. Supersedes the previous regulations approved April 23, 1987. The current revision reflects a change in policy with respect to the cycle of site visits; previously, such visits were required "at least every 4 years," whereas the policy now is for onsite inspections "at least every 6 years" supplemented by written reports from the training program at least every 3 years. Copyright © 1998, American Society of Health System Pharmacists, Inc. All rights reserved.

G-2: ASHP Accreditation Standard for Pharmacy Technician Training Programs

Part I—Administrative Responsibility for the Training Program

A. Pharmacy technician training programs may be conducted by either health care organizations or academic institutions. These training facilities must be accredited, when applicable, by the appropriate agency or agencies and shall be responsible for ensuring that the following requirements have been met:

1. The trainee's practical experience is obtained in qualified training site(s) that meet the requirements set forth in Parts II and III.
2. The program director shall meet the requirements set forth in Part IV.

B. When requested, the health care or academic institution shall provide the trainee applicant with information regarding the purpose of the training program, prospects for employment, realistic salary expectations, and regulatory issues.

C. A program director shall be named whose authority and responsibilities are commensurate with those of other allied health, technical, or vocational training programs offered by the institution. This individual shall have appropriate authority to direct all aspects of training. The director need not be a pharmacist; however, there must be a sufficient complement of

pharmacists on the faculty to meet all instructional objectives.

D. An advisory committee comprising a broad-based group of pharmacists, faculty, and pharmacy technicians must be established and have specific authority for the following:

1. Determining that the curriculum makes possible the attainment of all learning objectives set forth in Part VI.
2. Approving practice training sites.
3. Validating admission criteria.
4. Validating criteria for successful completion of the program.

E. Nothing in this standard shall prevent individual training programs from establishing more stringent requirements than those specified herein. Further, in instances where more stringent requirements have been established or adopted by state law, regulation, or governmental agency, those requirements will take precedence for the purposes of accreditation by ASHP of programs within the corresponding state or jurisdiction.

Part II—Qualifications of the Training Site

A. A health system facility that offers, or participates in offering, a technician training program shall be accredited by the Joint Commission on Accreditation of Healthcare Organizations, the

American Osteopathic Association, or the National Committee for Quality Assurance.

B. Other practice sites (e.g., community pharmacies and pharmaceutical companies) that participate in technician training shall have demonstrated substantial conformance with applicable professionally developed and nationally applied practice standards.

C. All practice sites shall comply with all federal, state, and local laws, codes, statutes, regulations, and licensing requirements.

D. Technician training sites shall conduct the practice component of the program in such a way as to ensure that any services the technician trainee is required to provide complement, rather than compete with, the educational and experiential objectives of the program.

Part III—Qualifications of the Pharmacy Service

A. All pharmacies involved in technician training shall be organized in accordance with the principles of good management under the direction of a legally qualified pharmacist and with sufficient appropriate personnel to provide a broad scope of pharmaceutical services to all patients served by the facility.

B. The training site(s) used for experiential training shall have adequate facilities to carry out services that meet, when applicable, the intent of the ASHP Guidelines: Minimum Standard for Pharmacies in Hospitals[1] or the ASHP Guidelines on Pharmaceutical Services for Ambulatory Patients.[2] It is necessary that practice experience be part of regular, ongoing services; hence, it is not sufficient to create artificial situations in which trainees can obtain this experience.

C. Pharmacies involved in technician training must be neat and orderly and must project a highly professional image.

Part IV—Qualifications of the Program Director and Preceptors

A. The technician training program shall be subject to similar general administrative control and guidance employed by the institution for other allied health care training programs. If the program is conducted by an academic institution, the program director must ensure that pharmacists or designees oversee and guide all experiential training of the pharmacy technician trainees at the practice site.

B. The program director shall be a member of a national pharmacy organization and the corresponding state affiliate. All other program faculty and preceptors should also hold active membership in these organizations.

C. The program director shall have considerable latitude in delegating preceptorial responsibilities for the technician training program to others on staff. Each individual designated as an instructor must have demonstrated competence in one or more related areas of pharmacy practice and possess an ability to teach. The program director, or designee, is ultimately accountable for the overall quality of the trainee's practical experience.

D. Persons who supervise experiential training must meet the following qualifications:

1. The program director, or designee, shall supervise experiential health system pharmacy training. This individual shall have had at least 5 years' experience in a pharmacy that meets the requirements of the ASHP Guidelines: Minimum Standard for Pharmacies in Hospitals.[1]

2. All experiential training that occurs outside the health system setting must be coordinated by a pharmacist or designee with sufficient knowledge and skills to provide a sound educational experience. Further, this individual must have demonstrated sufficient contribution and commitment to pharmacy practice and patient care.

Part V—Qualifications and Selection of the Applicant

A. The applicant must be a high school graduate or possess a high school equivalency certificate.

B. Final approval of the qualifications of the applicant for acceptance as a trainee shall be the responsibility of the director of the technician training program.

Part VI—Technician Training Program

A. The technician training program must include didactic, laboratory, and practice components structured to allow trainees to achieve program goals and objectives. The Model Curriculum for Pharmacy Technician Training (available from the American Society of Health System Pharmacists)[a] was developed to reflect current pharmacy technician functions and responsibilities. While not intended to be prescriptive, the Model Curriculum for Pharmacy Technician Training provides a comprehensive list of objectives that may be utilized to complement the designated program goals. Goals for the technician training program shall be in writing and shall be provided to each trainee at the beginning of the program. The training program should be based on the following goals:

- Assist the pharmacist in collecting, organizing, and evaluating information for direct patient care, drug-use review, and departmental management.
- Receive and screen prescriptions or medication orders for completeness and accuracy.
- Use pharmaceutical and medical terms, abbreviations, and symbols appropriately.
- Prepare and distribute medications in a variety of health system settings.
- Perform arithmetical calculations required for usual dosage determinations and solution preparation.
- Use knowledge of general chemical and physical properties of drugs in manufacturing and packaging operations.
- Use knowledge of proper aseptic technique and packaging in the preparation of medications.
- Collect payment or initiate billing for pharmacy services and goods.
- Purchase pharmaceuticals, devices, and supplies according to an established plan in a variety of health systems.
- Control the inventory of medications, equipment, and devices according to an established plan in a variety of health systems.
- Maintain pharmacy equipment used in preparing, storing, and distributing investigational drug products.
- Assist the pharmacist in monitoring the practice site or service area for compliance with federal, state, and local laws and regulations, and professional standards.
- Assist the pharmacist in preparing, storing, and distributing investigational drug products.

- Assist the pharmacist in the monitoring of drug therapy.
- Assist the pharmacist in the identification of patients who desire counseling on the use of medications, equipment, and devices.
- Understand the use and side effects of prescription and nonprescription drugs used to treat common disease states.
- Display compassion for patients and their caregivers.
- Take personal responsibility for assisting the pharmacist in improving the pharmaceutical care of patients.
- Understand the scope of pharmaceutical care delivery systems.
- Understand the importance of and resources for staying current with changes in pharmacy practice.
- Appreciate the need to adapt the delivery of pharmacy services for the culturally diverse.
- Maintain confidentiality of patient information.
- Communicate clearly orally and in writing.
- Use computers to perform pharmacy functions.
- Maintain an image appropriate for the profession of pharmacy.
- Demonstrate ethical conduct in all activities related to the delivery of pharmacy services.
- Appreciate the benefits of active involvement in local, state, and national technician and other pharmacy organizations.
- Appreciate the value of obtaining technician certification.
- Maintain confidentiality of patient information.
- Efficiently manage one's work whether performed alone or as a part of a team.
- Efficiently solve problems commonly encountered in one's own work.
- Understand principles for managing change.
- Establish and maintain effective interpersonal working relationships with other members of the health care team.

B. Appropriate laboratory exercises, including computerized application of record-keeping and drug distribution systems, shall be used to reinforce classroom instruction before on-site experiential training commences.

C. All instructors and trainees must be thoroughly familiar with the requirements of this standard.

D. Each trainee's activities shall be scheduled in advance and shall be planned to enable the trainee to attain the predetermined objectives. The training schedule shall consist of a minimum of 600 hours of training (contact) time, extending over a period of 15 weeks or longer. Programs may need to lengthen training schedules to provide more in-depth coverage of goals and objectives to meet the market needs of the health system community.

E. A broad plan for each student shall be developed and documented at the beginning of the program.

F. Records of training activities that clearly delineate the scope and period of training shall be maintained. The program director shall keep these records on file.

G. The program director shall arrange for formalized and regularly scheduled evaluation of the trainee's achievement in terms of the objectives previously established.

Part VII—Experimentation and Innovation

A. Experimental and innovative approaches to developing and implementing pharmacy technician training programs and alternative methods for meeting this standard shall be encouraged.

B. These experimental and innovative activities must be adequately planned and coupled with an appropriate evaluation system.

Part VIII—Certificate

A. The accredited program shall recognize those pharmacy technicians who have completed successfully the pharmacy technician training program by awarding an appropriate certificate or diploma.

B. No certificate shall be issued to any individual who has failed to complete the prescribed program or to meet the intent of this standard.

References

1. American Society of Health System Pharmacists. (1995). ASHP guidelines: Minimum standard for pharmacies in hospitals. *Am J Health-Syst Pharm, 52,* 2711–2717.
2. American Society of Hospital Pharmacists. (1991). ASHP guidelines: On pharmaceutical services for ambulatory patients. *Am J Hosp Pharm, 48,* 311–315.

[a]The Model Curriculum for Pharmacy Technician Training is recommended as a guide.

Approved by the ASHP Board of Directors, September 26, 1997. Developed by the ASHP Commission on Credentialing. Supersedes the previous accreditation standard approved September 23, 1992, and revised November 17–18, 1983, and November 20–21, 1985. For existing programs this revision of the accreditation standard takes effect July 1, 1998. Copyright © 1998, American Society of Health System Pharmacists, Inc. All rights reserved.

G–3: ASHP Technical Assistance Bulletin on Outcome Competencies and Training Guidelines for Institutional Pharmacy Technician Training Programs

Preamble

Definitions
The term "supportive personnel" has been recommended as standard nomenclature to be used in referring collectively to all nonprofessional hospital pharmacy personnel. This document describes the training outcome competencies for those supportive personnel designated "pharmacy technicians." A technician may be defined as a person skilled in the technique of a particular art (technique being the mechanical ability required to perform an activity).

For purposes of this document, a pharmacy technician shall be defined as someone who, under the supervision of a licensed pharmacist, assists in the various activities of the pharmacy department not requiring the professional judgment of the pharmacist. Such duties include, but need not be limited to: maintaining patient records; setting up, packaging, and labeling medication doses; filling and dispensing routine orders for stock supplies of patient-care areas; maintaining inventories of drug supplies; and mixing drugs with parenteral fluids. Technicians function in strict accordance with standard, written procedures and guidelines, any deviation from which must be approved by the supervising pharmacist.

Supportive personnel primarily engaged in duties *not* associated with the techniques of preparing and dispensing medications (e.g., secretaries, clerks, typists, and delivery personnel) are not considered "pharmacy technicians" and their competencies are not covered in this document. Likewise, competencies of supportive personnel who administer medication ("medication technicians") are also excluded. This document addresses the training of a "generalist" technician, one who can function appropriately in most hospitals, both small and large, in the kinds of activities for which there is generally the greatest need for supportive personnel manpower.

Application of the Outcome Competencies

The competencies described in this document are representative ones, and no attempt has been made to develop an exhaustive listing. It is believed that any technician who can demonstrate attainment of these competencies should be able to perform satisfactorily in any organized health care setting after a reasonable period of orientation. It is not expected, however, that all institutional pharmacy technicians will, in fact, possess these competencies.

The competencies are described in behavioral terms; thus, it should be possible to evaluate the trainee's attainment of each competency in the manner described in each statement. In some instances, this can be by paper and pencil tests; in other instances, it can be by oral statement; and in yet other cases, it can be by actually performing the activity or function under the observation of the evaluator. In the latter instances, it is extremely important that the evaluator judges the trainee's performance strictly on the basis of the objectives

previously established for the respective training activity relating to the competency.

Omitted from most of the competency statements are references to time or error limits. Obviously, they must be taken into account in the evaluation process. It is suggested that reasonable time and error limits be imposed where indicated, based on the evaluator's experience.

The training guidelines following the list of competencies for each objective statement consist of suggested topics to be covered in the didactic portion of the training program. Again, these are not exhaustive lists; every training institution is expected to add or delete topics as it deems necessary.

The training guidelines do not include training activities necessary for the development of manipulative skills. These are clearly implied in the statements listed under the competencies for each of the eleven objectives.

The qualifications of applicants to be admitted to the training program are discussed in Appendix A. Suggestions for the training program format are given in Appendix B.

Objective I

The technician should demonstrate appropriate knowledge and understanding of the health care institution and its pharmacy department.

Competencies

The technician should be able to:

1. Interpret the institution's organizational chart in terms of the name and title of the administrative person to whom the director of pharmacy reports and the administrative and professional relationship of the pharmacy department to any other departments in the institution.

2. Describe the general responsibilities and job status of personnel in other institutional departments with whom the technician will have contact in carrying out assigned duties and activities.

3. Interpret the organizational chart for the pharmacy department in terms of names and general responsibilities of all departmental supervisory and administrative personnel.

4. Describe the location of the major hospital departments and service units, and escort another person to any department or unit.

5. State at least three reasons why information about patients must be kept confidential.
6. State at least five reasons for initiation of a disciplinary action in the institution (e.g., absenteeism, incompetency, and dishonesty).

Training Guidelines
Suggested topics include:

1. Organization, functions, and responsibilities of the hospital.
2. Organization, functions, and responsibilities of the pharmacy.
3. Hospital and departmental policies and procedures.

Objective II

The technician should demonstrate a thorough knowledge and understanding of the duties and responsibilities of his/her position, including standards of ethics governing pharmacy practice.

Competencies
The technician should be able to:

1. State all of the technician's primary job responsibilities, the duties falling under each, and how they differ from the primary responsibilities of the pharmacist.
2. State the institutional and departmental policies applicable to each of the primary job responsibilities, and describe the procedures for each.
3. Define what is meant by "a decision requiring a pharmacist's judgment," and cite at least ten examples.
4. Demonstrate the use of correct telephone communication technique and protocol, both in receiving and in initiating calls.
5. Demonstrate the use of correct written communication by drafting a memorandum to the supervisor requesting a change in work assignment schedule to take care of personal business.
6. State the general requirements of any local, state, or federal laws that specifically affect any of the technician's responsibilities.

Training Guidelines
Suggested topics include:

1. Orientation to technician duties (job description).
2. Relationship of technicians to pharmacists, hospital staff, and patients.
3. Communication principles and techniques.

4. Legal aspects of technician functions such as:
   a. Accountability.
   b. Pharmacy regulations.
   c. Use and storage of controlled substances.

Objective III

The technician should have a working knowledge of the pharmaceutical-medical terms, abbreviations, and symbols commonly used in the prescribing, dispensing, and charting of medications in the institution.

Competencies
The technician should be able to:

1. Transcribe without error any twelve inpatient medication orders selected at random from at least four different patient units in the institution.
2. Define in lay terms the meaning of names of all clinical, diagnostic, and treatment units and services in the institution.

Training Guidelines
Suggested topics include:

1. Pharmaceutical-medical terminology.
2. Pharmaceutical-medical abbreviations and symbols.
3. Drug classification systems and drug nomenclature.

Objective IV

The technician should have a working knowledge of the general chemical and physical properties of all drugs handled in manufacturing and packaging operations in the pharmacy department.

Competencies
The technician should be able to:

1. Designate from a list of fifty drug names those that are light sensitive and those that must be refrigerated.
2. State what precautions and procedures must be used in handling caustic, poisonous, and flammable substances.
3. List the titles of at least four reference books where stability information on drug compounds can be found.

Training Guidelines
Suggested topics include:

1. Pharmaceutical solutes, solvents, and basic solution theory.

2. Basic principles of stability (effects of heat, cold, light, and moisture on drugs and chemicals).
3. Storage requirements for drugs and chemicals.
4. Safety considerations regarding:
   a. Toxic and caustic substances.
   b. Flammable chemicals and drugs.
   c. Operating pharmacy equipment.
   d. Control of microbiological contamination.
   e. Cleaning and housekeeping.
   f. Control records.

Objective V

The technician should demonstrate an ability to carry out the calculations required for the usual dosage determinations and solutions preparation, using weight and volume equivalents in both the metric and apothecary systems.

Competencies
The technician should be able to:

1. List without error the metric equivalents for the apothecary doses and for household doses written in twelve randomly selected medication orders.
2. Convert without error all metric or apothecary weights and volumes to the other system in at least four manufacturing formulas.
3. Perform the calculations necessary to prepare weight-in-volume and volume-in-volume solutions.

Training Guidelines
Suggested topics include:

1. Weights and measures (apothecary and metric systems, household measures, potency units and strengths, equivalents, and conversions).
2. Review of fractions, decimals, ratios, and percentages.
3. Dosage calculations and preparation of solutions.

Objective VI

The technician should demonstrate the ability to perform the essential functions relating to drug purchasing and inventory control.

Competencies
The technician should be able to:

1. Prepare a written report of a physical inventory of a representative stock of pharmacy drugs and supplies using prepared forms and records.
2. Determine from existing reorder levels which inventoried items should be ordered and in what quantity.
3. Demonstrate an ability to check in a drug shipment by using the packing list or invoice and purchase order, completing the receiving report, and adding the items to the inventory.
4. Demonstrate the ability to retrieve from the drug storeroom at least ten randomly designated drug items.
5. Describe the procedure for returning outdated drugs to the manufacturer.

Training Guidelines
Suggested topics include:

1. Inventory and purchasing procedures and records.
2. Maintaining controlled substances records.
3. Inspection of nursing unit drug supplies.
4. Use of computer terminals.

Objective VII

The technician should demonstrate a working knowledge of drug dosages, routes of administration, and dosage forms.

Competencies
The technician should be able to:

1. List at least:
   a. Six routes of drug administration.
   b. Ten dosage forms of drugs and their respective routes.
2. State the lumen size, length, and primary use for each of five different needles.
3. Identify, by name and use, each of five different syringes.

Training Guidelines
Suggested topics include:

1. Sources of drugs.
2. Rationales for drug use (preventive, curative and restorative, and limiting disease processes).
3. Dose-response relationships.
4. Absorption, biotransformation, and excretion of drugs.
5. Risk-benefit ratios.

6. Patient variables and drug therapy (age, weight, pathological conditions, and genetic factors).
7. Local administration (to skin and mucous membranes, to ears and eyes, and irrigations).
8. Systemic administration (oral, sublingual-buccal, inhalation, rectal, and parenteral).
9. Dosage forms (tablets, capsules, solutions, suspensions, ointments, suppositories, powders, and injectables).

Objective VIII

The technician should have a working knowledge of the procedures and operations relating to the manufacturing, packaging, and labeling of drug products.

Competencies
The technician should be able to:

1. Repackage and label twenty-five unit doses from a bulk supply of drugs and correctly complete all necessary control records.
2. Demonstrate for each of five randomly selected formulation and packaging requests:
   a. Correct selection of necessary equipment.
   b. Proper assembly and use of the equipment.
   c. Proper cleaning and storing of the equipment.
   d. Proper selection of each ingredient.
   e. Accurate calculation and measurement of each ingredient.
   f. Proper completion of worksheet record of weights and volumes, manufacturers' lot numbers, and other required information.
   g. Correct procedure for mixing and preparing product.
   h. Proper selection and preparation of packages/containers and closures.
   i. Proper packaging technique.
   j. Correct selection and preparation of labels.
   k. Proper quarantine procedure.
3. Identify from a list of ten different steps in manufacturing and packaging operations those functions that must be performed by a pharmacist only.

Training Guidelines
Suggested topics include:

1. Measurements of quantity (weights, volumes, and numbers).

2. Use, assembly, and maintenance of equipment and apparatus.
3. Control and recordkeeping procedures (formula mastersheets, worksheets and batch records, labeling and label control, quarantine, and product testing and monitoring).
4. Packaging considerations (drug containers and closures).
5. Storage and inventory control.

Objective IX

The technician should have a working knowledge of the procedures and techniques relating to aseptic compounding and parenteral admixture operations.

Competencies
The technician should be able to:

1. List five different possibilities for contamination of an injectable solution during its preparation and for each possibility a precaution that would prevent the contamination.
2. Demonstrate the proper technique for using a syringe and needle for aseptic withdrawal of the contents of:
   a. A rubber-capped vial.
   b. A glass ampul.
3. Demonstrate the proper technique for aseptic reconstitution of an antibiotic injection.
4. Describe the occasions when handwashing is required, and demonstrate the proper technique.
5. Demonstrate the correct techniques and procedures for preparing at least three parenteral admixtures, including the proper preparation of the label and completion of the control records.
6. Identify the major components of a laminar-flow hood, and state their functions.
7. Define or describe:
   a. Microbial growth and transmission.
   b. Origin, pharmacologic effect, and prevention of pyrogens.
   c. Sterility.
   d. Heat sterilization.
   e. "Cold" sterilization.
8. Designate from a list of ten different sterile preparations those that may be safely heat sterilized.
9. Demonstrate the proper technique for visual inspection of parenteral solutions.

Training Guidelines
Suggested topics include:

1. Parenteral routes of administration (rationale, precautions, and problems; routes; and methods of parenteral administration).
2. Equipment and systems used in parenteral administration (needles and syringes, administration sets, fluid containers, filters, and pumps).
3. Equipment used to prepare parenteral admixtures (laminar-flow hoods, filters, pumps, vacuum sets, and drug additive systems).
4. Aseptic compounding techniques (specific to the fluid system in use and including the prefilling of syringes, preparing ophthalmic solutions, etc.)
5. Labeling and recordkeeping (bottle labels, fluid orders and profiles, and compounding records).
6. Incompatibilities (visual and chemical incompatibilities, pH and concentration effects, and reference sources).
7. Quality control (particulate matter inspection and monitoring of contamination).

Objective X

The technician should demonstrate the ability to perform the usual technician functions associated with an institutional drug distribution system.

Competencies
The technician should be able to:

1. Prepare the drug profile for five newly admitted patients.
2. Pick all doses for one patient unit, and complete the necessary dispensing records.
3. Describe the special dispensing and recordkeeping procedures that apply to the dispensing of:
   a. Controlled drugs.
   b. Investigational drugs.
   c. Nonformulary drugs.
4. List for each of 30 commonly prescribed trade-name drugs:
   a. The generic name.
   b. The usual dose.

Training Guidelines
Suggested topics include:

1. Physicians' order sheets and patient medication profiles.
2. Setting up doses for patients.

3. Checking doses.
4. Delivery and exchange of medications.

Objective XI

The technician should demonstrate the ability to perform manipulative and recordkeeping functions associated with the dispensing of prescriptions for ambulatory patients.

Competencies
The technician should be able to:

1. Carry out the following functions for ten randomly selected ambulatory patient prescriptions:
   a. Correctly type the label.
   b. Select the proper drug from the dispensing stock.
   c. Accurately count or measure the product, and place it in the proper container.
   d. Complete the necessary records and documents.
   e. Calculate the charge for the prescription.
2. Describe the special procedures and documentation required in dispensing ambulatory patient prescriptions for:
   a. Controlled drugs.
   b. Investigational drugs.
   c. Nonprescription drugs.
3. Designate from a list of ten steps involved in ambulatory patient prescription dispensing those functions that only a pharmacist may carry out.

Training Guidelines
Suggested topics include:

1. Prescriptions and patient profiles.
2. Preparing prescription labels.
3. Counting and measuring drugs.

Appendix A: Qualifications for Training Program Applicants

Applicants to the technician training program should have certain demonstrated abilities as evidenced by successful completion of relevant high school courses or other appropriate educational programs or by acceptable grades on a written entrance examination. These abilities and knowledge include general basic chemistry, arithmetic, basic algebra, reading, and writing. Other requirements are adequate command of the English language; ability to acquire skill in the use of pharmaceutical apparatus, instruments, and equipment; ability to work with sustained attention and care on routine repetitive tasks; ability to follow oral and written instructions with accuracy, precision, and dependability; and ability to distinguish routine functions from those requiring a pharmacist's judgment. These requirements should be clearly understood by applicants to the program.

Appendix B: Training Program Format

The training course should consist of lectures, informal discussions, and practical experience sessions. The ratio of lecture material to practical experience sessions can vary, depending on the specific goals and design of the program. The course may be split into several options, with each trainee entering one of the options (e.g., parenteral admixture compounding). Alternatively, a single, more generalized course through which all trainees pass may be offered.

Each trainee should receive a course manual containing the following information:

1. General information about the hospital and hospital pharmacy (goals, organizational structures, personnel policy, etc.).
2. General information about the training program (attendance requirements, graduation requirements, and a complete schedule).
3. Detailed outline of each section of the program.
4. Detailed learning objectives in terms of behavioral outcomes for each didactic and practical training activity.
5. Other appropriate material such as pharmacy forms, lists of abbreviations, and explanatory notes.

It is suggested that topics that apply to several areas of study (e.g., safety considerations) be presented in the beginning of the course and then elaborated on as necessary for each individual section.

Approved by the ASHP Board of Directors, November 19–20, 1981. Copyright© 1982, American Society of Hospital Pharmacists, Inc. All rights reserved. Reprinted from the *Am J Hosp Pharm, 39,* 317–320 (1982).

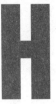
Body Surface Area Nomogram

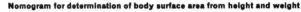

Nomogram for determination of body surface area from height and weight

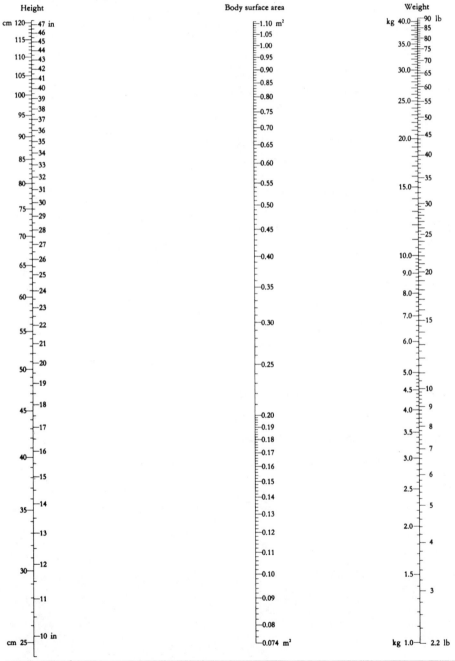

From the formula of Du Bois and Du Bois, *Arch. intern. Med.*, 17, 863 (1916): $S = W^{0.425} \times H^{0.725} \times 71.84$, or
$\log S = \log W \times 0.425 + \log H \times 0.725 + 1.8564$ (S = body surface in cm², W = weight in kg, H = height in cm)

Glossary

accreditation—the process by which an agency or organization evaluates and recognizes a program of study or an institution as meeting predetermined qualifications

achlorhydria—absence of hydrochloric acid in the stomach

action plan—a concise, written document listing the objectives an employee will accomplish in a specific period of time, such as 1 year. The objectives are mutually agreed upon by the employee and the supervisor and should be clear, measurable, and obtainable

active transport—movement of drug molecules against a concentration gradient (i.e., from an area of low concentration to an area of higher concentration)

acute illness—an illness with severe symptoms and of short duration

administer—give a patient medication, once it is checked for accuracy

administration (or route of administration)—refers to how a drug or therapy is introduced into the body. Systemic administration means that the drug goes throughout the body (usually carried in the bloodstream), and includes oral administration (by mouth) and intravenous administration (injection into the vein). Local administration means that the drug is applied or introduced into a specific area affected by disease (e.g., application directly onto the affected skin surface, called topical administration). The effects of most therapies depend upon the ability of the drug to reach the affected area, thus the route of administration and consequent distribution of a drug in the body is an important determinant of its effectiveness

administrative section—that part of the manual containing the policies and procedures that pertain to the operation of the department

admixture—term used to denote one or more active ingredients in a large-volume parenteral solution

ADT—computer program for admission/discharge and transfer which provides significant demographic and clinical information for each patient

adverse drug reaction—any unexpected obvious change in a patient's condition that the physician suspects may be due to a drug

aerosol—finely nebulized medication for inhalation therapy

AIDS—acquired immune deficiency syndrome

alkaloid—a nitrogenous basic substance found in plants or synthetic substances with structures similar to plant structures (e.g., atropine, caffeine, morphine)

allergy—a disorder in which the body becomes hypersensitive to a particular antigen (called an *allergen*)

allopathy—treatment of diseases with drugs that cause the opposite effect (e.g., antipyretics to reduce fever)

almshouse—a home for the poor and indigent

ambulatory care—care provided to persons who do not require either an acute care (hospital) or chronic care (skilled nursing facility) setting

American Council on Pharmaceutical Education—the accrediting body for colleges of pharmacy by which high educational standards are established and monitored

American Druggist Blue Book—provides prices and other miscellaneous information about prescription drugs, over-the-counter products, cosmetics, toiletries, and other items sold in pharmacy stores

American Society of Health System Pharmacists (ASHP)—a national organization established in 1942 and presently includes pharmacists in various institutional health care settings; presently contains a section for pharmacy technicians

analgesic—an agent that relieves pain without causing loss of consciousness (e.g., codeine)

anaphylaxis—severe allergenic reaction caused by a drug or biological

angiotensin-converting enzyme (ACE)—helps inhibit the renal mechanism for blood elevation

anhydrous—containing no water

anionic—carrying a negative charge

antagonist—a drug that opposes the action of another drug or a natural body chemical

antianginal—drug used to relieve chest pain

antiarrhythmic—agent that restores normal heart rhythm

antibiotic—medication that is derived from living cells or synthetic compounds and is antagonistic to other forms of life, especially bacteria; a soluble substance derived from a mold or bacterium that inhibits the growth of other organisms and is used to combat disease and infection

anticholinergic—a drug that blocks the passage of impulses through parasympathetic nerve fibers

antidote—a remedy for counteracting a poison

antiemetic—controls nausea and vomiting

antihypertensive—an agent that reduces blood pressure

antineoplastic agent—chemotherapy agent or cancer drug

antiseptic—a substance used to destroy pathogenic organisms

apothecary—early American or European term for a pharmacist

apparent volume of distribution—the apparent volume of plasma that would be required to account for all the drug in the body; rarely corresponds to a real volume space in the body

application software—referred to as programs, accepting data from the user; it calculates, stores user-specific data, and presents information according to the prescribed instructions

arrhythmia—any deviation from normal heartbeat

arteriosclerosis—disorder characterized by thickening, loss of elasticity, and calcification of the walls of the arteries

aseptic—a condition in which there are no living microorganisms; free from infection

asylum—an institution for the relief or care of the destitute or afflicted and especially the insane

automated pharmacy systems—mechanical systems that perform operations and activities, other than compounding and drug administration, relative to storage, packaging, dispensing, and distribution of medications and that collect, control, and maintain transaction information

backup systems—alternate procedures in the event the computer system should fail

bar coding—a series of vertical bars and spaces of varying thicknesses and heights to represent information

beta blocker—a drug that selectively blocks beta receptors in the autonomic nervous system

bile—a fluid secreted by the liver

bile salts—naturally occurring surface-active agents secreted by the gall bladder into the small intestine

bioavailability—term used to indicate the rate and relative amount of administered drug that reaches the circulatory system intact

biodegradable—can be broken down by living organisms

bioengineered therapies—the process used in the manufacture of therapeutic agents through recombinant DNA (deoxyribonucleic acid) technology

biological equivalents—those chemical equivalents that, when administered in the same amounts, will provide the same biological or physiological availability

biological fluids—includes blood, serum, plasma, lymph, etc.

biologicals—medicinal preparations made from living organisms or their products; include serums, vaccines, antigens, and antitoxins

biopharmaceutics—the branch of pharmaceutics that concerns itself with the relationship between physicochemical properties of a drug in a dosage form, and the pharmacologic, toxicologic, or clinical responses observed after drug administration

biotech drugs—genetically engineered therapeutic agents

biotechnology—the application of biological systems and organisms to technical and industrial processes

black plague—a worldwide epidemic of the fourteenth century in which some 60 million persons are said to have died; descriptions indicate that it was pneumonic plague, also called *black death* or *the plague*

blending—mixing

blister packages—cardboard and plastic material that is heat-sealed to individually package medication

board of trustees/directors—body responsible for governing the hospital in the community's best interest

bolus—an injection directly from the syringe barrel into a vein, also call *I.V. push*

botany—the science of plants, including structure, functions of parts, and classification

brand-name drugs—drugs that are research-developed, patented, manufactured, and distributed by a drug firm

B.S. degree—bachelor of science degree; an initial entry degree originally required for admission to a state board examination to obtain a license to practice as a pharmacist

budget—the projected costs allocated on a yearly basis for personnel, supplies, construction, and operating expenses

buffer—offers a resistance to pH change

calibrate—standardization of the graduations of a quantitative measuring device

candida—a yeast organism that normally lives in the intestines, but can flourish in other parts of the body at times of immune suppression

caplet—tablet shaped like a capsule

capsule—soluble container enclosing medicine

cardiotonic—an agent that has the effect of producing or restoring normal heart activity

carminative—a medicine that relieves stomach/intestinal gas

cataract—loss of transparency of the lens of the eye

cathartic—an agent that causes bowel evacuation

catheter—a tubular device used for the drainage or injection of fluids through a body passage; made of silicone, rubber, plastic, or other materials

cationic—carrying a positive charge

central processing unit (CPU)—the unit of the computer that accomplishes the processing or execution of given calculations or instructions

centralized system—a system of distribution in which all functions, processing, preparation, and distribution occur in a main area (e.g., the main pharmacy)

chelating—making a complex formation

chemical equivalents—those multiple-source drug products that contain identical amounts of the identical active ingredient in identical dosage forms

chemotherapy—the treatment of an illness with medication; commonly refers to the treatment of malignancy with agents that are cytotoxic (i.e., the medication kills cells); more specifically, use of chemicals to treat cancer

cholinergic—a drug that is stimulated, activated, or transmitted by acetylcholine

chronic illness—a disturbance in health that persists for a long time, usually showing little change or slow progression over time

Class A prescription balance—a sensitive balance scale with a range of 6 mg to 650 mg

clinical—involving direct observation of the patient

clinical pharmacokinetics—that branch of pharmaceutics that deals with the application of pharmacokinetics to the safe and effective therapeutic management of the individual patient

clinical pharmacy—patient-oriented pharmacy practice that is concerned with health care through rational drug use

clinical pharmacy practice—the application of knowledge about drugs and drug therapy to the care and treatment of patients

clinical section—that section of a policy and procedure manual describing patient-related monitoring activities

commission on credentialing—the body appointed to formulate and recommend standards and administer programs for accreditation of pharmacy personnel training programs

community pharmacy—pharmacy service provided in pharmacy health care; sometimes called the "family drug store" in which ambulatory individuals are provided prescription and nonprescription drugs and other health-related supplies

community relations and fund development—a department that communicates with and markets hospital programs with the local community

compliance—act of adhering to prescribed directions

compliance rate—an indicator of how many times out of a hundred (expressed as a percent) that a quality event occurs or fails to occur

compounding—preparation of a pharmaceutical that contains more than one ingredient according to a prescription or formula

computer—a programmable electronic device used to store, process, or communicate information

computer application—a series of computer programs written for a particular function (e.g., inventory management)

computer file—collection of like elements of information stored under a common name (e.g., Hospital Formulary)

computer network—the technology that supports the connection of multiple computers including application, processors, printers and microcomputers

computer server—a computer which collects and stores information for use by other computers

computer system—a combination of hardware and software working together to perform specific functions

computer terminal—a device that contains a keyboard and screen; functions as both the inpatient and outpatient device

consultant pharmacist—responsible for monitoring drug usage and drug therapy of residents in nursing homes

contaminated—unclean; microorganisms introduced into an area where they had not previously been present

continuous infusion—administration of an intravenous drug at a constant rate over a prolonged time period

contraindicate—to indicate against; to indicate the inappropriateness of a form of treatment or a drug for a specific disease

control—any method used to eliminate or reduce the potential harm of the distributed medication

control documents—forms, such as records, sheets, logs, or checklists, that track conformance with standards that have been established to reduce the likelihood of an error or negative outcome

controlled substances—drugs, controlled by the federal and/or state Drug Enforcement Administration, that can produce dependence or be abused (e.g., narcotics, select psychotropics, steroids)

Controlled Substances Act—federal law regulating the manufacture, distribution, and sale of drugs that have the potential for abuse

counter balance—a double-pan balance capable of weighing relatively large quantities

counterirritant—an agent, such as mustard plaster, that is applied locally to produce an inflammatory reaction for the purpose of affecting some other part, usually adjacent to or underlying the surface irritated

CPU—central processing unit of computer hardware; the brain of the computer

cream—water-based, semisolid external dosage form

credentialling—a process in which a formal, organized agency recognizes and documents the competencies and abilities performed by an individual or an organization

criteria—a set of statements that define quality

cyber—cultural revolution; computerization and telecommunication that transport information through fiber optics, CD-ROM, satellites, and the Internet

cytotoxic—a substance that causes cellular deterioration

data entry—the input function that involves recording, coding, or converting data to a form that the computer can recognize

decentralized system—a system of distribution in which all functions (processing, preparation, and distribution) occur on or near the nursing unit (e.g., satellite pharmacy)

dedicated—limited to processing information for one area

defenses—legal arguments that are raised by defendants in support of their case

deinstitutionalization—discharge of persons with a history of long-term mental health care in a hospital back to the community

Delphi Study—a futuristic study employed to gain insight into desirable courses of action to achieve the mission of the group

density—weight per unit volume

deposition—out-of-court sworn testimony, made in response to questioning by an attorney and recorded by a court reporter

diabetes mellitus—a metabolic disorder in which faulty pancreatic activity decreases the oxidation of carbohydrates

diagnosis—the determination of the nature of a disease or symptom through physical examination and clinical tests

diagnosis-related group (DRG))—utilized by Medicare, Medicaid, and other third-party payers to reimburse hospitals a predetermined fee for each patient based on the patient's diagnosis, irrespective of the quantity or cost of the care. Costs over this predetermined fee are not reimbursed by the government but are allocated to the hospital. The intent of implementing the DRG system was to regulate and control Medicare's health care expenditure. *See also* **prospective payment system (PPS)**

diagnostic equipment—articles or implements used to detect physical conditions that may be related to disease or biological changes; usually used at home by one patient

didactic instruction—formalized, structured, lecture-type education program

differentiated manpower—the distinction of responsibilities among available personnel to achieve the overall purpose of the entire group

discharge planning—a program developed to ensure continued appropriate care after the patient leaves the hospital

discovery—the formal pretrial process by which evidence is obtained by one party from another party to a litigation

disinfectant—a substance used to destroy pathogens; generally used on objects rather than on humans

dispensatory—a treatise on the quality and composition of medicine

dispensing—the process of selecting, preparing, checking, and delivering prescribed medication and associated information; must be under the supervision of a pharmacist

dissolution—the act of dissolving

distributional section—the part of a policy and procedure manual that presents those policies and procedures that deal with the appropriate storage, ordering, dispensing, documentation, and disposition of drugs and supplies

diuresis—increased excretion of urine

diuretic—an agent that causes an increase in the excretion of urine

dosage—the determination and regulation of the size, frequency, and number of doses

dosage forms—the various pharmaceutical forms whereby drugs are made available (e.g., capsules, patches, injections)

dosage schedule—the frequency, interval, and length of time a medicine is to be given

dosage strength—the quantity of a drug in a given dosage form

dose—a quantity of a drug or radiation to be given at one time

DRG—*see* **diagnostic-related group**

drug—any substance to treat or prevent disease

drug administration—process by which a drug enters the body by ingestion, injection, application, inhalation, instillation, etc.

drug disposition—all processes that occur to the drug after absorption and that can be subdivided into distribution and elimination

drug distribution—the process of reversible transfer of a drug to and from the site of measurement, usually the blood

drug elimination—the irreversible loss of a drug from the site of measurement, usually subdivided into metabolism and/or excretion

drug formulary—a list of medicinal agents selected by the medical staff considered to be the most useful in patient care

druggist—historically a person who compounds, dispenses, and sells drugs and medicine

drug information—information about drugs and the effects of drugs on people, the provision of which is a part of each pharmacist's practice

drug label—information placed on a drug container that includes data required by drug regulations

drug misadventures—what can go wrong in the "therapeutic adventure" of using a medication; encompass errors in prescribing judgment, system errors in the process of bringing drug products to the ultimate users, and idiosyncratic (individual and unusual sensitivity that is not dose related) responses to medication

drug order—a course of medication therapy ordered by the physician or dental practitioner in an organized health care setting

drug recalls—voluntary recall of a drug because of a health hazard potential

drug regimen review—process to provide appropriate drug therapy for patients as part of the health care team

drugs of choice—the preferred or best drug therapy that can be prescribed for a specific disease state, based upon majority medical opinion

Drug Topics Red Book—reference guide listing all pharmaceuticals, medicinals, and sundries sold in drug stores, with currently available prices

drug-use control—the system of knowledge, understanding, judgments, procedures, skills, controls, and ethics that ensures optimal safety in the distribution and use of medication

drug-use process—the series of steps necessary to move a drug product from purchase to patient use

duodenum—that area of the small intestine that is the first 25 cm after the stomach, responsible for significant drug absorption

durable medical equipment (DME)—includes health-related equipment that is used for long periods of time, is not disposable, and is rented or sold to clients for home care, such as wheelchairs, hospital beds, walkers, canes, crutches; *also see* **home medical equipment**

elastomer—an elastometric substance

elastometric—a polymer material with elastic properties

electrolytes—naturally occurring ions in the body that play an essential role in cellular function, maintaining fluid balance and establishing acid-base balance; an ionizable substance in solution (e.g., sodium, potassium chloride)

electronic mail (e-mail)—a form of transmitting, storing, and distributing text in electronic form via a communications network

electrostatic copying machine—a photocopier

embolism—obstruction or occlusion of a blood vessel by a transported blood clot

emesis—clinical term for vomiting

emetic—an agent that causes vomiting

emphysema—lung disease caused by constriction of airway passages

employee performance evaluations— a routine, formal process by the supervisor to provide feedback on the employee's performance versus the expected performance listed in the employee's action plan

emulsifying agent—a substance used in preparing an emulsion

endogenously—originating within the organism

enforcement—the process of making sure that policies and procedures are carefully and consistently followed

enteral—liquid nutrient solution administered by mouth or through feeding tube into stomach or intestines

enteric-coated tablet—a special tablet coating that prevents the release of a drug until it enters the intestine

enterohepatic cycling—drug taken up by the bile, secreted into the small intestine, and may be reabsorbed back to the blood

epidemic—a disease that attacks many people in the same region at the same time

epidural—infusion therapy directly into spinal cord fluid

etiology—the study of all the factors that may be involved in the development of disease

excretion—the process whereby the undigested residue of food and the waste products of metabolism are eliminated

expectorant—a substance that promotes the ejection of mucus or an exudate from the lungs, bronchi, and trachea

expiration date—the last date of sale as determined by the manufacturer. Any sale after this date is unethical and may result in a levy of fines by pharmacy and or health inspectors.

extemporaneous—prepared at the time it is required, with materials on hand

extended-release capsules—capsules that are formulated in such a way as to gradually release the drug over a predetermined time period

facsimile equipment—fax machine; sends order over telephone lines

FDA—*see* **Food and Drug Administration**

federal and state statutes—laws enacted by a legislative body that dictate the conduct of persons or organizations subject to the law

Federal Food, Drug and Cosmetic Act—the federal statute through which the FDA promulgates its rules and regulations

first pass effect—occurs when a drug is rapidly metabolized in the liver after oral administration with minimum bioavailability

floor stock—medications provided to the nursing unit for administration to the patient by the nurse, who is responsible for preparation and administration

fluidextract—a liquid preparation of a herb containing alcohol as a solvent or preservative

Food and Drug Administration (FDA)—promulgates rules, regulations, and standards; inspects drug and food facilities to ensure public safety regarding drug products

format—standardized method of documentation for consistency

franchise—authorization by a manufacturer to a distributor to sell a product

galenical—a standard preparation containing one or several organic ingredients (e.g., elixir)

gargle—a substance used to rinse or medicate the mucous membrane of the throat and mouth (e.g., Listerine™)

generic drugs—drugs labeled by their "official" name and manufactured by a drug firm after the original patent expires

genetically engineered drugs—exact duplication of a substance already available in the human body

geriatric pharmacy practice—pharmacy practice that focuses on the medical and pharmaceutical care of the elderly

glycoside—a compound containing a sugar molecule (e.g., digitalis)

graduate—a marked (or graduated) conical or cylindrical vessel used for measuring liquids

habituation—acquired tolerance for a drug

hard copy—information on a printed sheet

hardware—equipment, software, and sets of instructions that control and coordinate the activities of the hardware and direct the processing of data; refers to the actual computer system (e.g., IBM, Digital)

health care delivery—organized programs developed to provide physical, mental, and emotional health care in institutions for home-bound and ambulatory patients

health maintenance organization (HMO)—a prepaid health insurance plan that provides comprehensive health care for subscribers, with emphasis on the prevention and early detection of disease and continuity of care. HMOs are either not-for-profit or for-profit, are designated as either an independent practice association (IPA) or a staff model, and are often owned and operated by insurance carriers. HMOs were developed as a means to control health care delivery, access, and cost.

hemodialysis—procedure by which impurities or wastes are removed from the blood

hemophilia—hereditary blood-coagulation disorder

HEN—home enteral therapy

herb—a leafy plant used as a healing remedy or a flavoring agent

high efficiency particulate air (HEPA)—used in laminar flow hoods

Hippocrates—a Greek physician, called the "Father of Medicine"

HIS—*see* **hospital information system**

HIV—human immunodeficiency virus

home medical equipment (**HME**)—equipment used at home (e.g., hospital beds, crutches); *see* **durable medical equipment**

home health care—provision of health care services to a patient in his or her place of residence

home infusion—intravenous drug therapy provided in patient's own home

home pharmaceutical service—dispensing and delivery of medications to patients who have their clinical status monitored at home

homeostasis—a tendency toward stability in the internal body environment, a state of equilibrium

homogeneous—of uniform composition throughout

horizontal hospital integration—situation in which a number of hospitals share administrative, clinical, and technological functions

hormone—a chemical substance, produced by cells or an organ, that has a specific regulatory effect in the body

hospice—an institution that provides a program of palliative and supportive services to terminally ill patients and their families in the form of physical, psychological, social, and spiritual care

hospital—a network of health care services for treatment, care of the sick, study of disease, therapy, and the training of health care professionals

hospital information systems (**HIS**)—systems that integrate information from many parts of the hospital

human genome initiative—program of research that studies all human genes

humor—a fluid or semifluid substance in the body; originally phlegm, blood, bile (e.g., aqueous humor is a fluid produced in the eye—not tears)

hydration therapy—replaces fluid loss

hydroalcoholic—mixture of water and alcohol

hydrolysis—any reaction in which water is one of the reactants

hydrophilic—water loving

hydrophilic drug molecules—drug molecules that are polar and water loving

hydrophobic drugs—drugs whose molecules are nonpolar and lipid loving or water hating

hygroscopic—moisture absorbing

hyperalimentation—*see* **total parenteral nutrition**

hyperglycemia—high blood glucose level

hypersensitivity—excessive response of the immune system to a sensitizing antigen

hypertension—disorder characterized by elevated blood pressure

hypoglycemic—a drug that lowers the level of glucose in the blood; used primarily by diabetics

hypolipodemic—an agent to reduce lipids (fat) in the blood

hypometabolic—low basic metabolic rate

ideal drug therapy—safe, effective, timely, and cost-conscious medication use

immunity—the condition of being resistant to a particular disease (e.g., polio)

immunomodulators—agents that adjust the immune system to a desired level

incompatibility—lack of compatibility; an undesirable effect when two or more substances are mixed together

independent pharmacy—privately owned pharmacy

infection—the state or condition in which the body (or part of it) is invaded by an agent (microorganism or virus) that multiplies and produces an injurious effect (active infection)

infection control—the use of appropriate procedures and education to minimize the transfer of infections from one to another

infiltration—occurs when an intravenous solution is infused into the surrounding tissues instead of directly into the vein as intended

infusion—the introduction of a solution into a vein by gravity or by an infusion control device or pump

infusion pump—regulates the flow of an intravenous solution

infusion therapy—introduction of fluid into the body usually by intravenous route

in-house pharmacy—pharmacy located within the facility

injection—the introduction of a fluid substance into the body by means of a needle and syringe

inoculum—microorganism or other material introduced into a system

input devices—keyboards, light pens, optical scanners, bar code readers

institutional pharmacy—pharmacy services provided in hospitals, nursing homes, health maintenance organizations, prisons, mental retardation facilities, or other settings wherein groups of patients are provided formal, structured pharmacy programs

intermittent injection—repeated intravenous administration of a drug at specified time intervals

intoxication—state of being poisoned by a drug or being inebriated with alcohol

intraocular—within the eye

intrasynovial(I.S.)—injection directly into joint fluid

intrathecal(I.T.)—infusion into fluid surrounding brain

intravenous (I.V.)—within a vein; administering drugs or fluids directly into the vein to obtain a rapid or complete effect from the drug

inventory—a complete listing of the exact amounts of all the drugs in stock at a particular time

investigational drugs—drugs that have not received approval for marketing by the Food and Drug Administration

iontophoresis—use of an electric current to cause an ionized drug to pass through the skin into the system circulation

isotonic—having the osmotic pressure

job description—a guideline written by the employer for the employee that outlines the requirements and limits of the job

Joint Commission on Accreditation of Healthcare Organization (JCAHO)—not-for-profit organization whose standards are set to ensure effective quality services (e.g., optimal standards for the operation of hospitals)

judge—the trier of law (and of fact if there is no jury)

jury—generally composed of from six to twelve persons. The jury is the trier of facts.

lacrimal fluids—tears

leaching—effect of removing a soluble substance from a solution

levigation—mixing of particles with a base vehicle, in which they are insoluble, to produce a smooth dispersion of the drug by rubbing with a spatula on a tile

liability—that responsibility imposed upon a party who breaches a duty owed to another person

lipophilic—lipid loving

liposome—a small membrane that entraps and later releases an active ingredient

local area networks (LAN)—permit different systems (mainframe, minicomputers, and microcomputers), as well as computers made by different manufacturers, to communicate and share data

long-term care—health care provided in an organized medical facility for patients requiring chronic or extended treatment

long-term care facility—for individuals who do not need hospital care but are in need of a wide range of medical, nursing, and related health and social services

lotions—liquid preparations intended for external application

mainframe—the largest, most powerful type of computer system; is able to service many users at once and process several programs simultaneously; has large primary and secondary storage capacities

Maimonides—Rabbi Moses ben Maimon, Spanish-born teacher and physician

malaria—an infectious fever-producing disease, transmitted by infected mosquitos

malfeasance—commission of a substandard act

malpractice—a deviation from the standard of care that arises out of a professional relationship; also called *professional negligence*

managed care—provision of health care services in the most cost-effective way

materia medica—the branch of pharmacy that deals with drugs and their source, preparation, and use

materials management—the division of a hospital pharmacy responsible for the procurement, control, storage, and distribution of drugs and pharmaceutical products

matrix management—an organizational concept that emphasizes the interrelationship between departments and the common area of decision making

Medicaid—a state health care coverage program with some federal funding assistance for persons with low income, minimal assets, and no health care coverage as mandated by Title XIX of the Social Security Act. Medicaid may go by different names in different states; often known as *medical assistance programs.*

medical records—the hospital department responsible for the maintenance and review of patients' medical charts

Medicare—a federal health care coverage program for those 65 years of age and over, certain disabled persons, and persons with end-stage renal disease as mandated by Title XVIII of the Social Security Act of 1965. Medicare includes Part A and Part B, which cover both hospital care and outpatient services.

medication administration record (MAR)—the document used by the nursing department to chart the medication administered to the patient

medication administrator—person who administers or gives medication to patients; *see also* **medication technician**

medication technician—same as **medication administrator**

medium—solvent used in dissolution testing

memory—the storage of both data and instructions internally in the computer

meniscus—the outer surface of a liquid having a concave or crescent shape, caused by surface tension

metabolism—the conversion of one chemical specified to another in the body

micronized drug particles—very small drug particles that have a diameter in the smallest size range

microorganism—a microscopic plant or animal

Millis Study Commission—published a report in 1975 titled "Pharmacist for the Future." Its main premise stated that pharmacy is a knowledge profession.

milling—reducing the particle size

minicomputer, microcomputer, or personal computer systems—systems used for well-defined and specialized applications

mnemonic codes—short entries that are easy to remember and represent a longer instruction used to assist in the entry of data

moiety—a part of a molecule that exhibits a particular set of chemical and pharmacologic characteristics

monastery—the dwelling place for persons under religious vows who live in ascetic simplicity

morbidity—a disease state; the ratio of the sick to the well in a given area

mortality—occurrence of death; the ratio of deaths to the living in a given area

multiple sclerosis—a degenerative disease of the central nervous system

narcotic antagonists—agents that oppose or overcome effects of a narcotic

neurosonology—laboratory section of the neurology department specifically referring to EEG, EMG, carotid doppler, brain mapping, etc.

NAHC—National Association for Home Care

NKA—no known allergies

nosocomial—a disease or infection originating in the hospital

objective—the purpose or goal toward which effort is directed

Occupational and Safety Act—federal law that assures every working man and woman in the nation safe and healthful working conditions; established the Occupational Safety and Health Administration (OSHA)

ointment—oil-based, semisolid, external dosage form, usually containing a medicine substance

oleaginous—resembling or having the properties of oil

oncology—the study or knowledge of tumors; commonly refers to the study of cancer and related diseases

one-compartment model—the simplest case in pharmacokinetics in which the body is thought to behave as a single homogeneous compartment

operational manual—lists only those policies and procedures that affect the internal working of the pharmacy department

osteoporosis—disorder characterized by abnormal porosity of bone, usually in older women

ostomy—an artificial opening into the gastrointestinal tract

outcome competency—the measurable, desired ability, knowledge, and skill achieved upon completion of program

output devices—video display terminal (VDT), cathode ray tubes (CRT), printers, and plotters

pandemic—a global epidemic disease

parenteral—a sterile, injectable medication; introduction of a drug or nutrient into a vein, muscle, subcutaneous tissue, artery, or spinal column; often refers to intravenous infusions of nutritional solutions; *see also* **total parenteral nutrition**

passive diffusion—movement of drug molecules from an area of high concentration to one of a lower concentration

pathology—study of the characteristics, causes, and effects of disease

patient package insert—an informational leaflet written for the lay public describing the benefits and risks of medications

patient profile—a document that is used to incorporate patient information, allergies, sensitivities, and all medications the patient is receiving, both active and discontinued

Patient's Bill of Rights—a declaration ensuring that all patients, inpatients, outpatients, and emergency service patients are afforded their rights in a health care institution

PC—personal computer

PCA—patient controlled analgesia

peptides—a compound of two or more amino acids

percutaneous—through the skin

peripheral devices—sent to a computer for processing and receive information from the CPU once the data have been processed

Pharm. D. degree—the doctor of pharmacy degree earned after a 6- or 7-year course of study; emphasizes clinical (patient-oriented) professional skills

pharmaceutical alternates—drug products that contain the same therapeutic moiety and strength but differ in the salt, ester, or dosage form

pharmaceutical care—the responsible provision of drug therapy to achieve definite outcomes that improve a patient's quality of life

pharmaceutical services—focus on rational drug therapy and include the essential administrative, clinical, and technical functions to meet this goal

pharmaceutics—that area of the pharmaceutical sciences that deals with the chemical, physical, and physiological properties of drugs and dosage forms and drug-delivery systems

pharmacist—a person who has (1) completed 5, 6, or 7 years of formal education in a pharmacy school and (2) is licensed to prepare and distribute drugs and counsel on the use of medication in the state in which he/she practices

pharmacognosy—the study of the biologic and biochemical features of natural drugs

pharmacokinetics—that branch of pharmaceutics that deals with a mathematical description of drug absorption, distribution, metabolism, and excretion and their relationship to the dosage form

pharmacology—the science that deals with the origin, nature, chemistry, effects, and uses of drugs

pharmacopeia—an authorative treatise on drugs and their purity, preparation, and standards

pharmacotherapy—the treatment of disease with medications

pharmacy—the professional practice of discovering, preparing, dispensing, monitoring, and educating about drugs

Pharmacy and Therapeutics Committee—the liaison between the department of pharmacy and the medical staff. Consisting of physicians who represent the various clinical aspects, this committee selects the drugs to be used in the hospital. The pharmacy director is the secretary and a voting member of this committee.

Pharmacy Code of Ethics—rules established for the profession by pharmacists that guide proper conduct for pharmacists

pharmacy mission—to help people make the best use of medication

pharmacy service—(1) the procurement, distribution, and control of all pharmaceuticals used within the facility; (2) the evaluation and dissemination of comprehensive information about drugs and their use; and (3) the monitoring, evaluation, and assurance of the quality of drug use

pharmacy technician—a person skilled in various pharmacy service activities not requiring the professional judgment of the pharmacist; has received formal or informal skill training to participate in numerous pharmacy activities in concert with and under the supervision of a registered pharmacist

phlebitis—inflammation of a vein

phlegm—viscous mucus secreted orally

physician—an authorized practitioner of medicine

physician assistant—an authorized practitioner of medicine who works under the responsible supervision of a licensed physician

phytochemist—person who studies plant chemistry and applies these chemicals to science

PICC—peripherally inserted central catheter

piggyback—refers to a small-volume I.V. solution (25-250 mL) that is run into an existing I.V. line over a brief period of time; (e.g., 50 mL over fifteen minutes)

pill—a small globular or oval medicated mass intended for oral administration

pleadings—the initial court papers; generally the summons, complaint, and answer

pneumatic tube—a method of sending medication orders through the hospital by placing it in a "tube" and sending it to a dispatcher who then forwards it to the specific location

pneumonia—inflammation of lungs usually due to infection

podiatrist—a specialist in foot care

Poison Prevention Packaging Act—federal law mandating special packaging requirements that make it difficult for children under the age of 5 to open the package or container

policy—a defined course to guide and determine present and future decisions; established by an organization or employer who guides the employee to act in a manner consistent with management philosophy

polymer—a high-molecular-weight substance made up of identical base units

polymorphic state—a condition in which a substance occurs in more than one crystalline form

polyurethanes—substances sometimes used for linkage in elastomers

purified protein derivative (**PPD)**—skin test for tuberculosis

PPN—peripheral parenteral nutrition

practice plan—an agreed-upon guide, written by pharmacists, on how pharmacy will be practiced in a particular setting

preferred provider organization (PPO)—an insurance plan that provides comprehensive health care through contracted providers

preferred vendor—the drug firm selected as the wholesaler

preponderance of the evidence—the burden of proof (greater than 50 percent) that a plaintiff has to meet in a civil case to obtain a favorable verdict

prescriber—a person in health care who is permitted by law to order drugs that legally require a prescription; includes physicians, physician assistants, podiatrists, dentists

prescription—permission granted orally or in writing from a physician for a patient to receive a certain medication on an outpatient basis that will help relieve or eliminate the patient's problem

preservatives—substances used to prevent the growth of microorganisms

prime vendor—drug wholesaler who contracts directly with hospital pharmacies for the purpose of their high-volume pharmaceuticals

PRN (pro res natum)—drug to be given as needed when a clinical situation arises

procedures—guidelines on the preferred way to perform a certain function; particular actions to be taken to carry out a policy

product line management—an organization concept that emphasizes the end product or category of services being delivered

programs—instructions for a computer

propellent—substance used to help expel the contents of a pressurized container

prophylaxis—prevention of or protection against disease

prospective payment system (PPS)—a method of third-party reimbursement with predetermined reimbursement rates; *see also* **diagnosis-related group (DRG)**

proteins—macromolecules consisting of amino acids

protocol—a written description of how an activity, procedure, or function is to be accomplished

psychiatric—relating to the medical treatment of mental disorders

psychotropic—a drug used to treat mental and emotional disorders

quality assurance—a method of monitoring actual versus desired results in an effort to ensure a certain level of quality that meets predetermined criteria

quality assurance program—a format that elaborates special basic quality assurance steps

quality of life—a meaningful life for the patient at the optimum level of functioning for as long as possible

quality standards—the minimum results needed to achieve a desired level of quality

quasi-legal standards—recognized standards that are similar to law

radiopaque—having the property of absorbing X rays

reconstitute—add a sterile solvent to a sterile active ingredient for injectable purposes

Red Cross–Red Crescent—an international health-oriented institution that provides emergency and ongoing assistance in situations of need

regulation—an authoritative rule dealing with details of procedure

regulatory law—the area of law that deals with governmental agencies and how they enforce the intent of the statutes under which they operate

residents' rights—refers to those rights that residents have within the long-term care facility, such as confidentiality and maintenance of dignity

robotics—technology based on a mechanical device, programmed by remote control to accomplish manual activities such as picking medications according to a patient's computerized profile

rules and regulations—promulgated by government agencies at the local, state, and federal levels

rule of three—the process of pharmacy personnel checking a medication being prepared and dispensed three times before it is administered to the patient

sanitarium—an institution for the treatment of chronic disease such as tuberculosis or nervous disorders

satellite pharmacy—where distribution occurs from a decentralized pharmacy staffed by at least a pharmacist and technician. The satellite usually handles all the needs of the units for which they are responsible.

scanners—optical recognition devices that can read preprinted characters or codes

secondary storage—data and programs maintained on tapes or discs

sepsis—presence of pathogenic organisms in the blood

site survey—the visit by representatives of ASHP to review the training program to ascertain compliance with the standards

soft copy—visual display units

software—the actual programs for the computer system

solution—a homogeneous mixture of one or more substances dispersed in a dissolving solvent; clear liquid with all components completely dissolved

solution balance—single unequal arm balance used for weighing large amounts

solvation—process by which a solute is incorporated into the solvent

stability—a condition that resists change; for example a drug maintains potency

standard—a reference to be used in evaluating institutional programs and services

standard of care—the acceptable level of professional practice that exists by which the actions of a professional are judged

standards of practice—rules that pharmacists establish for the profession that represent the preferred way to practice

staphylococcus (plural staphylococci)—microorganism of the family *Micrococcaceae* that is the most common cause of localized suppurative infections

stat—(*statim*) to be given immediately

state board of pharmacy—body established to ensure that the public is well served professionally by pharmacists

sterile—free from microorganisms

stop order—stop medication. An automatic stop order requires a physician's renewal order for the medication, and after review by the pharmacist, should be discontinued.

structure criteria—specify necessary resources (e.g., equipment)

subcutaneously—under the skin; introduced beneath the skin (e.g., subcataneous injections)

sudorific—a substance that causes sweating; also called a *diaphoretic*

supportive pharmacy personnel—another term for **pharmacy technician**

suppositories—solid dosage forms for insertion into body cavities (e.g., rectum, vagina, urethra) where they melt at body temperature

surface active agents—substances that lower the surface tension of liquids

surfactants—surface active agents, commonly known as *wetting agents*

suspending agents—chemical additive used in suspensions to "thicken" the liquid and retard settling of particles

suspension—liquid containing finely divided drug particles uniformly distributed

synergies—groups working together in cooperation

synthesize—to produce by bringing elements together to form a chemical compound

syrup—a concentrated sugar solution that may have an added medicinal

system software—contains the operating system that includes master programs for coordinating the activities of the hardware and software in a computer system

systemic—relating to the body as a whole, rather than individual parts or organs

systemic action—affects the body as a whole

systemic side effect—an effect on the whole body, but secondary to the intended effect

table of contents—an index for easy referral to the appropriate policies and procedures

tablet—a solid dosage form of varying weight, size, and shape that contains a medicinal substance

tare—a weight used to counterbalance the container holding the substance being weighed

tax-free alcohol—ethyl alcohol obtained at cost under applicable federal regulations to be used only for diagnostic and therapeutic purposes

teratogenic—substance that interferes with normal prenatal development

therapeutic—provision of treatment of a disease, infirmity, or symptom by various methods

therapeutic alternates—drug products that contain different therapeutic moieties but that are of the same pharmacologic and/or therapeutic class

therapeutic effect—a healing, curative, or ameliorating effect

therapeutic equivalent—a drug product that, when administered in the same amount, will provide the same therapeutic effect and pharmacokinetic characteristics as another drug to which it is compared

therapeutic substitution—the substitution of one drug product with another that differs in composition but is considered to have the same or very similar pharmacologic and therapeutic activity

therapy—treatment of disease

thrombosis—development or presence of a blood clot

tincture—an alcoholic or hydroalcoholic solution containing a medicinal substance

title—indicates the subject that is covered

T.O.—abbreviation for telephone order; sometimes referred to as V.O. (verbal order)

tocolytic—substance that delays or prolongs birth process

topical—pertaining to the surface of a part of the body

total parenteral nutrition (TPN)—intravenous nutrition comprised of any or all of the following: amino acids, dextrose, lipids, vitamins, minerals, trace elements, electrolytes, and water in a prepared sterile solution that infuses into a large central venous blood vessel. TPN provides all of the essential nutrients needed for patients to survive if they are unable to ingest nutrients. *See also* **parenteral.**

toxic effect—acute or chronic poisoning through use of pharmaceuticals

toxicity—degree to which something is poisonous

toxicology—the scientific study of poisons and their actions, detection, and treatment of conditions caused by them

toxin—a poison

TPN—total parenteral nutrition

training program—the whole course of study (didactic, laboratory, and experiential) to prepare the student for a career

transdermal—entering through the dermis or skin, as in administration of a drug applied to the skin in ointment or patch form

triturate—to reduce particle size and mix one powder with another

troche—a small tablet intended to dissolve in the mouth to deliver medication to the mouth or throat

unit dose—a single-use package of a drug. In a unit-dose distribution system, a single dose of each medication is dispensed prior to the time of administration.

universal claim form (UCF)—a pharmacy prescription claim form that is utilized to serve as the basis for reimbursement of prescriptions dispensed

USP—*United States Pharmacopeia*

utilization review—work of committee that determines how use of resources meets criteria and standards

vaccination—introduction of a vaccine into the body to produce immunity to a particular disease (e.g., smallpox inoculation)

vaccine—a suspension of attenuated or killed bacteria, viruses, or rickettsiae administered for the prevention, amelioration, or treatment of infectious diseases (e.g., tetanus)

vascular—related to or containing blood vessels

vasoconstrictor—a process, drug, or substance that causes constriction of blood vessels

vasodilator—an agent or drug that causes dilitation of the blood vessels; increases the caliber of the blood vessels

verified—reviewed and approved as true and authentic

vertical health integration—a process that provides a continuum of care for the patient from hospital to ambulatory care, to home care, to long-term care

vertical hood—biological containment hood used to prepare cancer and other selective injectables

vertical laminar flow hood—an air filter process to maintain a particulate-free environment

video display terminal (VDT)—displays computer activities; sometimes referred to as *CRT* (cathode ray tube)

V.O.—voice order

volatile—evaporates at low temperature

volumetric check—an accuracy check for the rate of flow for an intravenous infusion

Index